ESSENTIAL IMMUNOLOGY

SIXTH EDITION

ESSENTIAL IMMUNOLOGY

Ivan M. Roitt

MA, DSc(Oxon), FRCPath, Hon MRCP (Lond), FRS
Professor and Head of
Departments of Immunology and Rheumatology Research
University College and Middlesex School of Medicine
University College
London W1P 9PG

BLACKWELL SCIENTIFIC PUBLICATIONS

OXFORD LONDON EDINBURGH

BOSTON PALO ALTO MELBOURNE

First published 1971
Reprinted 1972 (twice), 1973 (twice)
Second edition 1974, Reprinted 1975
Third edition 1977, Reprinted 1978, 1979
Fourth edition 1980, Reprinted, 1982, 1983
Fifth edition 1984
Sixth edition 1988

Spanish editions 1972, 1975, 1978, 1982
Italian editions 1973, 1975, 1979
Portuguese editions 1973, 1976
French editions 1975, 1979
Dutch editions 1975, 1978, 1982
Japanese editions 1976, 1978, 1982, 1986
German editions 1977, 1984
Polish edition 1977
Greek edition 1978
Slovak edition 1981
Indonesian edition 1985
ELBS editions 1978, 1982

DISTRIBUTORS

USA
  Year Book Medical Publishers
  35 East Wacker Drive
  Chicago, Illinois 60601
  (*Orders*: Tel. 312 726-9733)

Canada
  The C.V. Mosby Company
  5240 Finch Avenue East,
  Scarborough, Ontario
  (*Orders*: Tel. 416-298-1588)

Australia
  Blackwell Scientific Publications
  (Australia) Pty Ltd
  107 Barry Street
  Carlton, Victoria 3053
  (*Orders*: Tel. (03) 347 0300)

British Library
Cataloguing in Publication Data

Roitt, Ivan M.
  Essential immunology. — 6th ed.
  1. Immunology
  I. Title
  616.07'9   QR181

  ISBN 0-632-01994-8

Set by Setrite Ltd, Hong Kong
Printed and bound by
Dah Hua Printing Press Co Ltd, Hong Kong

CONTENTS

4 · THE RECOGNITION OF ANTIGEN
I — Primary Interaction

5 · THE RECOGNITION OF ANTIGEN
II — Detection and Application

6 · THE ACQUIRED IMMUNE RESPONSE
I — Consequences of Antigen Recognition

7 · THE ACQUIRED IMMUNE RESPONSE
II — Production of Effectors

CONTENTS

11 · IMMUNITY TO INFECTION
II — Prophylaxis and Immunodeficiency

12 · HYPERSENSITIVITY

13 · TRANSPLANTATION

14 · AUTOIMMUNE DISEASES
I — Scope and Aetiology

15 · AUTOIMMUNE DISEASES
II — Pathogenesis, Diagnosis and Treatment

ix

PREFACE

As one writes new editions of a book, one tends to fit the new advances into the overall structure of the first edition, not wishing to 'savage' the baby too severely. However, in the 17 years since the first edition appeared, my broad perception of the field has changed so much that an utterly radical reshaping of the book's structure now seemed inescapable. Thus, in many aspects this may be looked upon as a new book.

From the physiological standpoint, immunological systems evolved to provide protection against infection and it is logical therefore to begin with an account of the principal mechanisms which constitute the phylogenetically earlier innate immune system, phagocytosis, complement and other soluble microbicidal factors, and non-specific killer cells. The second chapter then shows how this innate immune system can be unbelievably improved by the operation of an adaptive or acquired system based upon lymphocytes. We note also that this sytem may occasionally produce unwanted effects and give rise to immunopathology. Thus, the first two chapters provide a general overview of the subject.

Another major decision was to treat B- and T-cell activities in parallel. Thus, Chapter 3, which is concerned with molecules involved in the recognition of antigen, includes not only immunoglobulins, but also the T-cell receptor and perforce the major histocompatibility complex; this also seemed the right place to discuss the generation of diversity in receptors. Chapter 4 deals with the nature of the primary antigen recognition process with an extended discussion of what the T-cell 'sees'. The detection of this recognition process and the technical applications to which this gives rise are covered in the following chapter.

The next four chapters deal with the acquired immune response as a consequence of antigen recognition. Chapter 6 discusses the early activation of lymphocytes and the anatomy of the lymphoid system where this occurs, while Chapter 7 goes on to cover the production of effectors — maturation to antibody-forming cells, monoclonal antibodies, T-cell lymphokines affecting B-cell and macrophage responses, and cytotoxic T-cells — all involving considerable updating. The next chapter looks at control of the acquired response by antibody, T-cells and idiotype networks and extends the discussion to networks linking the neurological and endocrine systems. A far more expanded account of the ontogeny of B- and T-cells is given in Chapter 9 and a large new section on lymphoproliferative disorders arising as unregulated developments of lymphoid cells is now included; finally, a discussion of phylogeny draws attention to the large family of recognition molecules based on the immunoglobulin domain ancestral gene.

Immunity to infection in Chapter 10 is examined from the point of view of the adversarial strategies of host and microbe engaged in unremitting warfare. Newer approaches to vaccines based on recombinant DNA technology, synthetic peptides and anti-idiotypes are looked at in Chapter 11, with the section on immunodeficiency including a far more expansive account of AIDS than the last edition, as might be expected.

Turning to immunopathology, the newer advances in our knowledge of IgE receptors, the biochemistry of mast cell activation and the importance of late reactions in atopic allergy are incorporated in the chapter on hypersensitivity. In the transplantation chapter (13), I highlight some of the work on T-cell anti-idiotypic suppression of allograft reactivity and on the increasing importance of cyclosporin; the developments in cancer immunotherapy based on biological response modifiers such as IL-2, inter-ferons and colony stimulating factors are also given a good run. Autoimmunity is split into two chapters and is structured more positively. A full account of the pathogenesis of rheumatoid arthritis focuses on recent work concerning glycosylation defects in the IgG molecule which raises the issue of oligosac-charide changes as a possible factor in the causation of other disorders.

The new two-column format should make the book easier to read. The diagrams have been greatly improved by the consultant art designer, Mike Rubens, and further colour plates have been added. I hope the reader will enjoy this new edition.

ACKNOWLEDGEMENTS

With great pleasure I acknowledge my gratitude to J.R. Batchelor, P.C.L. Beverley, J. Brostoff, A. Cooke, M. Feldmann, J.W. Hadden, F.C. Hay, P.G. Isaacson, P.M. Lydyard, D.K. Male, D.Y. Mason, J.H.L. Playfair, J. Taverne, N. Woolf for invaluable discussions and M.D. Cooper, H.M. Geysen, T. Ishisaka, H. Metzgar, G. Mitchell, S.A. Rosenberg, G.L. Smith, J.W. Yewdell for sending preprints of their articles. I am indebted also to my co-editors, J. Brostoff and D.K. Male, the publishers Gower Medical Publishing Ltd. and the following individuals for permission to utilize or modify their figures which have appeared in *Immunology*: J. Brostoff and T. Hall for Figs 1.12, 1.14 and 11.10, F.C. Hay for Figs 3.24, 3.27 and 12.18, J. Horton for Fig. 9.16, J. Howard for Fig. 8.18, D.K. Male and D.L. Brown for Figs 1.12 and 11.10, D.K. Male for Fig. 2.14, G. Rook for Figs 10.1 and 10.5, M. Steward for Fig. 4.8, J. Taverne for Figs 10.9, 10.14, 10.16 and Table 10.2.

I am especially grateful to Mike Rubens for his creative design work on the figures, to Mary-Clare Swatman for her friendly, excellent and unflappable editorship and John Robson for his expert overall supervision. My particular gratitude goes to my secretary, Christine Meats, who was just incredibly fast, accurate and so cheerful, and to my wife, Margaret, who supported me so ably and lovingly for what must have seemed an interminable time!

USER GUIDE

Throughout the illustrations standard forms have been used for commonly-occurring cells and pathways. A key to these is given in the figure below.

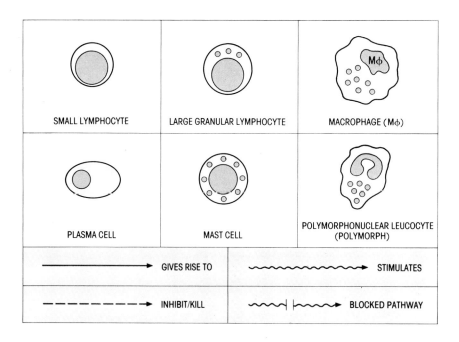

THE BASIS OF IMMUNOLOGY
1 – Innate Immunity

We live in a potentially hostile world filled with a bewildering array of infectious agents (figure 1.1) of diverse shape, size, composition and subversive character which would very happily use us as rich sanctuaries for propagating their 'selfish genes' had we not also developed a series of defence mechanisms at least their equal in effectiveness and ingenuity (except in the case of many parasitic infections where the situation is best described as an uneasy and often unsatisfactory truce). It is these defence mechanisms which can establish a state of immunity against infection (Latin *immunitas*, freedom from) and whose operation provides the basis for the delightful subject called 'Immunology'.

Aside from ill-understood constitutional factors which make one species innately susceptible and another resistant to certain infections, a number of non-specific anti-microbial systems (e.g. phagocytosis) have been recognized which are '*innate*' in the sense that they are not intrinsically affected by

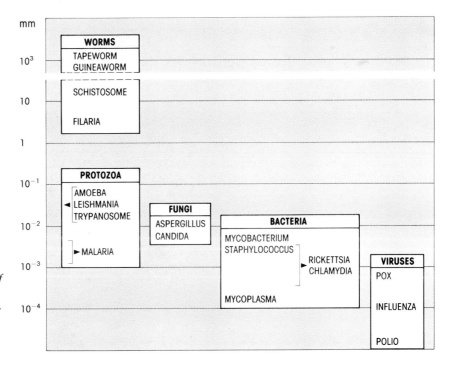

Figure 1.1. *The formidable range of infectious agents which confront the immune system. Although not normally classified as such because of their lack of a cell wall, the mycoplasmas are included under bacteria for convenience. Fungi adopt many forms and approximate values for some of the smallest forms are given.*

prior contact with the infectious agent. We shall discuss these systems and examine how, in the state of *specific acquired immunity*, their effectiveness can be greatly increased.

Barriers against infection

The simplest way to avoid infection is to prevent the micro-organisms from gaining access to the body (figure 1.2). The major line of defence is of course the skin which, when intact, is impermeable to most infectious agents; when there is skin loss, as for example in burns, infection becomes a major problem. Additionally, most bacteria fail to survive for long on the skin because of the direct inhibitory effects of lactic acid and fatty acids in sweat and sebaceous secretions and the low pH which they generate. An exception is *Staphylococcus aureus* which often infects the relatively vulnerable hair follicles and glands.

Figure 1.2. *The first lines of defence against infection: protection at the external body surfaces.*

Mucus, secreted by the membranes lining the inner surfaces of the body, acts as a protective barrier to block the adherence of bacteria to epithelial cells. Microbial and other foreign particles trapped within the adhesive mucus are removed by mechanical stratagems such as ciliary movement, coughing and sneezing. Among other mechanical factors which help protect the epithelial surfaces, one should also include the washing action of tears,

Figure 1.3 continued

neutrophil (below). (j) Mast cells from bone marrow. Round central nucleus surrounded by large darkly staining granules. Two small red cell precursors are shown at the bottom. Romanowsky stain. (k) Tissue mast cells in skin stained with Toluidine Blue. The intracellular granules are metachromatic and stain reddish purple. Note the clustering in relation to

saliva and urine. Many of the secreted body fluids contain bactericidal components, such as acid in gastric juice, spermine and zinc in semen, lactoperoxidase in milk and lysozyme in tears, nasal secretions and saliva.

A totally different mechanism is that of microbial antagonism associated with the normal bacterial flora of the body. These suppress the growth of many potentially pathogenic bacteria and fungi at superficial sites by competition for essential nutrients or by production of inhibitory substances such as colicins or acid. To give one example, pathogen invasion is limited by lactic acid produced by particular species of commensal bacteria which metabolize glycogen secreted by the vaginal epithelium. When protective commensals are disturbed by antibiotics, susceptibility to opportunistic infections by *Candida* and *Clostridium difficile* is increased.

If micro-organisms do penetrate the body, two main defensive operations come into play, the destructive effect of soluble chemical factors such as bactericidal enzymes and the mechanism of phagocytosis—literally 'eating' by the cell.

Phagocytic cells kill micro-organisms

'Professional' phagocytes

The engulfment and digestion of micro-organisms is assigned to two major cell types recognized by Metchnikoff at the turn of the century as *micro-* and *macrophages.*

The polymorphonuclear neutrophil

This cell, the smaller of the two, shares a common haemopoietic stem cell precursor with the other formed elements of the blood and is the dominant white cell in the bloodstream. It is a non-dividing short-lived cell with a multilobed nucleus and an array of granules which are virtually unstained by histological dyes such as haematoxylin and eosin, unlike those structures in the closely related eosinophil and basophil (figures 1.3 and 1.5). The neutrophil granules are of three types, the primary

dermal capillaries. The slides from which illustrations (a), (b), (d), (e), (f), (i) and (j) were reproduced were very kindly provided by Mr M. Watts of the Dept. Haematology, Middlesex Hospital Medical School; (c) was kindly supplied by Prof. J.J. Owen, (g) by Drs P. Lydyard and G. Rook, (h) by Dr Meryl Griffiths and (k) by Prof. N. Woolf.

Figure 1.3. *Cells involved in innate immunity. (a) Monocyte, showing 'horseshoe-shaped' nucleus and moderately abundant pale cytoplasm. Note the three multilobed polymorphonuclear neutrophils and the small lymphocyte (bottom left). Romanowsky stain. (b) Two monocytes stained for non-specific esterase with α-naphthyl acetate. Note the vacuolated cytoplasm. The small cell with focal staining at the top is a T-lymphocyte. (c) Four polymorphonuclear leucocytes (neutrophils) and one eosinophil. The multilobed nuclei and the cytoplasmic granules are clearly shown, those of the eosinophil being heavily stained. (d) Polymorphonuclear neutrophil showing cytoplasmic granules stained for alkaline phosphatase. (e) Early neutrophils in bone marrow. The primary azurophilic granules (PG) originally clustered near*
the nucleus, move towards the periphery where the neutrophil-specific granules are generated by the Golgi apparatus as the cell matures. The nucleus gradually becomes lobular (LN). Giemsa. (f) Inflammatory cells from the site of a brain haemorrhage showing the large active macrophage in the centre with phagocytosed red cells and prominent vacuoles. To the right is a monocyte with horseshoe-shaped nucleus and cytoplasmic bilirubin crystals (haematoidin). Several multilobed neutrophils are clearly delineated. Giemsa. (g) Macrophages in monolayer cultures after phagocytosis of mycobacteria (stained red). Carbol-Fuchsin counterstained with Malachite Green. (h) Numerous plump alveolar macrophages within air spaces in the lung. (i) Basophil with heavily staining granules compared with a

Figure 1.4. *The mononuclear phagocyte system (previously included with endothelial cells and polymorphs under the term 'the reticuloendothelial system' or RES). Promonocyte precursors in the bone marrow develop into circulating blood monocytes which eventually become distributed throughout the body as mature macrophages (Mφ) as shown. The other major phagocytic cell, the polymorphonuclear neutrophil, is largely confined to the bloodstream except when recruited into sites of acute inflammation.*

azurophilic granule containing myeloperoxidase, some lysozyme and a family of cationic proteins, the secondary 'specific' granules holding lactoferrin, lysozyme and a B_{12}-binding protein and tertiary granules akin to the conventional lysosomes with acid hydrolases. The abundant glycogen stores can be utilized by glycolysis enabling the cells to function under anaerobic conditions.

The macrophage

These cells derive from bone marrow promonocytes which, after differentiation to blood monocytes, finally settle in the tissues as mature macrophages where they constitute the *mononuclear phagocyte system* (figure 1.4). They are present throughout the connective tissue and around the basement membrane of small blood vessels and are particularly concentrated in the lung (alveolar macrophages), liver (Kupffer cells), and lining of spleen sinuosoids and lymph node medullary sinuses where they are strategically placed to filter off foreign material. Other examples are mesangial cells in the kidney glomerulus, brain microglia and osteoclasts in bone. Unlike the polymorphs, they are long-lived cells with significant rough-surfaced endoplasmic reticulum and mitochondria (figure 1.5) and whereas

the polymorphs provide the major defence against pyogenic (pus-forming) bacteria, as a rough generalization it may be said that macrophages are at their best in combating those bacteria (figure 1.3g), viruses and protozoa which are capable of living within the cells of the host.

Phagocytosis

Before phagocytosis can occur, the microbe must first adhere to the surface of the polymorph or macrophage, an event mediated by some rather primitive recognition mechanism likely to involve carbohydrate elements. Depending on its nature, a particle attached to the surface membrane may initiate the ingestion phase by activating an actin—myosin contractile system which extends pseudopods around the particle (figures 1.6 and 1.7); as adjacent receptors sequentially attach to the surface of the microbe, the plasma membrane is pulled around the particle just like a 'zipper' until it is completely enclosed in a vacuole (phagosome; figures 1.6 and 1.8). Events are now moving smartly and within one minute the cytoplasmic granules fuse with the phagosome and discharge their contents around the imprisoned micro-organism (figure 1.8) which is subject to a formidable battery of microbicidal mechanisms.

Killing

Oxygen-dependent mechanisms

Trouble starts for the invader from the moment phagocytosis is initiated. There is a dramatic increase in activity of the hexose monophosphate shunt generating NADPH. This is utilized ultimately to reduce molecular oxygen bound to a unique plasma-membrane cytochrome (cyt b_{-245}) causing a burst of oxygen consumption. As a result, oxygen is converted to superoxide anion, hydrogen peroxide, singlet O_2 and hydroxyl radicals, all of which are powerful microbicidal agents. Furthermore, the combination of peroxide, myeloperoxidase and halide ions constitutes a potent halogenating system capable of killing both bacteria and viruses (table 1.1).

Oxygen-independent mechanisms

It can also be seen from table 1.1 that the dismutation of superoxide consumes hydrogen ions and raises the pH gently so allowing the family of cationic proteins to function optimally. Although not

Specific granules

Azurophil granules

1 μm

(a)

(b)

Figure 1.5. *Ultrastructure of phagocytic cells. (a) Neutrophil. The multi-lobed nucleus and cytoplasmic granules are well displayed. (Courtesy of Dr D. McLaren.) (b) Monocyte (× 10 000). 'Horseshoe' nucleus. Phagocytic and pinocytic vesicles, lysosomal granules, mitochondria and isolated profiles of rough-surfaced endoplasmic reticulum are evident.*

fully characterized yet; they damage bacterial membranes both by neutral proteinase (cathepsin G) action and by direct transfer to the microbial surface. Low pH, lysozyme and lactoferrin constitute bactericidal or bacteriostatic factors which are oxygen independent and can function under anaerobic circumstances. Finally, the killed organisms are digested by hydrolytic enzymes and the degradation products released to the exterior (figure 1.7).

By now, the reader may be excused a little smugness as she or he shelters behind the impressive anti-microbial potential of the phagocytic cells. But there are snags to consider; our formidable array of weaponry is useless unless the phagocyte can (i) 'home onto' the micro-organism, (ii) adhere to it, and (iii) respond by the membrane activation which initiates engulfment. Some bacteria do produce chemical substances which directionally attract

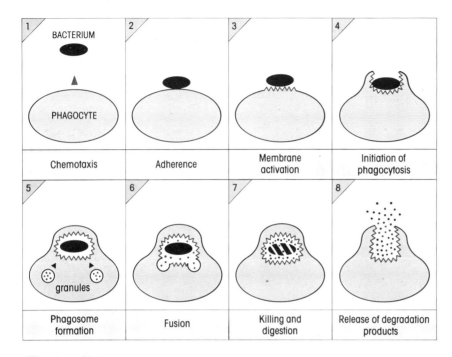

Figure 1.6. *Phagocytosis and killing of a bacterium.*

(a)

(b)

Figure 1.7. *Adherence and phagocytosis.*
(a) Phagocytosis of **Candida albicans** *by a polymorphonuclear leucocyte (neutrophil). Adherence to the surface initiates enclosure of the fungal particle within arms of cytoplasm. Lysosomal granules are abundant but mitochondria are rare (×15 000). (b) Phagocytosis of C. albicans by a monocyte showing near completion of phagosome formation (arrowed) around one organism and complete ingestion of two others (× 5000). (Courtesy of Dr H. Valdimarsson.)*

(a)

(b)

Figure 1.8. *Phagolysosome formation.*
(a) Neutrophil 30 minutes after ingestion of **C. albicans.** *The cytoplasm is already partly degranulated and two lysosomal granules (arrowed) are fusing with the phagocytic vacuole. Two lobes of the nucleus are evident (× 5000). (b) Higher magnification of (a) showing fusing granules discharging their contents into the phagocytic vacuole (arrowed). (× 33 000; courtesy of Dr H. Valdimarsson.)*

OXYGEN-DEPENDENT MECHANISMS:

Glucose + NADP$^+$	$\xrightarrow[\text{shunt}]{\text{hexose monophosphate}}$	pentose phosphate + NADPH	O_2 burst + generation of superoxide anion
NADPH + O_2	$\xrightarrow{\text{cytochrome b}_{-245}}$	NADP$^+$ + **O_2^-**	
$2O_2^- + 2H^+$	$\xrightarrow[\text{dismutation}]{\text{spontaneous}}$	**H_2O_2** + **$^1O_2$**	Spontaneous formation of further microbicidal agents
$O_2^- + H_2O_2$	$\longrightarrow$	**.OH** + OH$^-$ + **$^1O_2$**	
$H_2O_2 + Cl^-$	$\xrightarrow{\text{myeloperoxidase}}$	**OCl$^-$** + H_2O	Myeloperoxidase generation of micro-bicidal molecules
OCl$^-$ + H_2O	$\longrightarrow$	**$^1O_2$** + Cl$^-$ + H_2O	
$2O_2^- + 2H^+$	$\xrightarrow[\text{dismutase}]{\text{superoxide}}$	$O_2 + H_2O_2$	Protective mechanisms used by host + many microbes
$2H_2O_2$	$\xrightarrow{\text{catalase}}$	$2H_2O + O_2$	

OXYGEN-INDEPENDENT MECHANISMS:

Cationic proteins (incl. cathepsin G)	Damage to microbial membranes
Lysozyme	Splits mucopeptide in bacterial cell wall
Lactoferrin	Deprives proliferating bacteria of iron
Proteolytic enzymes Variety of other hydrolytic enzymes	Digestion of killed organisms

Table 1.1. *Anti-microbial systems in phagocytic vacuoles. Microbicidal species in bold letters. O_2^- superoxide anion; $^1O_2$, singlet (activated) oxygen; OH, hydroxyl free radical.*

leucocytes, a process known as chemotaxis; some organisms do adhere to the phagocyte surface and some do spontaneously provide the appropriate membrane initiation signal. However, our teeming microbial adversaries are continually mutating to produce new species which may outwit the defences by doing none of these. What then? The body has solved these problems with the effortless ease that comes with a few million years of evolution by developing the complement system.

Complement facilitates phagocytosis

Complement and its activation

Complement is the name given to a complex series of some 20 proteins which, along with blood clotting, fibrinolysis and kinin formation, forms one of the triggered enzyme systems found in plasma. These systems characteristically produce a rapid, highly amplified response to a trigger stimulus mediated by a cascade phenomenon where the product of one reaction is the enzymic catalyst of the next.

Some of the complement components are designated by the letter 'C' followed by a number which is related more to the chronology of its discovery than to its position in the reaction sequence. The most abundant and the most pivotal component is C3 which has a molecular weight of 195 kD and is present in plasma at a concentration of around 1.2 mg/ml.

The C3 cleavage mechanism

Under normal circumstances, the internal thioester bond in C3 becomes activated at a very slow rate either through reaction with water or with trace amounts of a plasma proteolytic enzyme to form a reactive intermediate, either the split product C3b, or a functionally similar molecule. In the presence of Mg^{++}, this can complex with another complement component, factor B, which then undergoes cleavage by a normal plasma enzyme (factor D) to generate $\overline{\text{C3bBb}}$. Note that conventionally, a bar over a complex denotes enzymic activity and that on cleavage of a complement component, the larger product is generally given the suffix 'b' and the smaller 'a'.

INNATE IMMUNITY

C3bBb has an important new enzymic activity: it is a 'C3 convertase' which can split C3 to give C3a and C3b. We will shortly discuss the important biological consequences of C3 cleavage in relation to microbial defences, but under normal conditions there must be some mechanism to restrain this process to a 'tick-over' level since it can also give rise to more C3bBb, that is, we are dealing with a potentially runaway positive-feedback circuit (figure 1.9). As with all potentially explosive triggered cascades, there are powerful regulatory mechanisms.

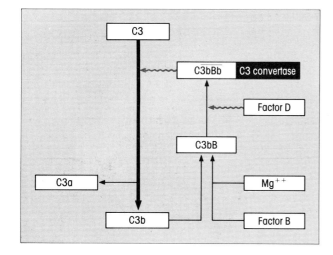

Figure 1.9. *The C3 convertase loop.* ∿∿➤ *represents an activation process. The horizontal bar above a component designates its activation.*

The control of C3b levels

In solution, the C3bBb convertase is unstable and factor B is readily displaced by another component, factor H, to form a complex which is susceptible to attack by the C3b inactivator, factor I (figure 1.10). The inactivated C3bi is biologically inactive and undergoes further degradation by trypsin-like enzymes in the body fluids.

Activation of the C3 cleavage mechanism

A number of micro-organisms can activate the C3bBb convertase to generate large amounts of C3 cleavage products by stabilizing the enzyme on their (carbohydrate) surfaces thereby protecting the C3b from factor H. Another protein, properdin, acts subsequently on this bound convertase to stabilize it even further. As C3 is split by the surface membrane-bound enzyme, its internal thioester bond

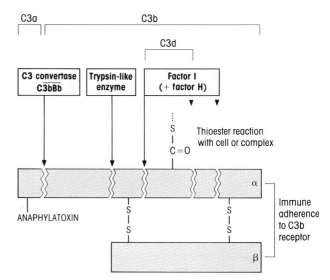

Figure 1.10. *Structural basis for the cleavage of C3. The β-chain together with the disulphide-linked fragments remaining after factor I cleavage is termed C3c.*

becomes activated and the reactive intermediate binds covalently to the membrane. Each catalytic site thereby leads to the deposition of large numbers of C3b molecules on the micro-organism. This series of reactions leading to C3 breakdown provoked directly by microbes has been called '*the alternative pathway*' of complement activation (figure 1.11).

The post-C3 pathway

The next component to be activated is C5 which on complexing with membrane-bound C3b becomes a substrate for C3bBb and is cleaved to release a small polypeptide, C5a, leaving the larger fragment, C5b, on the membrane. This binds C6, C7 and then C8 to form a complex which induces a critical orientation between two or more molecules of the terminal component C9. This leads to unfolding of C9, insertion into the lipid bilayer and polymerization to an annular 'membrane attack complex' (MAC; figures 1.12 and 2.2) forming a transmembrane channel fully permeable to electrolytes and water. Due to the high internal colloid osmotic pressure of cells, there is a net influx of Na^+ and water frequently leading to lysis.

Complement has a range of biological functions

These can be grouped conveniently under three headings:

8

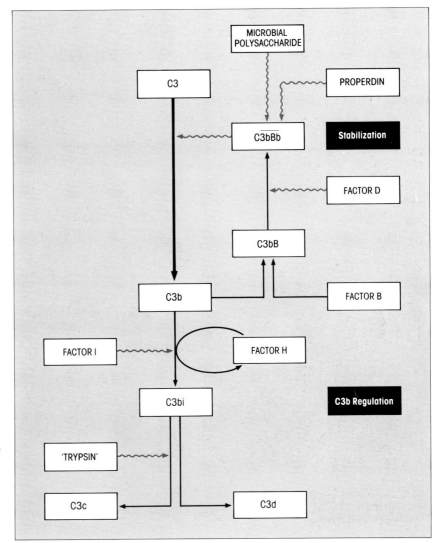

MICROBIAL
POLYSACCHARIDE

C3

PROPERDIN

C3bBb — Stabilization

FACTOR D

C3bB

C3b — FACTOR B

FACTOR I — FACTOR H

C3bi — C3b Regulation

'TRYPSIN'

C3c — C3d

9

Figure 1.11. *Microbial activation of the alternative complement pathway and its control by factors H and I. Although in phylogenetic terms this is the oldest pathway, it was discovered after a separate pathway to be discussed in the next chapter, and so has the confusing designation 'alternative'.*

1 Adherence reactions

Phagocytic cells have receptors for C3b and C3bi which facilitate the adherence of C3b-coated micro-organisms to the cell surface.

2 Biologically active fragments

C3a and C5a, the small peptides split from the parent molecules during complement activation, have several important actions. Both act directly on phagocytes, especially neutrophils, to stimulate the respiratory burst associated with production of oxygen metabolites. Also, both are 'anaphylatoxins' in that they are capable of triggering mediator release from mast cells (figures 1.3 and 1.13) and their circulating counterpart the basophil (figure 1.3), a phenomenon of such relevance to our present discussion that I have presented details of the media-

tors and their actions in figure 1.14; note in particular the chemotactic properties of these mediators and their effects on blood vessels. In its own right, C5a is a potent neutrophil chemotactic agent and has a striking ability to act directly on the capillary endothelial cells to produce vasodilatation and increased permeability, an effect which is prolonged by leukotriene B4 released by both mast cells and activated neutrophils.

3 Membrane lesions

As described above, the insertion of the membrane attack complex into a membrane may bring about cell lysis. Providentially, complement is relatively inefficient at lysing the cell membranes of the autologous host.

(a)

a

(b)

b

Figure 1.12. *Post C3 pathway generating C5a and the C5b−9 membrane attack complex. (a) Cartoon of molecular assembly. (b) Electron micrograph of a membrane C5b−9 complex incorporated into liposomal membranes clearly showing the annular structure. The cylindrical complex is seen from the side inserted into the membrane of the liposome on the left, and end-on in that on the right (courtesy Prof. J. Tranum-Jensen and Dr S. Bhakdi).*

Figure 1.13. *The mast cell. (a) A resting cell containing many membrane-bound granules containing pre-formed mediators. (b) A triggered mast cell. Note that the granules have released their contents and are morphologically altered, being larger and less electron dense. Although most of the altered granules remain within the circumference of the cell, they are open to the extracellular space. (Electron micrographs × 5400; courtesy of Drs D. Lawson, C. Fewtrell, B. Gomperts and M. Raff: from* **J. Exp. Med. 1975, 142, 391.***)*

The complement-mediated acute inflammatory reaction

We can now put together an effectively orchestrated defensive scenario initiated by activation of the alternative complement pathway (figure 1.15).

In the first act, C3bBb is stabilized on the surface of the microbe and cleaves large amounts of C3. The C3a fragment is released but C3b molecules bind copiously to the microbe. These activate the next step in the sequence to generate C5a and the membrane attack complex (although many organisms will be resistant to its action).

The next act sees C3a and C5a, together with the mediators they trigger from the mast cell, acting to recruit polymorphonuclear neutrophils and further plasma complement components to the site of microbial invasion. The relaxation induced in arteriolar walls causes increased blood flow and dilatation of the small vessels while contraction of capillary endothelial cells allows exudation of plasma proteins. Neutrophils slow down and marginate to the walls of the capillaries where they pass through gaps between the endothelial cells (diapedesis) and move up the concentration gradient of chemotactic factors until they come face to face with the

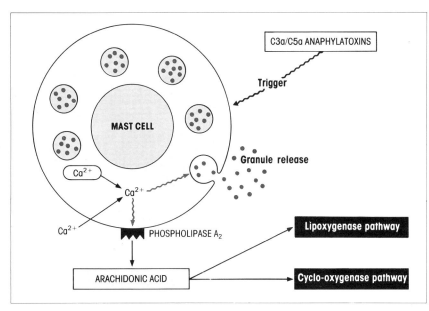

Figure 1.14. *Mast cell triggering leading to release of mediators by two major pathways: (i) release of pre-formed mediators present in the granules, and (ii) the metabolism of arachidonic acid produced through activation of a phospholipase. Intracellular Ca^{++} and cAMP are central to the initiation of these events but details are still unclear. (ECF = eosinophil chemotactic factor; NCF = neutrophil chemotactic factor. Chemotaxis refers to directed migration of granulocytes up the concentration gradient of the mediator while chemokinesis describes randomly increased motility of these cells.)*

Granule release	PRE-FORMED	EFFECT
	HISTAMINE	Vasodilation, incr. capillary permeability, chemokinesis, bronchoconstriction
	HEPARIN	Anti-coagulant
	TRYPTASE	Activates C3
	β-GLUCOSAMINIDASE	Splits off glucosamine
	ECF	Eosinophil chemotaxis
	NCF	Neutrophil chemotaxis
	PLATELET ACTIVATING FACTOR	Mediator release

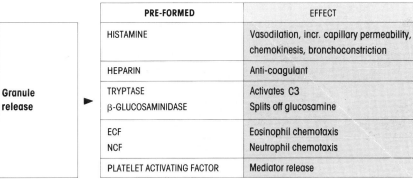

	NEWLY SYNTHESIZED	EFFECT
Lipoxygenase pathway	LEUKOTRIENES C_4 AND D_4 (SRS-A) LEUKOTRIENE B_4	Vasoactive, bronchoconstriction, chemotaxis and/or chemokinesis
Cyclo-oxygenase pathway	PROSTAGLANDINS THROMBOXANES	Affect bronchial muscle, platelet aggregation and vasodilation

C3b-coated microbe. Adherence to the neutrophil C3b-receptors then takes place, C3a and C5a activate the respiratory burst and, hey presto, the slaughter of the last act can begin!

The processes of capillary dilatation (redness), exudation of plasma proteins and also of fluid (oedema) due to hydrostatic and osmotic pressure changes, and accumulation of neutrophils are collectively termed *the acute inflammatory response*.

Humoral mechanisms provide a second defensive strategy

Turning now to those defence systems which are mediated entirely by soluble factors, we recollect that many microbes activate the complement system and may be lysed by the insert of the membrane attack complex. The spread of infection may be limited by enzymes released through tissue injury which activate the clotting system. Of the soluble bactericidal substances elaborated by the body, perhaps the most abundant and widespread is the enzyme lysozyme, a muramidase which splits the exposed peptidoglycan wall of susceptible bacteria (cf. figure 10.1).

Acute phase proteins

A number of plasma proteins collectively termed *acute phase proteins* show a dramatic increase in

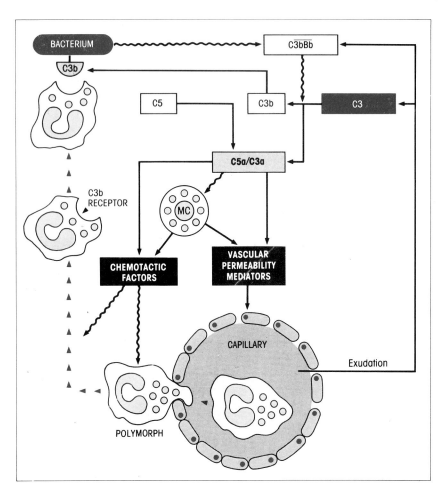

Figure 1.15. *The defensive strategy of the acute inflammatory reaction initiated by bacterial activation of the alternative C pathway. Directions: start with the activation of the C3bBb C3 convertase by the bacterium, notice the generation of C3b (which binds to the bacterium), C3a and C5a and recruitment of mast cell mediators, follow their effect on capillary dilatation and exudation of plasma proteins and their chemotactic attraction of polymorphs to the C3b-coated bacterium and triumph in their adherence and final activation for the kill.*

concentration in response to infection or tissue injury. These include C-reactive protein (CRP), serum amyloid A protein, α_1-anti-trypsin, α_2-macroglobulin, fibrinogen, caeruloplasmin, C9 and factor B.

As an example, during an infection, microbial products such as endotoxins stimulate the release of interleukin-1 (IL-1) which is an endogenous pyrogen (incidentally capable of improving our general defences by raising the body temperature). IL-1 in turn acts on the liver to increase the synthesis and secretion of CRP to such an extent that its plasma concentration may rise 1000-fold.

Human CRP is composed of five identical polypeptide units non-covalently arranged as a cyclic pentamer. This class of protein has been around in the animal kingdom for some time since a closely related homologue, limulin, is present in the haemolymph of the horseshoe crab, not exactly a close relative of *Homo sapiens*. A major property of CRP is its ability to bind, in a Ca-dependent fashion, to a number of micro-organisms which contain phosphorylcholine in their membranes, the complex having the useful property of activating complement (by the classical and not the alternative pathway with which we are at present familiar). This results in the deposition of C3b on the surface of the microbe which thus becomes opsonized (i.e. 'made ready for the table') for adherence to phagocytes.

Interferons

These are a family of broad-spectrum anti-viral agents present in birds, reptiles and fishes as well as the higher animals, and first recognized by the phenomenon of viral interference in which an animal infected with one virus resists superinfection by a second unrelated virus. Different molecular forms of interferon have been identified, all of which have been gene cloned. There are at least 14 different α-interferons (IFNα) produced by lymphocytes while fibroblasts, and probably all cell types, synthesize IFNβ. We will keep a third type (IFNγ), which is not directly induced by viruses, up our sleeves for the moment.

Cells synthesize interferon when infected by a virus and secrete it into the extracellular fluid whence it binds to specific receptors on uninfected neighbouring cells. The bound interferon now exerts its anti-viral effect in the following way. At least two genes are thought to be derepressed in the interferon-treated cell allowing the synthesis of two new enzymes. The first, a protein kinase, catalyses the phosphorylation of a ribosomal protein and an initiation factor necessary for protein synthesis, so greatly reducing mRNA translation. The other catalyses the formation of a short polymer of adenylic acid which activates a latent endonuclease; this in turn degrades both viral and host mRNA.

Whatever the precise mechanism of action ultimately proves to be, the net result is to establish a cordon of uninfectable cells around the site of virus infection so restraining its spread. The effectiveness of interferon *in vivo* may be inferred from experiments in which mice injected with an antiserum to murine interferons could be killed by several hundred times less virus than was needed to kill the controls. However, it must be presumed that interferon plays a significant role in the recovery from, as distinct from the prevention of, viral infections.

As a group, the interferons may prove to have a wider biological role than the control of viral infection. It will be clear, for example, that the induced enzymes described above would act to inhibit host cell division just as effectively as viral replication. The interferons may also modulate the activity of other cells such as the natural killer (NK) cells, to be discussed in the following section.

Extracellular killing

Natural killer (NK) cells

Viruses lack the apparatus for self-renewal so it is essential for them to penetrate the cells of the infected host in order to take over its replicative machinery. It is clearly in the interest of the host to find a way to kill such infected cells *before* the virus has had a chance to reproduce. NK cells appear to do just that when studied *in vitro*.

They are large granular lymphocytes (figure 1.3) with a characteristic morphology (figure 2.6b). They are thought to recognize structures on high molecular weight glycoproteins which appear on the surface of virally infected cells and which allow them to be differentiated from normal cells. This recognition occurs through receptors on the NK cell

surface which bring killer and target into close opposition. Activation of the NK cell ensues and leads to extracellular release of granule contents into the space between the two cells. Perhaps the most important of these is a *perforin* or *cytolysin* bearing some structural relationship to C9; like that protein, it can insert itself into the membrane of the target and associate to form a transmembrane pore with an annular structure, comparable to the complement membrane attack complex, which induces cell death. Antibodies made against the cytolysin inhibit this extracellular killing. The granules also contain two serine esterases which can function as NK cytotoxic factors but the time course of their action casts some doubt over the primacy of their role in NK-mediated lysis. Chondroitin sulphate A, a protease-resistant highly negatively charged proteoglycan, is also present and may subserve the function of protecting the NK cell from autolysis by its own lethal agents (figure 1.16).

The various interferons augment NK cytotoxicity and since interferons are produced by virally infected cells, we have a nicely integrated feedback defence system.

Eosinophils

Large parasites such as helminths cannot physically be phagocytosed and extracellular killing by eosinophils would seem to have evolved to help cope with

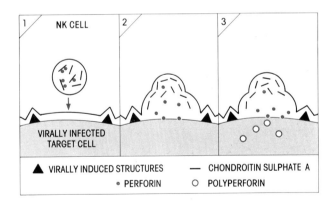

Figure 1.16. *Extracellular killing of virally infected cell by natural killer (NK) cell (following diagram by Tschopp J. & Conzelmann A. In* Immunology Today *1986, 7, 135). As the NK receptors bind to the surface of the virally infected cell, the granules release perforin molecules extracellularly; these polymerize to form transmembrane channels which bring about lysis of the target. Tschopp & Conzelmann have shown that chondroitin sulphate A binds to and inactivates the perforin particularly at the low pH within the granule and suggest that as the granule discharges, the higher pH dissociates the perforin which then acts to lyse the target cell.*

this situation. These polymorphonuclear 'cousins' of the neutrophil have distinctive granules which stain avidly with acid dyes (figure 1.3) and have a characteristic appearance in the electron microscope (figure 10.15). A major basic protein (MBP) is localized in the core of the granules while an eosinophilic cationic protein together with a peroxidase have been identified in the granule matrix. Other enzymes include arylsulphatase B, phospholipase D and histaminase. They have surface receptors for C3b and on activation produce a particularly impressive respiratory burst with concomitant generation of active oxygen metabolites. As if that were not enough, it has recently been demonstrated that one of the granule proteins can produce a transmembrane plug in the target membrane like C9 and the NK perforin.

Most helminths can activate the alternative complement pathway, but although resistant to C9 attack, their coating with C3b allows adherence of eosinophils through their C3b receptors. Upon activation, the eosinophil launches its extracellular attack which includes the release of MBP and especially the cationic protein which damages the parasite membrane.

14

THE BASIS OF IMMUNOLOGY
II – Specific Acquired Immunity

The need for specific immune mechanisms

Our microbial adversaries have tremendous opportunities through mutation to evolve strategies which evade our innate immune defences. For example, most of the *successful* parasites activate the alternative complement pathway and bind C3b, yet eosinophils which adhere are somehow not triggered into offensive action. The same holds true for many bacteria while some may so shape their exteriors as to avoid complement activation completely. The body obviously needed to 'devise' defence mechanisms which could be dovetailed individually to each of these organisms no matter how many there were. In other words *a very large number* of specific immune defences needed to be at the body's disposal. Quite a tall order!

Antibody—the specific adaptor

Evolutionary processes came up with what can only be described as a brilliant solution. This was to fashion an adaptor molecule which was intrinsically capable not only of activating the complement system *and* of stimulating phagocytic cells, but also of sticking to the offending microbe. The adaptor thus had three main regions, two concerned in communicating with complement and the phagocytes (the biological functions) and one devoted to binding to an individual micro-organism (the external recognition function). In most biological systems like hormones and receptors, and enzymes and substrates, recognition usually occurs through fairly accurate complementarity in shape allowing the ligands to approach so close to each other as to permit the normal intermolecular forces to become relatively strong. In the present case, each adaptor would have a recognition portion complementary in shape to some micro-organism to which it could then bind reasonably firmly. The part of the adaptor with biological function would be constant, but for each of hundreds of thousands of different organisms, a special recognition portion would be needed.

Thus the body has to make hundreds of thousands, or even millions, of adaptors with different recognition sites. The adaptor is of course the molecule we know affectionately as *antibody* (figure 2.1).

Antibody initiates a new complement pathway ('classical')

Antibody, when bound to a microbe, will link to and activate the first molecule in the so-called classical complement sequence, C1q. This molecule is polyvalent with respect to antibody binding and consists of a central collagen-like stem branching into six peptide chains each tipped by an antibody-binding subunit (resembling the blooms on a bunch of flowers). C1q is associated with two further subunits, C1r and C1s, in a Ca^{++} stabilized trimolecular complex and these are activated sequentially

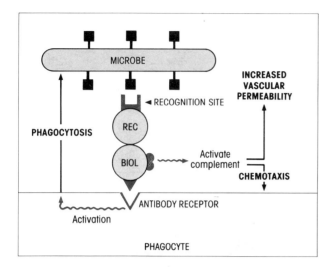

Figure 2.1. *The antibody adaptor molecule. The constant part with biological function (BIOL) activates complement and the phagocyte. The portion with the recognition unit for the foreign microbe (REC) varies from one antibody to another.*

with C1s acquiring proteolytic activity which allows it to act on the next component in the chain C4 (unfortunately components were numbered before the sequence was established). As expected in a multi-enzyme cascade, several molecules of C4 undergo cleavage, releasing a small C4a fragment and revealing a nascent but labile internal thioester bond in the residual $\overline{\text{C4b}}$ which may then bind either to the antibody-C1 complex or the surface of the microbe itself. In the presence of Mg^{++}, C2 can complex with the $\overline{\text{C4b}}$ to become a new substrate for the $\overline{\text{C1s}}$; the resulting product $\overline{\text{C4b2b}}$ now has the vital C3 convertase activity required to activate C3 with the same specificity as the $\overline{\text{C3bBb}}$ generated

by the alternative pathway. From then on things march along exactly in parallel to the post-C3 pathway with one molecule of C3b added to the $\overline{\text{C4b2b}}$ to make it into a C5-splitting enzyme with eventual production of the membrane attack complex (figure 2.2). Just as the alternative pathway C3 convertase is controlled by factors H and I, so the breakdown of $\overline{\text{C4b2b}}$ is brought about by either a C4 binding protein (C4bp) or a cell surface C3b receptor (CR1) in the presence of factor I.

The similarities between the two pathways are set out in figure 2.3 and show how antibody can supplement and even improve on the ability of the innate immune system to initiate acute inflammatory reactions. Antibody provides yet a further bonus in this respect; the class known as immunoglobulin E (see legend to figure 2.2) can sensitize mast cells through binding to their surface so that combination with antigen triggers mediator release independently of C3a or C5a, adding yet more flexibility to our defences.

Complexed antibody activates phagocytic cells

I drew attention to the fact that many C3b-coated organisms adhere to phagocytic cells yet avoid provoking their uptake. If small amounts of antibody are added the phagocyte springs into action. It does so through the recognition of two or more antibody molecules bound to the microbe, using specialized receptors on the cell surface.

A single antibody molecule complexed to the micro-organism is not enough because it cannot cause the cross-linking of antibody receptors in the

Figure 2.2. *Multiple lesions in cell wall of* **Escherichia coli** *bacterium caused by interaction with IgM antibody and complement. (Human antibodies are divided into five main classes, immunoglobulin M— shortened to IgM—IgG, IgA, IgE and IgD, which differ in the specialization of their 'rear ends' for different biological functions such as complement activation or mast cell sensitization.) Each lesion is caused by a single IgM molecule and shows as a 'dark pit' due to penetration by the 'negative stain'. This is somewhat of an illusion since in reality these 'pits' are like volcano craters standing proud of the surface, and are each single 'membrane attack' complexes. Comparable results may be obtained in the absence of antibody since the cell wall endotoxin can activate the alternative pathway in the presence of higher concentrations of serum. Magnification × 400 000. (Courtesy of Drs R. Dourmashkin and J.H. Humphrey.)*

Figure 2.3. *Comparison of the alternative and classical complement pathways. The classical pathway with odd*

exceptions such as C-reactive protein, is antibody dependent, the alternative pathway is not.

phagocyte surface membrane which is required to activate the cell. There is a further consideration connected with what is often called 'the bonus effect of multivalency'; for thermodynamic reasons, which will be touched on in Chapter 4, the association constant of ligands which use several rather than a single bond to react with receptors is increased geometrically rather than arithmetically. For example, three antibodies bound close together on a bacterium could be attracted to a macrophage a

thousand times more strongly than a single antibody molecule (figure 2.4).

The cellular basis of antibody production

Antibodies are made by lymphocytes

The majority of resting lymphocytes are small cells with a darkly staining nucleus due to condensed

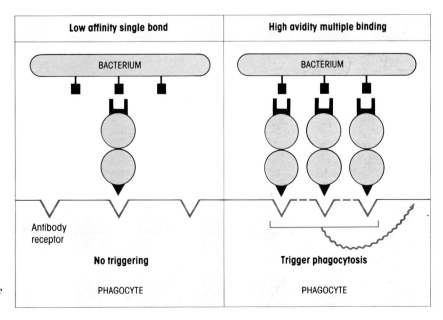

Figure 2.4. *Binding of bacterium to phagocyte by multiple antibodies gives strong association forces and triggers phagocytosis by cross-linking the surface receptors for antibody.*

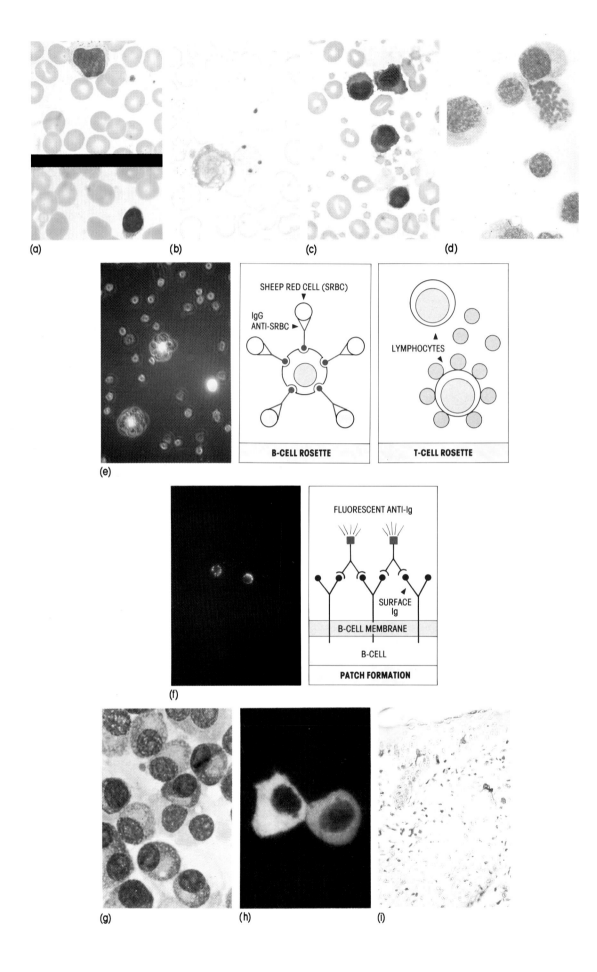

(a)

(b)

(c)

(d)

(e)

SHEEP RED CELL (SRBC)

IgG
ANTI-SRBC

B-CELL ROSETTE

LYMPHOCYTES

T-CELL ROSETTE

(f)

FLUORESCENT ANTI-Ig

SURFACE
Ig

B-CELL MEMBRANE

B-CELL

PATCH FORMATION

(g)

(h)

(i)

chromatin and relatively little cytoplasm containing the odd mitochondrion required for basic energy provision. Figures 2.5 and 2.6 compare the morphology of these cells with that of the minority population of large granular lymphocytes which includes the NK set referred to in Chapter 1.

The central role of the small lymphocyte in the production of antibody was established largely by the work of Gowans. He depleted rats of their lymphocytes by chronic drainage of lymph from the thoracic duct by an indwelling cannula, and showed that they had a grossly impaired ability to mount an antibody response to microbial challenge. The ability to form antibody could be restored by injecting thoracic duct lymphocytes obtained from another rat. The same effect could be obtained if, before injection, the thoracic duct cells were first incubated at 37°C for 24 hours under conditions which kill off large and medium sized cells and leave only the small lymphocytes. This shows that the small lymphocyte is necessary for the antibody response.

The small lymphocytes can be labelled if the donor rat is previously injected with tritiated thymidine; it then becomes possible to follow the fate of these lymphocytes when transferred to another rat of the same strain which is then injected with micro-organisms to produce an antibody response (figure 2.7). It transpires that after contact with the injected microbes, some of the transferred labelled lymphocytes develop into plasma cells (figures 2.5g and 2.8) which can be shown to contain (figure 2.5h) and secrete antibody.

Antigen selects the lymphocytes which make antibody

The molecules in the micro-organisms which evoke and react with antibodies are called *antigens* (*gener*ates *anti*bodies). It was originally envisaged that antibodies were derived from some master plastic molecule which could be moulded to the right shape by using the antigen as a template. Stimulated by the ideas of Jerne and Burnet and many others (not forgetting the incredible Ehrlich who foresaw it at the turn of the century, would you believe it?!), we now know that antibodies are formed before antigen is seen and that they are *selected for* by antigen.

It works in the following way. Each lymphocyte of a subset called the B-lymphocytes, because they differentiate in the bone marrow, is programmed to make one, and only one, antibody and it places this antibody on its outer surface to act as a receptor. This can be detected by using fluorescent probes and in figure 2.5f one can see the molecules of antibody on the surface of a human B-lymphocyte stained with a fluorescent rabbit antiserum raised against

Facing page

Figure 2.5. *Cells involved in the acquired immune response.*
(a) Small lymphocytes. Condensed chromatin gives rise to heavy staining of the nucleus. The cell on the bottom is a typical T-cell with receptors for IgM with a thin rim of cytoplasm. The upper nucleated cell is a large granular lymphocyte (LGL); it has more cytoplasm and azurophilic granules are evident. Isolated platelets are visible. B-lymphocytes range from small to intermediate in size and lack granules. Giemsa stain. (b) Small T-cells with characteristic cytoplasmic dot(s) in cytoplasm stained for acid esterase; compare with diffuse distribution in cytoplasm of monocyte above. (c) T-lymphocytes from buffy coat stained with a monoclonal anti-T using the alkaline phosphatase immunoenzymatic method (cf. figure 5.21). Note the single unstained non-T lymphocyte on the bottom. (d) Transformed lymphocytes (lymphoblasts) following stimulation of lymphocytes in culture with a polyclonal activator. The large lymphoblasts with their relatively high ratio of cytoplasm to nucleus may be compared in size with the isolated small lymphocyte. One cell is in mitosis. May–Grunewald–Giemsa. (e) Identification of lymphocytes by rosette formation with red cells visualized in U.V. light after staining with Acridine Orange which makes the lymphocyte nucleus fluorescent green. T-cell rosettes are formed by spontaneous binding to sheep erythrocytes. B-cell rosettes are developed through binding of IgG-coated

erythrocytes to specific cell surface receptors.
(f) Immunofluorescent staining of B-lymphocyte surface immunoglobulin using fluorescein-conjugated (■) anti-Ig. Provided the reaction is carried out in the cold to prevent pinocytosis, the labelled antibody cannot penetrate to the interior of the viable lymphocytes and reacts only with surface components. Patches of aggregated surface Ig are seen which are beginning to form a cap in the right-hand lymphocyte. During cap formation, submembranous myosin becomes redistributed in association with the surface Ig and induces locomotion of the previously sessile cell in a direction away from the cap. (g) Plasma cells. The nucleus is eccentric. The cytoplasm is strongly basophilic due to high RNA content. The juxta-nuclear lightly stained zone corresponds with the Golgi region. May–Grunewald–Giemsa. (h) Plasma cells stained to show intracellular immunoglobulin using a fluorescein-labelled anti-IgG (green) and a rhodamine-conjugated anti-IgM (red). (i) Langerhans cells in human epidermis in leprosy, increased in the sub-epidermal zone, possibly as a consequence of the disease process. Stained by the immunoperoxidase method with S-100 antibodies. Material for (a), (b) and (c) was kindly supplied by Mr M. Watts of the Dept. Haematology, Middlesex Hospital Medical School, (d), (e) and (f) by Dr P. Lydyard, (g) and (h) by Prof. C. Grossi and (i) by Dr Marian Ridley.

(a)

(b)

Figure 2.6. (a) Small T-lymphocyte with receptors for IgM. Indented nucleus with condensed chromatin, sparse cytoplasm: single mitochondrion shown and many free ribosomes but otherwise few organelles ($\times$ 13 000). B-lymphocytes are essentially similar with slightly more cytoplasm and occasional elements of rough-surfaced endoplasmic reticulum. (b) Large granular lymphocyte ($\times$ 7500). The more abundant cytoplasm contains several mitochondria (M), free ribosomes (R) with some elements of rough-surfaced endoplasmic reticulum (ER), prominent Golgi apparatus (Go) and characteristic membrane-bound electron-dense granules (Gr). The nuclear chromatin is less condensed than that of the T_M cell. (Courtesy of Drs A. Zicca and C.E. Grossi.)

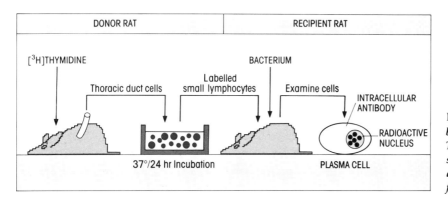

Figure 2.7. Labelled small lymphocytes become antibody-forming plasma cells. Transferred cell with radioactive nucleus shown by autoradiography. Intracellular antibody revealed by staining with fluorescent probes (cf. figure 2.5h).

CHAPTER 2

Figure 2.8. *Plasma cell* (× *10 000*). *Prominent rough-surfaced endoplasmic reticulum associated with the synthesis and secretion of Ig.*

a preparation of human antibodies. Each lymphocyte has of the order of 10^5 antibody molecules on its surface.

When an antigen enters the body, it is confronted by a dazzling array of lymphocytes all bearing different antibodies each with its own individual recognition site. The antigen will only bind to those receptors with which it makes a good fit. Lymphocytes whose receptors have bound antigen receive a triggering signal and develop into antibody-forming plasma cells and since the lymphocytes are programmed to make only one antibody, that secreted by the plasma cell will be identical with that originally acting as the lymphocyte receptor, i.e. it will bind well to the antigen. In this way, antigen selects for the antibodies which recognize it effectively (figure 2.9).

The need for clonal expansion means humoral immunity must be acquired

Because we can make hundreds of thousands, maybe even millions, of different antibody molecules, it is not feasible for us to have too many lymphocytes producing each type of antibody; there just would not be enough room in the body to accommodate them. To compensate for this, lymphocytes which are triggered by contact with antigen undergo successive waves of proliferation (figure 2.5d) to build up a large clone of plasma cells which will be making antibody of the kind for which the parent lymphocyte was programmed. By this system of

clonal selection, large enough concentrations of antibody can be produced to combat infection effectively (figure 2.10).

The importance of proliferation for the development of a significant antibody response is highlighted by the ability of anti-mitotic drugs to abolish antibody production to a given antigen stimulus completely.

Because it takes time for the proliferating clone to build up its numbers sufficiently, it is usually several days before antibodies are detectable in the serum following primary contact with antigen. The newly formed antibodies are a consequence of antigen exposure and it is for this reason that we speak of the *acquired immune response*.

Acquired memory

When we make an antibody response to a given infectious agent, by definition that micro-organism must exist in our environment and we are likely to meet it again. It would make sense then for the immune mechanisms alerted by the first contact with antigen to leave behind some memory system which would enable the response to any subsequent exposure to be faster and greater in magnitude.

Our experience of many common infections tells us that this must be so. We rarely suffer twice from such diseases as measles, mumps, chicken-pox, whooping cough and so forth. The first contact clearly imprints some information, imparts some

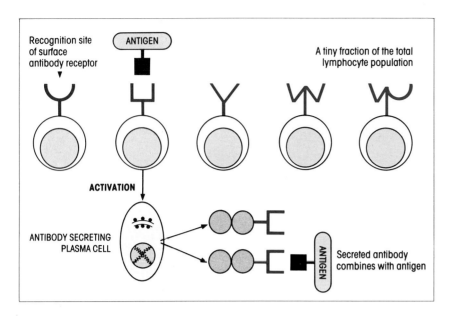

Figure 2.9. *Antigen activates those B-cells whose surface antibody receptors it can combine with firmly.*

Recognition site of surface antibody receptor ▼

ANTIGEN

A tiny fraction of the total lymphocyte population

ACTIVATION

ANTIBODY SECRETING PLASMA CELL

ANTIGEN

Secreted antibody combines with antigen

memory, so that the body is effectively prepared to repel any later invasion by that organism and a state of immunity is established.

Secondary antibody responses

By following the production of antibody on the first and second contacts with antigen we can see the basis for the development of immunity. For example, when we inject a bacterial product such as tetanus toxoid into a rabbit, for reasons already discussed, several days elapse before antibodies can be detected in the blood; these reach a peak and then fall (figure 2.11). If we now allow the animal to rest and then give a second injection of toxoid, the course of events is dramatically altered. Within two to three days the antibody level in the blood rises steeply to reach much higher values than were observed in the *primary response*. This *secondary response* then is characterized by a more rapid and more abundant production of antibody resulting from the 'tuning up' or priming of the antibody-forming system.

With our knowledge of lymphocyte function, it is perhaps not surprising to realize that these are the cells which provide memory. This can be demonstrated by adoptive transfer of lymphocytes to another animal, an experimental system frequently employed in immunology (cf. figure 2.7). In the present case, the immunological potential of the transferred cells is expressed in a recipient treated with X-rays which destroy its own lymphocyte population; thus any immune response will be of donor not recipient origin. In the experiment described in figure 2.12, small lymphocytes are taken from an animal given a primary injection of tetanus toxoid and transferred to an irradiated host which is then boosted with the antigen; a rapid, intense production of antibody characteristic of a secondary response is seen. To exclude the possibility that the first antigen injection might exert a *non-specific* stimulatory effect on the lymphocytes, the boosting injection includes influenza haemagglutinin as a control antigen. Furthermore, a 'criss-cross' control group primed with influenza haemagglutinin must also be included to ensure that this antigen is capable of giving a secondary booster response. I have explained the design of the experiment at some length to call attention to the need for careful selection of controls.

The higher response given by a primed lymphocyte population can be ascribed mainly to an expansion of the numbers of cells capable of being stimulated by the antigen (figure 2.13) although we shall see later that there are some qualitative differences in the cells as well.

The specificity of acquired immunity

The establishment of memory or immunity by one organism does not confer protection against another unrelated organism. After an attack of measles we are immune to further infection but are susceptible to other agents such as the polio or mumps viruses. Acquired immunity then shows *specificity*

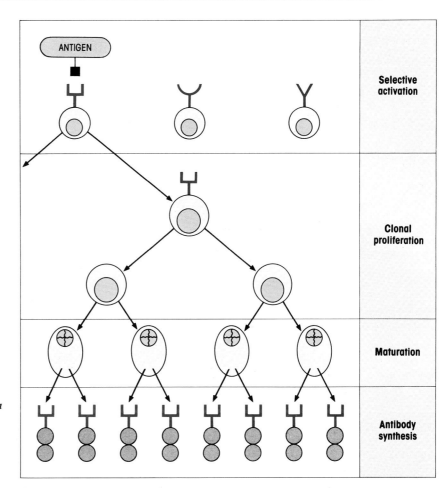

23

Figure 2.10. *Clonal selection. The cell selected by antigen undergoes many divisions during the clonal proliferation and the progeny mature to give an expanded population of antibody-forming cells. The antibody response is particularly vulnerable to anti-mitotic agents at the proliferation stage.*

Figure 2.11. *Primary and secondary response. A rabbit is injected on two separate occasions with tetanus toxoid. The antibody response on the second contact with antigen is more rapid and more intense.*

and the immune system can differentiate specifically between the two organisms. A more formal experimental demonstration of this discriminatory power was seen in figure 2.12 where priming with tetanus toxoid evoked memory for that antigen but not for influenza and vice versa.

The basis for this lies of course in the ability of the recognition sites of the antibody molecules to distinguish between antigens; antibodies which react with the toxoid do not bind to influenza and, *mutatis mutandis* as they say, anti-influenza is not particularly smitten with the toxoid.

This ability to recognize one antigen and distinguish it from another goes even further. The individual must also recognize what is foreign, i.e. what is '*non-self*'. The failure to discriminate between 'self' and 'non-self' could lead to the synthesis of antibodies directed against components of the subject's own body (*autoantibodies*) which in principle could prove to be highly embarrassing. On purely theoretical grounds it seemed to Burnet and Fenner that the body must develop some mechanism whereby 'self' and 'non-self' could be distinguished, and they postulated that those circulating body components which were able to reach the developing lymphoid system in the perinatal period could in some way be 'learnt' as 'self'. A permanent

1st injection of antigen ►	Transfer small lymphocytes to irradiated recipient ►	Boost with **Mixture** of both antigens ►	Measure antibody response to:	
			TOXOID	INFLUENZA
TETANUS TOXOID ▼	⊗		SECONDARY	PRIMARY
INFLUENZA HAEMAGGLUTININ ▼	⊗		PRIMARY	SECONDARY

Figure 2.12. *Memory for a primary response can be transferred by small lymphocytes. Recipients are treated with a dose of X-rays which directly kill lymphocytes (highly sensitive to radiation) but only affect other body cells when they divide; the recipient thus functions as a living 'test-tube' which permits the function of the donor cells to be followed.*

The reasons for the design of the experiment are given in the text. In practice, because of the possibility of interference between the two antigens, it would be wiser to split each of the primary antigen-injected groups into two, giving a separate boosting antigen to each to avoid using a mixture.

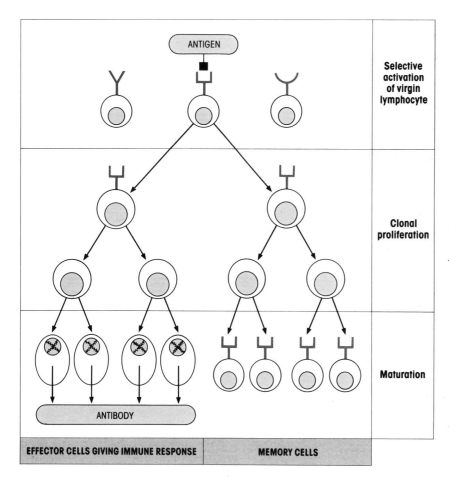

Figure 2.13. *The cellular basis for the generation of effector and memory cells after primary contact with antigen. A fraction of the progeny of the original antigen-reactive lymphocytes become non-dividing memory cells and others the effector cells of humoral or, as we shall see subsequently, cell-mediated immunity. Memory cells require fewer cycles before they develop into effectors and this shortens the reaction time for the secondary response. The expanded clone of cells with memory for the original antigen provides the basis for the greater secondary relative to the primary immune response. Priming with low doses of antigen can often stimulate effective memory without producing very adequate antibody synthesis.*

unresponsiveness or tolerance would then be created so that as immunological maturity was reached there would normally be an inability to respond to 'self' components. As we shall see later, these predictions have been amply verified.

Vaccination

Nearly 200 years ago, Edward Jenner carried out the remarkable studies which mark the beginning of immunology as a systematic subject. Noting the pretty pox-free skin of the milkmaids, he reasoned that deliberate exposure to the pox virus of the cow, which is not virulent for the human, might confer protection against the related human smallpox organism. Accordingly, he inoculated a small boy with cowpox and was delighted—and I hope relieved—to observe that he was now protected against a subsequent exposure to smallpox (what would today's ethical committees have said about that?!). By injecting a harmless form of a disease organism, Jenner had utilized the specificity and memory of the acquired immune response to lay the foundations for modern vaccination (Latin *vacca*, cow).

The essential strategy is to prepare an innocuous form of the infectious organism or its toxins which still substantially retains the antigens responsible for establishing protective immunity. This has been done by using killed or live attenuated organisms, purified microbial components or chemically modified antigens (figure 2.14).

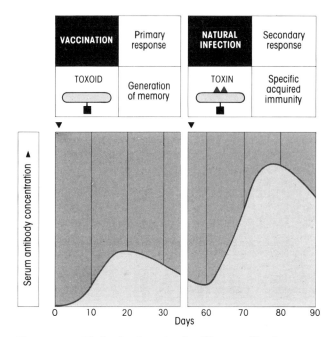

Figure 2.14. *The basis of vaccination illustrated by the response to tetanus toxoid. Treatment of the bacterial toxin with formaldehyde destroys its toxicity (associated with ▲▲) but retains antigenicity. Exposure to toxin in a subsequent natural infection boosts the memory cells producing high levels of neutralizing antibody which are protective.*

Cell-mediated immunity protects against intracellular organisms

Many micro-organisms live inside host cells where it is impossible for humoral antibody to reach them. Obligate intracellular parasites like viruses *have* to replicate inside cells; facultative intracellular parasites like mycobacteria and leishmania can replicate within cells, particularly macrophages, but *don't have to*; they like the intracellular life because of the protection it affords. A totally separate acquired immunity system has evolved to deal with this situation based on a distinct lymphocyte subpopulation made up of T-cells, designated thus because, unlike the B-lymphocytes, they differentiate within the milieu of the thymus gland. Because they are specialized to operate against cells bearing intracellular organisms, T-cells only recognize antigen when it is on the surface of a body cell. Accordingly, its surface receptors, which are different from the antibody molecules used by B-lymphocytes, recognize antigen *plus* a surface marker which informs the T-lymphocyte that it is making contact with another cell. These cell markers belong to an important group of molecules known as the major histocompatibility complex (MHC) identified originally through their ability to evoke powerful transplantation reactions in other members of the same species.

Lymphokine-producing T-cells help macrophages to kill intracellular parasites

These organisms only survive inside macrophages through their ability to subvert the innate killing mechanisms of these cells. None the less, they cannot prevent the macrophage from processing small antigenic fragments (possibly of organisms which have spontaneously died) and placing them on the host cell surface. A subpopulation of T-lymphocytes called T-helper cells, if primed to that antigen, will recognize and bind to the combination of antigen with class II MHC molecules on the macrophage surface and produce a variety of soluble factors called *lymphokines*. These include γ-interferon and other macrophage activating factors which switch on the previously subverted microbicidal mechanisms of the macrophage and bring about the death of the intracellular micro-organisms (figure 2.15).

Killing of virally infected cells by cytotoxic T-cells

We have already discussed the advantage to the host of killing virally infected cells before the virus begins to replicate and have seen that large granular lymphocytes with NK activity (p. 13) can subserve a

1	2	3
Infection by intracellular facultative organisms	Macrophage activation	Death of intracellular microbes

Figure 2.15. *Intracellular killing of micro-organisms by macrophages activated by lymphokines released from T-helpers binding to surface microbial antigen (●) complexed with class II MHC molecules (■).*

cytotoxic function. However, NK cells have a limited range of specificities and in order to improve their efficacy, this range needs to be expanded.

One way in which this can be achieved is by coating the target cell with antibodies specific for the virally coded surface antigens because NK cells have receptors for the constant part of the antibody molecule, rather like phagocytic cells. Thus antibodies will bring the NK cell very close to the target by forming a bridge, and the NK cell being activated by the complexed antibody molecules is able to kill the virally infected cell by its extracellular mechanisms (figure 2.16). This system, termed 'antibody-dependent cell-mediated cytotoxicity' (ADCC) is very impressive when studied *in vitro* but it has proved difficult to establish to what extent it operates within the body.

On the other hand, a subset of cytotoxic T-cells has evolved for which there is evidence of *in vivo* activity. These cells have a very wide range of antigen specificities because they clonally express a large number of different surface receptors similar to, but not identical with, the surface antibody receptors on the B-lymphocytes. Again, each lymphocyte is programmed to make only one receptor and, like the T-helper cell, recognizes antigen only in association with a cell marker, in this case class I MHC molecules (figure 2.16). Through this recognition of surface antigen, the cytotoxic cell comes into intimate contact with its target and administers the 'kiss of death'. It also releases γ-interferon which would help to reduce the spread of virus to adjacent cells, particularly in cases where the virus itself may prove to be a weak inducer of IFNα or β.

In an entirely analogous fashion to the B-cell, T-cells are selected and activated by combination with antigen, expanded by clonal proliferation and mature to give T-helper and cytotoxic T-effectors together with an enlarged population of memory cells. Thus both T- and B-cells provide specific acquired immunity with a variety of mechanisms which in most cases operate to extend the range of effectiveness of innate immunity and confer the valuable advantage that a first infection prepares us to withstand further contact with the same micro-organism.

Figure 2.16. *Killing virally infected cells. The non-specific killing mechanism of the NK cell can be focused on the target by antibody to produce antibody-dependent cell-mediated cytotoxicity (ADCC). The cytotoxic T-cell homes onto its target specifically through receptor recognition of surface antigen in association with MHC class I molecules.*

Immunopathology

The immune system is clearly 'a good thing', but like mercenary armies, it can turn to bite the hand that feeds it, and cause damage to the host.

Thus where there is an especially heightened response or persistent exposure to exogenous antigens, tissue damaging or *hypersensitivity* reactions may result. Examples are allergy to grass pollens, blood dyscrasias associated with certain drugs, immune complex glomerulonephritis occurring after streptococcal infection, and chronic granulomas produced during tuberculosis or schistosomiasis.

In other cases, the ability to maintain non-reactivity against self-components may break down giving rise to a wide variety of diseases with an *autoimmune* component, such as thyrotoxicosis, myasthenia gravis and many of the rheumatological disorders.

Another immunopathological reaction of some consequence is *transplant rejection* where the major histocompatibility complex antigens on the donor graft may well provoke a fierce reaction. Lastly, one should consider the by no means infrequent occurrence of inadequate functioning of the immune system—immunodeficiency. I would like to think that at this stage the reader would have no difficulty in predicting that the major problems in this condition relate to persistent infection, the type of infection being related to the elements of the immune system which are defective.

SUMMARY

A wide range of innate immune mechanisms operate which do not improve with repeated exposure to infection. Micro-organisms are kept out of the body by the skin, the secretion of mucus, ciliary action, the lavaging action of bactericidal fluids (e.g. tears), gastric acid and microbial antagonism. If penetration occurs, bacteria are destroyed by soluble factors such as lysozyme and by phagocytosis with intracellular digestion.

The main phagocytic cells are polymorphonuclear neutrophils and macrophages. Organisms adhere to their surface, activate the engulfment process and are taken inside the cell where they fuse with cytoplasmic granules. A formidable array of oxygen-dependent and oxygen-independent microbicidal mechanisms then come into play.

The complement system, a multicomponent triggered enzyme cascade, is used to attract phagocytic cells to the microbes and engulf them. The most abundant component, C3, is split by a convertase enzyme formed from its own cleavage product C3b and factor B and stabilized against breakdown caused by factors H and I, through association with the microbial surface. As it is formed, C3b becomes linked covalently to the micro-organism. The next component, C5, is activated yielding a small peptide, C5a; the residual C5b binds to the surface and assembles the terminal components C6−9 into a membrane attack complex which is freely permeable to solutes and can lead to osmotic lysis. C5a is a potent chemotactic agent for polymorphs and greatly increases capillary permeability. C3a and C5a act on mast cells causing the release of further mediators such as histamine and leukotriene B4 with effects on capillary permeability and neutrophil chemotaxis; they also activate neutrophils. The neutrophils bind to the C3b-coated microbes by their surface C3b receptors. The influx of polymorphs and the increase in vascular permeability constitute the potent anti-microbial *acute inflammatory response* (figure 2.17).

Other humoral defences involve the acute phase proteins such as C-reactive protein.

Recovery from viral infections can be effected by the interferons which block viral replication. Virally infected cells can be killed by large granular lymphocytes with natural killer (NK) activity.

Extracellular killing by C3b-bound eosinophils may be responsible for the failure of many large parasites to establish a foothold in potential hosts.

The antibody molecule evolved as a specific adaptor to attach to micro-organisms which either fail to activate the alternative complement pathway or prevent activation of the phagocytic cells. The antibody fixes to the antigen by its specific recognition site and its constant structure regions activate complement through the classical pathway (binding C1 and generating a $\overline{C4b2b}$ convertase to split C3) and phagocytes through their antibody receptors. This supplementary route into the acute inflammatory reaction is enhanced by antibodies which sensitize mast cells (figure 2.17).

Antibodies are made by plasma cells derived from B-lymphocytes each of which is programmed to make only one antibody which is placed on the cell surface as a receptor. Antigen binds to the cell with a complementary antibody, activates it and causes clonal proliferation and finally maturation to antibody-forming cells and memory cells. Thus the antigen brings about clonal selection of the cells making antibody to itself. The increase in memory

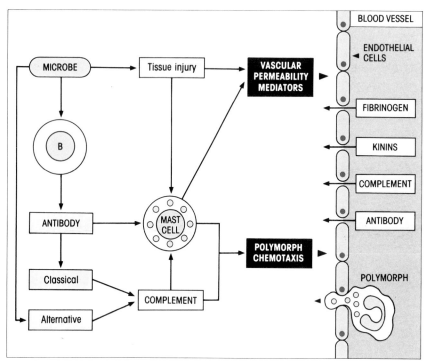

Figure 2.17. *Production of a protective acute inflammatory reaction by microbes either (i) through tissue injury (e.g. bacterial toxin) or direct activation of the alternative complement pathway or (ii) by antibody-dependent triggering of the classical complement pathway or mast cell degranulation (a special type of antibody does this).*

cells after priming means that the acquired secondary response is faster and greater providing the basis for vaccination, using a harmless form of the infective agent for the initial injection.

Another class of lymphocyte, the T-cell, is concerned with control of intracellular infections. Like the B-cell, each T-cell has its individual antigen receptor (although it differs structurally from antibody) which recognizes antigen and undergoes clonal expansion to form effector and memory cells providing specific acquired immunity. The T-cell recognizes cell surface antigens in association with molecules of the major histocompatibility complex (MHC).

T-helper cells which see antigen with class II MHC on the surface of macrophages, release γ-interferon to activate the macrophage and enable it to kill intracellular parasites. Cytotoxic T-cells recognize antigen plus class I MHC on the surface of virally infected cells which are killed before the virus replicates. They also release γ-interferon which can make surrounding cells resistant to viral spread (figure 2.18).

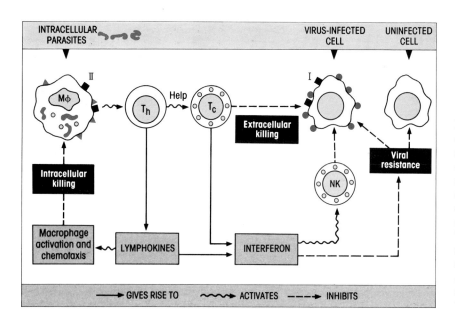

Figure 2.18. *T-cells link with the innate immune system to resist intracellular infection. Class I and class II major histocompatibility molecules (■) are important for T-cell recognition of surface antigen. The T-helper cells (T$_h$) cooperate in the development of cytotoxic T-cells (T$_c$) from precursors. The macrophage (Mφ) microbicidal mechanisms are switched on by macrophage activating lymphokines. Interferon inhibits viral replication and stimulates NK cells which together with T$_c$ kill virus-infected cells.*

Although the innate mechanisms do not improve with repeated exposure to infection as do the acquired, they play a vital role since they are intimately linked to the acquired systems in two different 'trinities' which all but encapsulate the whole of immunology. Antibody, complement and polymorphs give protection against most extracellular organisms while T-cells, soluble cytokines and macrophages deal with intracellular infections (figure 2.19).

Immunopathologically-mediated tissue damage can occur as a result of inappropriate hypersensitivity reactions to exogenous antigens, loss of tolerance to self-giving autoimmune disease and reaction to foreign grafts. Immunodeficiency leaves the individual susceptible to infection.

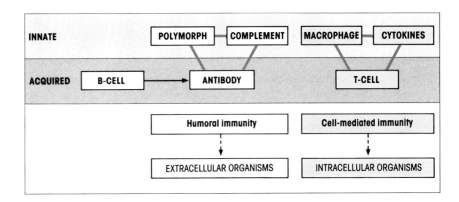

Figure 2.19. *The two trinities linking innate and acquired immunity.*

29

Further reading

Golub E.S. (1981) *The Cellular Basis of the Immune Response.* Sinauer Assoc., Mass., USA.
Herberman R.B., Reynolds C.W. & Ortaldo J. (1986) Mechanisms of cytotoxicity by NK cells. *Ann. Rev. Immunol.,* **4**, 651.
Joiner K.A., Brown E.J. & Frank M.M. (1984) Complement and bacteria. *Ann. Rev. Immunol.,* **2**, 461.
Lewis G.P. (1986) *Mediators of Inflammation.* Wright, Bristol.
Mims C.A. & White D.O. (1984) *Viral Pathogenesis and Immunology.* Blackwell Scientific Publications, Oxford.
Porter R.R., Lachmann P.J. & Reid K.B.M. (1984) A discussion on the biochemistry and genetics of complement. *Phil. Trans. Roy. Soc.(B),* **306**, no. 1129.

General reading

Herbert W.J., Wilkinson P.C. & Stott D.I. (eds) (1985) *Dictionary of Immunology,* 3rd edn. Blackwell Scientific Publications, Oxford.
Hood L.E., Weissman I.L., Wood W.B. & Wilson J.H. (1984) *Immunology,* 2nd edn. Benjamin/Cummings, California, USA. (A very good, in-depth textbook of fundamental immunology in which concepts are extended by numerous mind-bending problems, many of which are based on original data. Thin on clinical side.)
Klein J. (1982) *Immunology: the Science of Self-Nonself Discrimination.* Wiley, N.Y. (In-depth textbook of basic immunology on the grand scale.)
McConnell I., Munro A. & Waldmann H. (1981) *The Immune System: a Course on the Molecular and Cellular Basis of Immunity,* 2nd edn. Blackwell Scientific Publications, Oxford. (An excellent text for further study of fundamental immunological principles, but a little dated.)
Playfair J.H.L. (1987) *Immunology at a Glance,* 4th edn. Blackwell Scientific Publications, Oxford. (Very useful for revision.)
Roitt I.M., Brostoff J. & Male D.K. (1985) *Immunology.* Gower Medical Publishing, London. (An extensively and colourfully illustrated textbook.)
Stites D.P., Stobo J.D., Fudenberg H.H. & Wells J.V. (1984) *Basic and Clinical Immunology,* 5th edn. Lange Medical Publications, California. (I find this of most use for reference purposes.)

Historical

Humphrey J.H. & White R.G. (1970) *Immunology for Students of Medicine,* 3rd edn. Blackwell Scientific Publications, Oxford. (Dated but scholarly.)
Landsteiner K. (1946) *The Specificity of Serological Reactions.* Harvard University Press (reprinted 1962 by Dover Publications, New York).
Metchnikoff E. (1893) *Comparative Pathology of Inflammation.* Transl. F.A. & E.H. Starling. Kegan Paul, Trench, Trübner & Co., London.
Parish H.J. (1968) *Victory with Vaccines.* Churchill Livingstone, Edinburgh.

Series for the advanced reader

* *Advances in Immunology* (Annual). Academic Press, London.
Ann. Rev. Immunology. Ann Reviews Inc., California.
Contemporary Topics in Molecular Immunology. Plenum Press, New York.
Contemporary Topics in Immunobiology. Plenum Press, New York.
* *Immunological Reviews* (ed. G. Moller). Munksgaard, Copenhagen.
Modern Trends in Immunology. Butterworth, London.

Progress in Allergy. S. Karger, Basle.

* *Progress in Immunology.* Academic Press, Orlando, USA. (Triennial proceedings of the international congresses in immunology with an up-to-date account of a wide range of subjects.)

Protides of the Biological Fluids. Pergamon Press, Oxford.

* In depth treatment.

Current information

Current Titles and Abstracts in Immunology, Transplantation & Allergy. Elsevier, Amsterdam. (Quick coverage of current literature.)

Immunology Today. Elsevier Science Publications, Amsterdam. (The immunologist's 'newspaper'.)

Major journals

Nature, Lancet, Science, J.Exp.Med., Immunology, J.Immunology, Clin.Exp.Immunology, Mol.Immunol., Immunopharmacology, Infect & Immunity, Int.Arch.Allergy, Cell.Immunology, European J.Immunology, Scand.J.Immunol., Clin.Immunol. & Immunopath., J.Clin.Immunol., J.Immunogenetics, J.Immunol.Methods, J.Reticuloendoth.Soc., Tissue Antigens, Immunogenetics, Human Immunol., Transplantation, Ann.d'Immunologie, Cancer Immunol.Immunotherapy, J.Allergy Clin. Immunol., Clin.Allergy, Ann. Allergy, J.Clin.Lab.Immunology, Parasitic Immunol.

30

MOLECULES WHICH RECOGNIZE ANTIGEN

THE IMMUNOGLOBULINS

The basic structure is a four-peptide unit

The antibody molecule is made up of two identical heavy and two identical light chains held together by interchain disulphide bonds (figure 3.1). These chains can be separated by reduction of the S–S bonds and acidification. The exposed hinge region is extended in structure due to the high proline content and is therefore vulnerable to proteolytic attack; thus the molecule is split by papain to yield two identical fragments, each with a single combining site for antigen (Fab; *fragment antigen binding*), and a third fragment which lacks the ability to bind antigen and is termed Fc (*fragment crystallizable*). Pepsin strikes at a different point and cleaves the Fc from the remainder of the molecule to leave a large 5S fragment which is formulated as F(ab′)$_2$ since it is still divalent with respect to antigen binding just like the parent antibody (figure 3.2).

The location of the antigen combining sites was elegantly demonstrated by a study of purified antibodies to the dinitrophenyl (DNP) group mixed with the compound:

DNP		DNP

$$NO_2-\bigcirc-NH-CH_2CH_2CH_2CH_2CH_2CH_2CH_2CH_2-NH-\bigcirc-NO_2$$
$$NO_2 \qquad\qquad\qquad\qquad\qquad\qquad\qquad\qquad NO_2$$

The two DNP groups are far enough apart not to interfere with each other's combination with antibody so that they can bring the antigen combining sites on two different antibodies together end to end. When viewed by negative staining in the electron microscope, a series of geometric forms are observed which represent the different structures to be expected if a Y-shaped hinged molecule with a combining site at the end of each of the two arms of

30

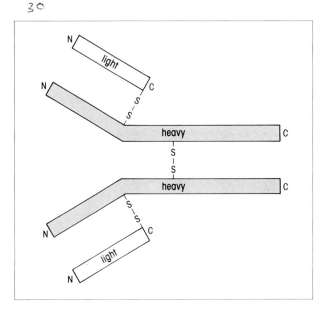

Figure 3.1. *Antibody model with two heavy and two light polypeptide chains held by interchain disulphide bonds. In the diagram the amino-terminal residue(N) is on the left for each chain.*

| IMMUNOGLOBULIN | IMMUNOGLOBULIN | IMMUNOGLOBULIN |

Antigen combining site

PAPAIN

PEPSIN

Reduce and acidify

Fab

Fab

Fc

F(ab')₂

pFc'

PAPAIN FRAGMENTS

PEPSIN FRAGMENTS

ISOLATED CHAINS

Figure 3.2. *Degradation of immunoglobulin to constituent peptide chains and to proteolytic fragments showing divalence of pepsin F(ab')₂ and univalence of the papain Fab. After pepsin digestion the pFc' fragment representing the C-terminal half of the Fc region is formed and is held together by non-covalent bonds. The portion of the heavy chain in the Fab fragment is given the symbol Fd.*

the Y were to complex with this divalent antigen. Triangular trimers, square tetramers and pentagonal pentamers may be readily discerned (figure 3.3). The way in which these polymeric forms arise is indicated in figure 3.4. The position of the Fc fragment and its lack of involvement in the combination with antigen are apparent from the shape of the polymers formed using the pepsin F(ab')₂ fragment (figure 3.3e).

Amino acid sequences reveal variations in immunoglobulin structure

For good reasons, the antibody population in any given individual is just incredibly heterogeneous, and this has meant that determination of amino acid sequences was utterly useless until it proved possible to obtain the homogeneous product of a single clone. The opportunity to do this first came from the study of *myeloma proteins*.

In the human disease known as multiple myeloma, one cell making one particular individual immunoglobulin divides over and over again in the uncontrolled way a cancer cell does, without regard for the overall requirement of the host. The patient then possesses enormous numbers of identical cells derived as a clone from the original cell and they all synthesize the same immunoglobulin—the myeloma or M-protein—which appears in the serum, sometimes in very high concentrations. By purification of the myeloma protein we can obtain a preparation of an immunoglobulin having a unique structure. Monoclonal antibodies can also be obtained by fusing individual antibody-forming cells with a B-cell tumour to produce a constantly dividing clone of cells dedicated to making the one antibody (cf. figures 2.10 and 7.10).

The sequencing of a number of such proteins has revealed that the N-terminal portions of both heavy and light chains show considerable variability whereas the remaining parts of the chains are relatively constant, being grouped into a restricted number of structures. It is conventional to speak of variable and constant regions of both heavy and light chains (figure 3.5).

Certain sequences in the variable regions show quite remarkable diversity and systematic analysis localizes these hypervariable sequences to three

Figure 3.3. *(a)−(d) Electron micrograph (×
1 000 000) of complexes formed on mixing the
divalent DNP hapten with rabbit anti-DNP
antibodies. The 'negative stain' phosphotungstic
acid is an electron-dense solution which penetrates
in the spaces between the protein molecules. Thus
the protein stands out as a 'light' structure in the
electron beam. The hapten links together the Y-
shaped antibody molecules to form (a) dimers, (b)
trimers, (c) tetramers and (d) pentamers (cf. figure
3.4). The flexibility of the molecule at the hinge
region is evident from the variation in angle of the
arms of the 'Y'.*

*(e) As in (b); trimers formed using the F(ab')₂
antibody fragment from which the Fc structures
have been digested by pepsin (× 500 000). The
trimers can be seen to lack the Fc projections at
each corner evident in (b). (After Valentine R.C. &
Green N.M. (1967) J.mol.Biol. 27, 615; courtesy of
Dr Green and with the permission of Academic
Press, New York.)*

segments on the light chain (figure 3.6) and three on
the heavy chain.

Isotypes

Based upon the structure of their heavy chain constant regions, immunoglobulins are classed into
major groups termed *classes* which may be further
subdivided into subclasses. In the human, for example, there are five classes: immunoglobulin G
(IgG), IgA, IgM, IgD and IgE. They may be differentiated not only by their sequences but also by the
antigenic structures to which these sequences give
rise. Thus, by injecting a human IgG myeloma protein into a rabbit, it is possible to raise an antiserum
which can be absorbed by mixtures of myelomas of

other classes to remove cross-reacting antibodies
and which will then be capable of reacting with
IgG, but not IgA, IgM, IgD or IgE (figure 3.7).

Since all the heavy chain constant region (C_H)
structures which give rise to classes and subclasses
are expressed together in the serum of a normal
subject, they are termed isotypic variants (table
3.1). Likewise, the light chain constant regions (C_L)
exist in isotypic forms known as κ and λ which are
associated with all heavy chain isotypes. Because
the light chains in a given antibody are identical,
immunoglobulins are either κ or λ but never mixed
(unless specially engineered in the laboratory).
Thus IgG exists as IgGκ *or* IgGλ, IgM as IgMκ or
IgMλ, and so on.

MOLECULES WHICH RECOGNIZE ANTIGEN

33

Figure 3.4. *Three DNP antibody molecules held together as a trimer by the divalent antigen (●——●). Compare figure 3.3b. When the Fc fragments are first removed by pepsin, the corner pieces are no longer visible (figure 3.3e).*

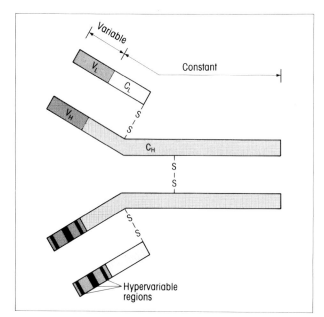

Figure 3.5. *Amino acid sequence variability in the antibody molecule. ■ hypervariable; ▨ variable; □ relatively constant. The terms 'V region' and 'C region' are used to designate the variable and constant regions respectively, 'V_L' and 'C_L' are generic terms for these regions on the light chain and 'V_H' and 'C_H' specify variable and constant regions on the heavy chain. As stressed previously, each pair of heavy chains are identical, as are each pair of light chains.*

Allotypes

This type of variation depends upon the existence of allelic forms (encoded by alleles or alternative

Figure 3.6. *Wu and Kabat plot of amino acid variability in the variable region of immunoglobulin heavy and light chains. The sequences of chains from a large number of myeloma monoclonal proteins are compared and variability at each position is computed as the number of different amino acids found divided by the frequency of the most common amino acid; obviously, the higher the number the greater the variability. The three hypervariable regions (blue) in the heavy (a) and light chains (b), sometimes referred to as Complementarity Determining Regions (CDR), are clearly defined. The intervening peptide sequences are termed framework regions. (Courtesy of Prof. E.A. Kabat.)*

genes at a single locus) which therefore provide genetic markers (table 3.1). In somewhat the same way as the red cells in genetically different individuals can differ in terms of the blood group antigen system A, B, O, so the Ig heavy chains differ in the expression of their allotypic groups. Typical allotypes are the Gm specificities on IgG (Gm = *marker* on IgG) which are recognizable by the ability of the individual's IgG to block agglutination of red cells coated with anti-rhesus D bearing the Gm allotype by sera from patients with rheumatoid arthritis containing the appropriate anti-Gm rheumatoid factors (figure

| IgG MYELOMA | ▶ | Immunize | ▶ | RABBIT ANTISERUM | ▶ | ABSORBED BY IgA MYELOMA | ▶ | SPECIFIC ANTIBODIES |

Figure 3.7. *The use of monoclonal myeloma proteins to produce antibodies specific for different Ig structures. The rabbit makes antibodies directed to different parts of the IgG myeloma. Antibodies to those parts which are common to other classes can be absorbed out with myelomas of those classes leaving antibodies reacting with class-specific G and variable region-specific (idiotype; Id) structures on the* original molecule. *By the same token, further absorption with other IgG myelomas will remove the common IgG specific antibodies leaving an antiserum directed to the idiotypic determinants alone. (In an attempt to simplify, I have ignored subclasses and allotypes, but the same principles can be extended to generating antisera specific for these variants.)*

3.8). Allotypic differences at a given Gm locus usually involve one or two amino acids in the peptide chain. Take, for example, the G1m(a) locus on IgG1 (table 3.1). An individual with this allotype would have the peptide sequence: Asp.Glu.Leu.Thr.Lys. on each of his IgG1 molecules. Another person whose IgG1 was a-negative would have the sequence *Glu*.Glu.*Met*.Thr.Lys., i.e. two amino acids different. To date, 25 Gm groups have been found on the γ-heavy chains and a further three (the Km—previously Inv groups) on the κ constant region.

Allotypic markers have also been found on the immunoglobulins of rabbits and of mice using re-agents prepared by immunizing one animal with an immune complex obtained with antibodies from another animal of the same species. As in other allelic systems, individuals may be homozygous or heterozygous for the genes encoding the markers; these are expressed co-dominantly and are inherited in simple Mendelian fashion. Take, for example, the b4, b5 allotypes on rabbit light chains: an animal of b^4b^4 genotype would express the b4 allotype whereas a rabbit of b^4b^5 genotype derived from b^4b^4 and b^5b^5 parents would express the b4 marker on one fraction and b5 on another fraction of its immunoglobulin molecules.

TYPE OF VARIATION	DISTRIBUTION	VARIANT	LOCATION	EXAMPLES
ISOTYPIC	All variants present in serum of a normal individual	Classes	C_H	IgM, IgE
		Subclasses	C_H	IgA1, IgA2
		Types	C_L	κ, λ
		Subgroups	C_L	λOz^+, λOz^-
		Subgroups	V_H/V_L	$V_{\kappa I}$ $V_{\kappa II}$ $V_{\kappa III}$ V_{HI} V_{HII} V_{HIII}
ALLOTYPIC	Alternative forms: genetically controlled so not present in all individuals	Allotypes	Mainly C_H/C_L sometimes V_H/V_L	Gm groups (human) b4, b5, b6, b9 (rabbit light chains) Igh-1ᵃ, Igh-1ᵇ (mouse γ_{2a} heavy chains)
IDIOTYPIC	Individually specific to each immuno-globulin molecule	Idiotypes	Variable regions	Probably one or more hypervariable regions forming the antigen-combining site

Table 3.1. *Summary of immunoglobulin variants.*

MOLECULES WHICH RECOGNIZE ANTIGEN

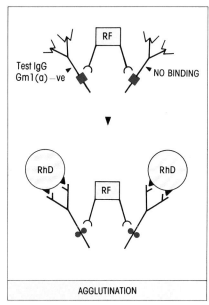

| AGGLUTINATION | NO AGGLUTINATION | AGGLUTINATION |

Figure 3.8. *Demonstration of allotypic specificity on IgG by agglutination inhibition. RhD red cells coated with anti-D bearing the allotype, are agglutinated by a rheumatoid arthritis serum selected for the ability of the rheumatoid factor (RF; anti-IgG) to combine with the allotype. If the test* *IgG added (drawn to show only one combining site and the backbone) bears the allotype in question, it will block the combining sites on RF which will no longer be able to agglutinate the red cells.*

Idiotypes

We have seen that it is possible to obtain antibodies that recognize isotypic and allotypic variants; it is also possible to raise antisera which are specific for individual antibody molecules and discriminate between one monoclonal antibody and another independently of isotypic or allotypic structures (figure 3.7). Such antisera define the individual determinants characteristic of each antibody, collectively termed the *idiotype* (Kunkel & Oudin). Not surprisingly, it turns out that the idiotypic determinants are located in the variable part of the antibody associated with the hypervariable regions (figure 3.9).

Anti-idiotypes which react with one antibody and no other are said to recognize *private* idiotypes and provide further support for the idea that each antibody has a unique structure. Frequently, antibody molecules of closely similar amino acid structure may, in addition, share idiotypes (e.g. MI04 and Hdex2 in figure 3.9) and we then speak of *public* or *cross-reacting* idiotypes.

Anti-idiotypic sera provide useful reagents for demonstrating the same V region on different heavy chains and on different cells, for identification of specific immune complexes in patients' sera, for recognition of V_L type amyloid in subjects excreting Bence-Jones' proteins, for detection of residual monoclonal protein after therapy and perhaps for selecting lymphocytes with certain surface receptors. The reader will (or should be) startled to learn that it is possible to raise *auto*anti-idiotypic sera since this means that individuals can make antibodies to their own idiotypes. This has quite momentous consequences as will become apparent when we discuss the Jerne network theory in Chapter 8.

Immunoglobulins are folded into globular domains which subserve different functions

Immunoglobulin domains have a characteristic structure

In addition to the *interchain* disulphide bonds which bridge heavy and light chains, there are internal, *intrachain* disulphide links which form loops in the peptide chain. As Edelman predicted, the loops are compactly folded to form globular domains (figure 3.10) which have a characteristic β-pleated sheet protein structure.

Significantly, the hypervariable sequences appear at one end of the variable domain where they form parts of the β-turn loops and are clustered close to each other in space.

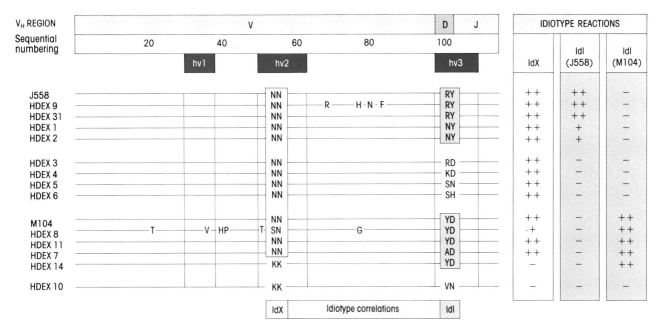

Figure 3.9. *Structural correlates of idiotopes (individual determinants on an idiotype) on antidextran antibodies. Amino acid sequences of variable heavy chain regions of mouse monoclonal antidextran antibodies are shown. All antibodies have λ_1 L chains. Lines indicate identity to the sequence of the first protein, J558; letters (Dayhoff code) show differences or regions correlated with idiotopes (central boxed areas). The cross-reacting idiotope (IdX) is associated with second hypervariable region (hv2) structures while the private idiotopes (IdI) are features of the hv3 region in these antibodies. The presence of the idiotopes on each antibody molecule is assessed by reaction with antisera specific for IdX, J558 IdI and M104 IdI (on the right). Cross-reacting idiotopes may also be associated with the hv3 region in other systems (from J.M. Davie et al. (1986)* **Ann. Rev. Immunol. 4, 147,** *with permission.* © *by Annual Reviews Inc.).*

37

Figure 3.10. *Structure of the globular domains of a light chain (from X-ray crystallographic studies of a Bence-Jones' protein by Schiffler et al. (1973)* **Biochemistry 12, 4620**). *One surface of each domain is composed essentially of four chains (grey arrows) arranged in an anti-parallel β-pleated structure stabilized by interchain H bonds between the amide CO. and NH. groups running along the peptide backbone, and the other surface of three such chains (blue arrows); the dark bar represents the intra-chain disulphide bond. This structure is characteristic of all immunoglobulin domains. Of particular interest is the location of the hypervariable regions (▬▬▬) in three separate loops which are closely disposed relative to each other and form the light chain contribution to the antigen binding site (cf. figure 3.11). One numbered residue from each complementary determinant is identified. To generate a Fab fragment (cf. figure 3.13), imagine a V_H–$V_H{}^1$ segment just like the V_L–C_L in the diagram, rotate it 180° around the axis of the arrow on the right of the figure and lay it on top of V_L–C_L segment (Dr A. Feinstein).*

The variable domain binds antigen

The clustering of the hypervariable loops at the tips of the variable regions where the antigen binding site is localized (figures 3.3 and 3.4) makes them the obvious candidates to subserve the function of antigen recognition (figure 3.11) and this has been confirmed by X-ray crystallographic analysis (cf. figure 4.6). The sequence heterogeneity of the three heavy and three light chain hypervariable loops ensures tremendous diversity in combining specificity for antigen through variation in the shape and nature of the surface they create. Thus each hypervariable region may be looked upon as an independent structure contributing to the complementarity of the binding site for antigen and perhaps one can speak of complementarity determinants.

That these variable regions of heavy and light chains both contribute to antibody specificity is suggested by experiments in which isolated chains were examined for their antigen combining power. In general, varying degrees of residual activity were associated with the heavy chains but relatively little with the light chains; on recombination, however, there was always a significant increase in antigen binding capacity.

Amino acids associated with the combining site can be identified by 'affinity labelling'. In this technique, a hapten (a well-defined chemical grouping to which antibodies can be formed, e.g. DNP in figure 3.3) is equipped with a chemically reactive side-chain which will form covalent links with adjacent amino acids after combination of the hapten with antibody, so labelling residues in the neighbourhood of the combining site. A modification introduced by Porter and his colleagues utilizes a 'flick-knife' principle. The hapten with an azide side-chain combines with its antibody and is then illuminated with ultraviolet light; this converts the azide to the reactive nitrene radical which will covalently link to almost any organic group with which it comes in contact (e.g. figure 3.12). The affinity label binds to both heavy and light chains *in the hypervariable regions*.

Constant region domains determine secondary biological function

The classes of antibody differ from each other in many respects: in their half-life, their distribution throughout the body, their ability to fix complement and their binding to cell surface Fc receptors. Since the classes all have the same κ and λ light

(a)

(b)

Figure 3.11. *(a) Idealized two-dimensional representation of an antigen binding site formed by spatial apposition of peptide loops containing the hypervariable regions (hot spots: ▫) on light and heavy chains. Numbers refer to amino acid residues. Glycine residues (Ⓖ) are invariably present at the positions indicated whatever the specificity or animal species of the immunoglobulin. They are of importance in allowing peptide chains to fold back and form β-pleated sheet structures which enable the hypervariable regions to lie close to each other (figure 3.10). Wu and Kabat have suggested that the flexibility of bond angle in this amino acid contributes to the effective formation of a binding site. On this basis the greater frequency of invariant glycines on the light chain might indicate that coarse specificity for antigen binding was provided by the heavy chain and 'fine tuning' by the light chain. Through binding to different combinations of hypervariable regions and to different residues within each of these regions, each antibody molecule can form a complex with a variety of antigenic determinants (with a comparable variety of affinities). (b) A simulated combining site formed by apposing the three middle fingers of each hand, each finger representing a hypervariable loop. (Photograph by B.N.A. Rice; inspired by A. Munro!)*

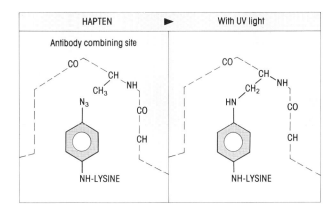

| HAPTEN | ▶ | With UV light |

Antibody combining site

Figure 3.12. *Affinity labelling: the hapten binds to its antibody and the azide group activated by ultraviolet light loses N_2 forming a reactive radical which combines with an adjacent amino acid—in this hypothetical example an alanine residue. Analysis of the protein after digestion would show the alanine to be labelled with the hapten and implicate this residue in the combining site. Studies by Fleet G.W.J., Porter R.R. & Knowles J.R.* (**Nature** *1969,* **224,** *511) indicate that the affinity label combines with heavy and light chains in a ratio of approximately 3.5:1 in their system.*

chains, and heavy and light variable region domains, these differences must lie in the heavy chain constant regions.

It has been possible to localize these biological activities to the various heavy chain domains by using myeloma proteins which have spontaneous domain deletions, or enzymic fragments produced by papain (Fc), pepsin (F(ab')$_2$ and pFc', the C-terminal portion of Fc) and plasmin (Facb from rabbit IgG lacks pFc' but retains the N-terminal half of Fc). Nowadays, of course, it can all be done by genetically engineered proteins.

A model of the IgG molecule is presented in figure 3.13 which indicates the spatial disposition and interaction of the domains in IgG and ascribes the various biological functions to the relevant structures. In principle, the V region domains form the recognition unit (cf. figure 2.1) and constant region domains mediate the secondary biological functions.

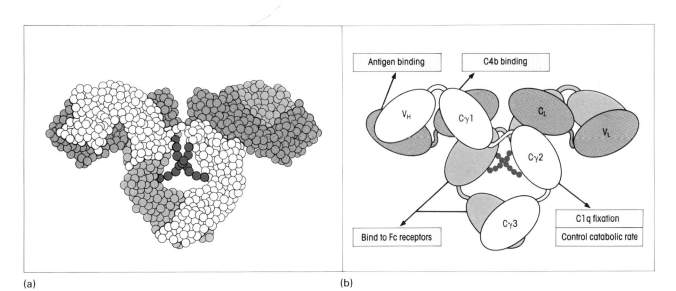

(a)   (b)

Figure 3.13. *The disposition, interaction and biological properties of the Ig domains in IgG. (a) Computer generated model of IgG. One heavy chain is depicted in mid blue, the other in light blue and the light chains in grey. Carbohydrate bound to and separating the Cγ2 domains is in dark blue. The structure was determined by Silverton E.W., Navia M.A. & Davies J.R. (1977)* Proc. Nat. Acad. Sci. 74, 5140, *and the figure generated by computer graphics using R.J. Feldmann's system (Nat. Inst. Health). (b) Diagram based on the model indicating the location of biological function and showing apposing domains making contact through hydrophobic regions (after Dr A. Feinstein). The structures of these contact frameworks are highly conserved, an essential feature if different V_H and V_L domains are to associate in order to* generate a wide variety of antibody specificities. These hydrophobic regions on the two complement fixing C_H2 (Cγ2) domains are partly masked by carbohydrate and remain independent so allowing the formation of a hinge region which is extremely flexible both with respect to variation in the angle of the Fab fragments and their rotation about the hinge peptide chain. Thus combining sites in IgG can be readily adapted to spatial variations in the presentation of the antigenic epitopes. The combined Cγ2 and Cγ3 domains bind to Fc receptors on phagocytic cells, NK cells and placental syncytiotrophoblast; also to staphylococcal protein A. (Note the IgG heavy chain is designated γ and the constant region domains Cγ1, Cγ2 and Cγ3.)*

MOLECULES WHICH RECOGNIZE ANTIGEN

Immunoglobulin classes and subclasses

The physical and biological characteristics of the five major immunoglobulin classes in the human are summarized in tables 3.2 and 3.3. The following comments are intended to supplement this information.

Immunoglobulin G

During the secondary response IgG is probably the major immunoglobulin to be synthesized. Through its ability to cross the placenta it provides a major line of defence against infection for the first few weeks of a baby's life which may be further reinforced by the transfer of colostral IgG across the gut mucosa in the neonate. IgG diffuses more readily than the other immunoglobulins into the extravascular body spaces where, as the predominant species, it carries the major burden of neutralizing bacterial toxins and of binding to micro-organisms to enhance their phagocytosis. The complexes of bacteria with IgG antibody activate complement thereby chemotactically attracting polymorphonuclear phagocytic cells (cf. p. 11) which adhere to the bacteria through surface receptors for complement and the Fc portion of IgG (Fcγ); binding to the Fc receptor then stimulates ingestion of micro-organisms through phagocytosis. In a similar way, the extracellular killing of target cells coated with IgG antibody is mediated largely through recognition of the surface Fcγ by NK cells bearing the appropriate receptors (cf. p. 26). The interaction of IgG complexes with platelet Fc receptors presumably leads to aggregation and vasoactive amine release but the physiological significance of Fcγ binding sites on other cell types, particularly lymphocytes, has not yet been clarified. Although unable to bind firmly to mast cells in human skin, IgG alone among the human immunoglobulins has the somewhat useless property of fixing to guinea-pig skin. The thesis that the biological individuality of different immunoglobulin classes is dependent on the heavy chain constant regions, particularly the Fc, is amply borne out in relationship to the activities we have discussed such as transplacental passage, complement fixation and binding to various cell types, where function has been shown to be mediated by the Fc part of the molecule.

With respect to overall regulation of IgG levels in the body, the catabolic rate appears to depend directly upon the total IgG concentration whereas synthesis is largely governed by antigen stimulation, so that in germ-free animals, for example, IgG levels are extremely low but rise rapidly on transfer to a normal environment.

Immunoglobulin A

IgA appears selectively in the sero-mucous secretions such as saliva, tears, nasal fluids, sweat, colostrum and secretions of the lung, genito-urinary and gastro-intestinal tracts where it clearly has the job of defending the exposed external surfaces of the

DESIGNATION	IgG	IgA	IgM	IgD	IgE
Sedimentation coefficient	7S	7S, 9S, 11S*	19S	7S	8S
Molecular weight	150 000	160 000 and dimer	900 000	185 000	200 000
Number of basic four-peptide units	1	1, 2*	5	1	1
Heavy chains	γ	α	μ	δ	ε
Light chains κ + λ	κ + λ	κ + λ	κ + λ	κ + λ	κ + λ
Molecular formula†	$\gamma_2\kappa_2, \gamma_2\lambda_2$	$(\alpha_2\kappa_2)_{1-2}$ $(\alpha_2\lambda)_{1-2}$ $(\alpha_2\kappa_2)_2 S$* $(\alpha_2\lambda_2)_2 S$*	$(\mu_2\kappa_2)_5$ $(\mu_2\lambda_2)_5$	$\delta_2\kappa_2(\delta_2\lambda_2?)$	$\epsilon_2\kappa_2, \epsilon_2\lambda_2$
Valency for antigen binding	2	2,4	5(10)	2	2
Concentration range in normal serum	8–16 mg/ml	1.4–4 mg/ml	0.5–2 mg/ml	0–0.4 mg/ml	17–450 ng/ml‡
% Total immunoglobulin	80	13	6	0–1	0.002
% Carbohydrate content	3	8	12	13	12

Table 3.2. *Physical properties of major human immunoglobulin classes.*
* Dimer in external secretions carries secretory component—S.
† IgA dimer and IgM contain J-chain.
‡ ng = 10^{-9} g.

	IgG	IgA	IgM	IgD	IgE
Major characteristics	Most abundant Ig of internal body fluids particularly extravascular where it combats micro-organisms and their toxins	Major Ig in sero-mucous secretions where it defends external body surfaces	Very effective agglutinator; produced early in immune response — effective first-line defence vs. bacteraemia	Most, if not all, present on lymphocyte surface	Protection of external body surfaces Recruits anti-microbial agents Raised in parasitic infections Responsible for symptoms of atopic allergy
Complement fixation Classical	++	−	+++	−	
Alternative	−	±	−	−	
Cross placenta	+	−	−	−	−
Fix to homologous mast cells and basophils	−	−	−	−	+
Binding to macrophages and polymorphs	+	±	−	−	−

Table 3.3. *Biological properties of major immunoglobulin classes in the human.*

body against attack by micro-organisms. It is present in these fluids as a dimer stabilized against proteolysis by combination with another protein—the secretory component which is synthesized by local epithelial cells and has a single peptide chain of molecular weight 60 000. The IgA is synthesized locally by plasma cells and dimerized intracellularly together with a cysteine-rich polypeptide called J-chain of molecular weight 15 000. If dimerization occurred randomly *after* secretion, dimers of mixed specificity would be formed which would not be as effective in combining with antigen as those of single specificity which would have a higher effective valency. The dimeric IgA binds strongly to the secretory component precursor present on the surface of the cell in which it was produced and the complex is then actively endocytosed, transported across the cytoplasm and secreted into the external body fluids (figure 3.14).

IgA antibodies function by inhibiting the adherence of coated micro-organisms to the surface of mucosal cells thereby preventing entry into the body tissues. Aggregated IgA binds to polymorphs and can also activate the alternative (figure 2.3), as distinct from the classical complement, pathway which probably accounts for reports of a synergism between IgA, complement and lysozyme in the killing of certain coliform organisms. Human plasma contains relatively high concentrations of monomeric IgA and its role is still something of a mystery.

Immunoglobulin M

Often referred to as the macroglobulin antibodies because of their high molecular weight, IgM molecules are polymers of five four-peptide subunits each bearing an extra C_H domain. As with IgA, polymerization of the subunits depends upon the presence of J-chain whose function may be to stabilize the Fc sulphydryl groups during Ig synthesis so that they remain available for cross-linking the subunits to give the structure shown in figure 3.15a. Under negative staining in the electron microscope, the free molecule in solution assumes a 'star' shape but when combined as an antibody with an antigenic surface membrane it can adopt a 'crab-like' configuration (figure 3.15b and c). The theoretical combining valency is of course 10 but this is only observed on interaction with small haptens; with larger antigens the effective valency falls to 5 and this must be attributed to some form of steric restriction due to lack of flexibility in the molecule. IgM antibodies tend to be of relatively low affinity as measured against single determinants (haptens) but, because of their high valency, they bind with quite respectable avidity to antigens with multiple epitopes (bonus effect of multivalency, p. 61).

For the same reason, these antibodies are extremely efficient agglutinating and cytolytic agents and since they appear early in the response to infection and are largely confined to the bloodstream, it is likely that they play a role of particular

MOLECULES WHICH RECOGNIZE ANTIGEN

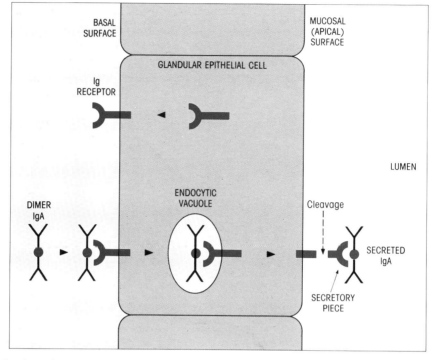

Figure 3.14. *The mechanism of IgA secretion at the mucosal surface. The mucosal cell synthesizes an Ig receptor which is inserted into the basal membrane. Dimeric IgA binds to this receptor and is transported via an endocytic vacuole to the apical surface. Cleavage of the receptor releases the IgA still attached to part of the receptor termed* **secretory piece.** *Transport of IgG across the placenta probably involves a similar mechanism utilizing surface IgG receptors.*

Figure 3.15. *The structure of IgM. The arrangement of domains in one of the five subunits showing how the pentamer is built up through the disulphide linkages between C_H3 and C terminal regions (after Hilschman & Feinstein). Without too much aggravation, I hope the reader will appreciate that the hinge region in IgG (cf. figure 3.13) is replaced by a rigid pair of extra domains (C_H2), while C_H3 and C_H4 domains in IgM are structurally equivalent to the C_H2 and C_H3 regions respectively in IgG. (a) As shown by electron microscopy of a human Waldenström's macroglobulin in free solution adopting a 'star'-shaped configuration. (b) As revealed in an*

E.M. preparation of specific sheep IgM antibody bound to **Salmonella paratyphi** *flagellum where the immunoglobulin has assumed a 'crab-like' conformation in establishing its links with antigen. With the $F(ab')_2$ arms bent out of the plane of the central Fc_5 region, the C_H3 complement binding domains are now readily accessible to the first component of complement (cf. p. 15). The Fc_5 constellation obtained by papain cleavage can activate complement directly. (Electron micrographs—kindly provided by Dr A. Feinstein and Dr E.A. Munn—are negatively stained preparations of magnification × 2 000 000, i.e. 1 mm represents 0.5 nm.)*

importance in cases of bacteraemia. The isohaem-agglutinins (anti-A, anti-B) and many of the 'natural' antibodies to micro-organisms are usually IgM; antibodies to the typhoid 'O' antigen (endotoxin) and the 'WR' antibodies in syphilis also tend to be found in this class. IgM would appear to precede IgG in the phylogeny of the immune response in vertebrates.

Monomeric IgM (i.e. a single four-peptide unit) with a hydrophobic sequence stitched into the C-terminal end of the heavy chain to anchor the molecule in the cell membrane, is the major antibody receptor used by B-lymphocytes to recognize antigen (cf. p. 19).

Immunoglobulin D

This class was recognized through the discovery of a myeloma protein which did not have the antigenic specificity of IgG, A or M, although it reacted with antibodies to immunoglobulin light chains and had the basic four-peptide structure. The hinge region is particularly extended and although protected to some degree by carbohydrate, it may be this feature which makes IgD, among the different immunoglobulin classes, uniquely susceptible to proteolytic degradation, and account for its short half-life in plasma (2.8 days). An exciting development has been the demonstration that nearly all the IgD is present, together with IgM, on the surface of a proportion of blood lymphocytes where it seems likely that they may operate as mutually interacting antigen receptors for the control of lymphocyte activation and suppression. The even greater susceptibility of IgD to proteolysis on combination with antigen could well be implicated in such a function.

Immunoglobulin E

Only very low concentrations of IgE are present in serum and only a very small proportion of the plasma cells in the body are synthesizing this immunoglobulin. It is not surprising, therefore, that so far only six cases of IgE myeloma have been recognized compared with tens of thousands of IgG paraproteinaemias. IgE antibodies remain firmly fixed for an extended period when injected into human skin where they are probably bound to mast cells. Contact with antigen leads to degranulation of the mast cells with release of vasoactive amines. This process is responsible for the symptoms of hay fever and of extrinsic asthma when patients with atopic allergy come into contact with the allergen, e.g. grass pollen.

The main *physiological* role of IgE would appear to be protection of the external mucosal surfaces of the body by local recruitment of plasma factors and effector cells through triggering an acute inflammatory reaction. Infectious agents penetrating the IgA defences would combine with specific IgE on the mast cell surface and trigger the release of vasoactive agents and factors chemotactic for granulocytes, so leading to an influx of plasma IgG, complement, polymorphs and eosinophils (cf. p. 156). In such a context, the ability of eosinophils to damage IgG-coated helminths and the generous IgE response to such parasites would constitute an effective defence.

Immunoglobulin subclasses

Antigenic analysis of IgG myelomas revealed further variation and showed that they could be grouped into four isotypic *subclasses* now termed IgG1, IgG2, IgG3 and IgG4. The differences all lie in the heavy chains which have been labelled γ1, γ2, γ3 and γ4 respectively. These heavy chains show considerable homology and have certain structures in common with each other—the ones which react with specific anti-IgG antisera—but each has one or more additional structures characteristic of its own subclass arising from differences in primary amino acid composition and in interchain disulphide bridging. These give rise to differences in biological behaviour which are summarized in table 3.4.

Two subclasses of IgA have also been found, of which IgA1 constitutes 80–90% of the total. The IgA2 subclass is unusual in that it lacks interchain disulphide bonds between heavy and light chains. Class and subclass variation is not restricted to human immunoglobulins but is a feature of all the higher mammals so far studied: monkey, sheep, rabbit, guinea-pig, rat and mouse.

THE MAJOR HISTOCOMPATIBILITY COMPLEX (MHC)

Molecules within this complex were originally recognized through their ability to provoke vigorous rejection of grafts exchanged between different members of a species. In Chapter 2, brief mention was made of the necessity for cell-surface antigens to be associated with class I or class II MHC molecules in order that they may be recognized by T-lymphocytes. The intention now is to give more insight into the nature of these molecules.

Class I and class II molecules are membrane-bound heterodimers

Class I molecules consist of a heavy peptide chain of 43 kD non-covalently linked to a smaller 11 kD peptide called β_2-microglobulin. The largest part of

	IgG1	IgG2	IgG3	IgG4
% Total IgG in normal serum	65	23	8	4
Electrophoretic mobility	slow	slow	slow	fast
Spontaneous aggregation	−	−	+ + +	−
Gm allotypes	a,z,f,x	n	b0,b1,b3, g,s,t, etc.	
Ga site reacting with rheumatoid factor*	+ + +	+ + +	−	+ + +
Combination with staphylococcal A protein	+ + +	+ + +	−	+ + +
Cross placenta	+ +	±	+ +	+ +
Complement fixation (Cl pathway)	+ + +	+ +	+ + + +	±
Binding to monocytes	+ + +	+	+ + +	±
Binding to heterologous skin	+ +	−	+ +	+ +
Blocking IgE binding	−	−	−	+
Antibody dominance	Anti-Rh	Anti-dextran Anti-levan	Anti-Rh	Anti-Factor VIII

Table 3.4. *Comparison of human IgG subclasses.*
* Other rheumatoid factors apparently react with Gm specific sites.

the heavy chain is organized into three globular domains (α_1, α_2 and α_3; figure 3.16) which protrude from the cell surface; a hydrophobic section anchors the molecule in the membrane and a short hydrophilic sequence carries the C-terminus into the cytoplasm. Both β_2-microglobulin and the α_3 section are like immunoglobulin domains with respect to sequence homology and presumably folding.

Class II MHC molecules are also transmembrane glycoproteins, in this case consisting of α and β polypeptide chains of molecular weight 34 kD and 28 kD respectively. Both chains are folded to give two domains, the ones nearest to the membrane having considerable sequence homology with β_2-microglobulin and the characteristic Ig domain (figure 3.16).

The genes coding for C4 and for the two products, C2 and factor B, which carry the active site for C3 convertase, have made their way into the MHC region and are referred to as class III genes.

Gene map of the major histocompatibility complex

The clusters of class I, II and III genes in the MHC of mouse and man are set out in figures 3.17 and 3.18.

There have been many furrowed brows concerning the nature of I-J, which is defined serologically, i.e. by an antibody, as a marker of suppressor T-cells which maps to the I-E region. The problem arises because there is no room in this region to code for polypeptides other than E_α and E_β. There is no doubting the genetic data and the most plausible explanation is that the I-E alleles mediate the selection of structurally related molecules indirectly,

perhaps through idiotypic interactions involving the T-cell receptor (see figure 8.4).

The genes of the MHC display remarkable polymorphism

Unlike the immunoglobulin system where, as we shall see, variability is achieved in each individual by a *multigenic* system, the MHC has evolved in terms of variability between individuals with a highly polymorphic system based on multiple alleles (i.e. alternative genes at each locus). The extent of this polymorphism is detailed in Chapter 13, but suffice to say here that it is very high in the classical class I molecules, HLA-A and -B (mainly in the α_1 and α_2 domains), and in DQ_α, DQ_β and DR_β (both very high) and DP_β (modestly high) in the class II of the human. As for the mouse, extensive polymorphism expressed through multiple alleles is clearly evident in α_1 and α_2 domains in H-2K and H-2D, and in the first domain of I-A$_\alpha$, I-A$_\beta$ and I-E$_\beta$.

As more class II sequences in the mouse have become available, Wu and Kabat type plots (cf. figure 3.6) of variability at different positions in the peptide chains have begun to reveal allelic diversity localized to 3−4 short sequences in the first domain (figure 3.16). These are also shown schematically in figure 3.16 to indicate, more in hope than anger, a potential clustering of variable loops to form a possible recognition site akin to that in the immunoglobulin molecule. However, these are still early days and X-ray crystallographic data is what is urgently required.

Multiple allelic forms can be generated by a variety of mechanisms: point mutations, recombina-

44

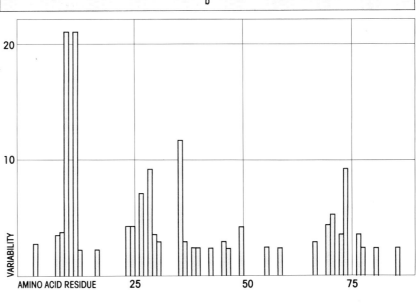

Figure 3.16. *Class I and class II major histocompatibility complex molecules. (a) Structure showing domains and transmembrane segments. The class I heavy chain is always non-covalently associated with β₂-microglobulin. The polymorphic regions are speculatively indicated by dotted lines. (b) Wu and Kabat type plot analysing HLA−DR_{β1} (1st exon) structures from different individuals showing regions of amino acid variability, presumably associated with polymorphic (allelic) variants. Note that, unlike immunoglobulins, there are no variations in the structure of MHC molecules expressed by a given haplotype. (Data kindly provided by Dr A. So.)*

Figure 3.17. *The genes in the major histocompatibility complex in the mouse. There are 17 Qa genes in the Qa region and 12 in the Tla region although most are silent.*

MOLECULES WHICH RECOGNIZE ANTIGEN

COMPLEX	HLA									
MHC CLASS	II			III				I		
GENES	DPα DPβ	(DQα DQβ)	(DRα DRβ)	C2	FB	C4A	C4B	B	C	A
GENE PRODUCTS	HLA - DP	HLA - DQ	HLA - DR	C2	FB	C4A	C4B	HLA - B	HLA - C	HLA - A

Figure 3.18. *The genes in the major histocompatibility complex of the human. Where the precise order is still uncertain, the genes are bracketed. The class III region also encodes two different 21-hydroxylase enzymes. The HLA complex is on chromosome 6.*

tion, homologous but unequal crossing over, and gene conversion.

The latter mechanism has been identified as an important contributory factor in the formation of a series of spontaneous mutations in the *H-2K* region of C57BL mice. Most of the mutations contain clusters of multiple amino acid substitutions and seem to arise by transfer of stretches of up to 95 nucleotides from class I *Qa* genes to the α_1 and α_2 domains of *H-2K*. These intriguing findings have fostered the view that the large number of seemingly functionless *Qa* genes may represent a stockpile of genetic information for the generation of polymorphic diversity in the 'working' class I molecules. Evidence for gene conversion has also been obtained for the class II genes and an example is given in figure 3.19.

Nomenclature

Since much of the experimental work relating to the MHC is based on experiments in our little laboratory friend, the mouse, it may be helpful to explain the nomenclature used to describe the allelic genes and their products. If someone says to you in a little-known language, 'I have kicked my commissar', you fail to understand, not because the idea is complicated but because you do not comprehend the language. It is much the same with the shorthand used to describe the H-2 system which looks unnecessarily frightening to the uninitiated. In order to identify and compare allelic genes within the H-2 complex in different strains, it is usual to start with certain pure inbred strains, obtained by successive brother–sister matings, to provide the prototypes. The collection of genes in the H-2 complex is called the haplotype and the haplotype of each prototypic strain will be allotted a given superscript. For example, the DBA strain haplotype is designated $H-2^d$ and the genes constituting the complex are therefore $H-2K^d$, $I-A^d_\alpha$, $I-A^d_\beta$, $H-2D^d$ and so on; their products will be $H-2K^d$, $I-A^d$ and $H-2D^d$ and so forth. When new strains are derived from these by genetic recombination during breeding, they are assigned new haplotypes but the individual genes are designated by the haplotype of the prototype strain from which they were derived. Thus the A/J strain produced by genetic cross-over during interbreeding between $(H-2^k \times H-2^d)$ F1 mice (cf. figure 3.20) is arbitrarily assigned the haplotype $H-2^a$, but table 3.5 shows that individual genes in the complex are identified by the haplotype symbol of the original parents.

46

Figure 3.19. *Evidence for gene conversion generating a class II mutant. A stretch of nucleotides from the parent strain E_β gene appears to have been transferred to A_β to produce the $A_\beta^{bm/2}$ mutant as shown by the comparison of DNA and amino acid sequences. The maximum and minimum possible sequences exchanged are indicated.*

STRAIN	CBA	F₁ HYBRID	DBA/2
H-2 GENOTYPE	k/k	k×d k/d	d/d
LYMPHOCYTES (H-2 PHENOTYPE)	k · · k	k · · d	d ■ ■ d
ANTI H-2ᵏ	Killing	Killing	—
ANTI-H-2ᵈ	—	Killing	Killing

Figure 3.20. *Inheritance and co-dominant expression of MHC genes. The first familial generation (F1) obtained by crossing the pure parental strains CBA (H-2ᵏ) and DBA/2 (H-2ᵈ) has the H-2 genotype k/d. Since 100% of F1 lymphocytes are killed in the presence of complement by antibodies to H-2ᵏ or to H-2ᵈ (raised by injecting H-2ᵏ lymphocytes into an H-2ᵈ animal and vice versa), the MHC molecules encoded by both parental genes must be expressed on every lymphocyte. The same holds true for other tissues in the body.*

Table 3.5. *The haplotypes of the H-2 complex of some commonly used mouse strains and recombinants derived from them.*

STRAIN	HAPLOTYPE	ORIGIN OF INDIVIDUAL REGIONS					
		K	A	(J)	E	S	D
C57BL	b	b	b	b	b	b	b
CBA	k	k	k	k	k	k	k
DBA/2	d	d	d	d	d	d	d
A/J	a	k	k	k	k*	d	d
B.10A(4R)	h4	k	k	b	b	b	b

A/J was derived by interbreeding (k × d) F1 mice, recombination occurring between E and S regions(*).

Inheritance of the MHC

Pure strain mice derived by prolonged brother—sister mating are homozygous for each pair of homologous chromosomes. Thus, in the present context, the haplotype of the MHC derived from the mother will be identical to that from the father and animals of the C57BL strain, for example, will each bear two chromosomes with the *H-2ᵇ* haplotype (cf. table 3.5).

Let us see how the MHC behaves when we cross two pure strains of haplotypes *H-2ᵏ* and *H-2ᵈ* respectively. We find that the lymphocytes of the offspring (the F1 generation) all display *both* H-2ᵏ and H-2ᵈ molecules on their surface, i.e. there is co-dominant expression (figure 3.20). If we go further and breed F1s together, the progeny have the genotypes *k*, *k/d* and *d* in the proportions to be expected if the haplotype segregates as a single Mendelian trait. This happens because the H-2 complex spans

0.5 centimorgans, equivalent to a recombination frequency between the *K* and *D* ends of 0.5%, and the haplotype tends to be inherited *en bloc*. Only the relatively infrequent recombinations caused by meiotic cross-over events, as described for the A/J strain above, reveal the complexity of the system.

The tissue distribution of MHC molecules

Essentially, all nucleated cells carry class I molecules. These are abundantly expressed on lymphoid cells, less so on liver, lung and kidney and only sparsely on brain and skeletal muscle. In the human, the surface of the villous trophoblast does not display HLA-A, B or C components. Class II molecules are more restricted being especially associated with B-cells, antigen-presenting cells and macrophages; however, when activated by agents such as γ-interferon, capillary endothelia and many epithelial cells can be stained for surface class II.

MHC functions

Although originally discovered through transplantation reactions, the MHC molecules are utilized for vital biological functions by the host. Their function as cell surface markers to signal cytotoxic and helper T-cells will be explored in depth in subsequent chapters. Aside from the potential role of Qa genes in the generation of polymorphism, molecules encoded by the Tla complex are involved in differentiation events particularly in the embryo and possibly also in the placenta.

The MHC has been implicated in a variety of non-immunological phenomena such as body weight in mice and egg production in chickens; many of these may have a hormonal basis and the evidence that class I molecules may also function as components of hormone receptors merits some consideration. For example, the Daudi tumour cell line which does not express surface class I because of a failure to synthesize β_2-microglobulin, lacks insulin receptors. If one strips class I, but not class II, from the cell surface by 'capping' with antibodies (see p. 141), the binding of insulin is significantly diminished. Last, if a cell binds photoaffinity-labelled insulin, chemical links with H-2K but not H-2D may be seen. Associations with receptors for glucagon, epidermal growth factor and γ-endorphin have also been described. Of course, one of the lessons to be learned is that we should never look at immunological events as phenomena isolated from the biology of the whole individual—and beyond (figure 3.21).

48

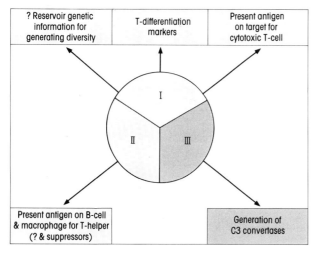

Figure 3.21. *The functions of MHC molecules.*

THE T-CELL RECEPTOR

Like the B-lymphocyte, the T-cell has a specific receptor for antigen recognition on its surface. But whereas the B-cell receptor is a membrane-bound immunoglobulin M monomer, the T-cell receptor is a heterodimer composed of an α and a β chain each of molecular weight 40−50 kD and which are clearly not products of immunoglobulin genes (figure 3.22). Each chain is folded into two domains, one having

a relatively invariant structure homologous to the famous 'Ig fold', the other exhibiting far more variability through its structure than the Ig variable domains. Thus while it is safe to assume that the variable region has the job of binding to antigen and MHC, we do not yet have the data to define the structural basis of that recognition process. In some way the broadening of hypervariability beyond the restricted clearly defined loops in the V_H and V_L domains must be linked to the more complicated process of recognizing the MHC molecule in addition to the antigen.

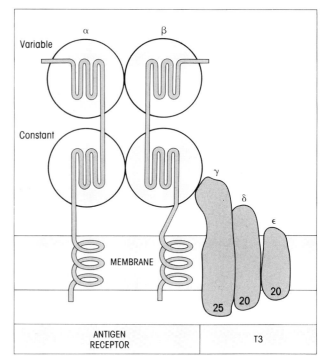

Figure 3.22. *The T-cell receptor. Antigen plus MHC is recognized by the disulphide-linked transmembrane heterodimer composed of an α and a β chain each having a variable and a constant domain. The receptor is intimately associated with the γ, δ and ε chains which form the T3 complex, each chain having the molecular weight in kD indicated. The γ chain becomes phosphorylated. The precise arrangement of the chains is still unknown.*

Both α and β chains are required for antigen specificity as shown by transfection of the T-receptor genes from a cytotoxic T-cell clone specific for fluorescein + H-2D^d to another clone of different specificity; when it expressed the new α and β genes, the transfected clone acquired the ability to lyse the fluoresceinated H-2D^d target cells. Another type of experiment utilized T-cell hybridomas formed by fusing single antigen-specific T-cells with T-cell tumours to achieve 'immortality'. A hybridoma recognizing chicken ovalbumin in association with I-A^d gave rise spontaneously to two variants, one of which lost the chromosome encoding the α chain, and the other, the β chain. Neither variant recognized antigen but when they were physically fused together, each supplied the complementary receptor chain and reactivity with antigen was restored.

In all immunocompetent T-cells, the antigen receptor is non-covalently but still intimately linked in a complex with T3, a molecule composed of three peptide chains (γ, δ and ε), which transduces the antigen recognition signal received by the α, β heterodimer to the inside of the cell. It really seems sensible to regard the complete receptor as a five-peptide complex of the heterodimer with T3 (figure 3.22).

A third polypeptide chain, γ, has been identified which behaves like a T-cell receptor gene in showing the same genetic rearrangements as the T-receptor α and β chains. It is transcribed at relatively high levels early in thymic ontogeny but only recently, by analysis of the T3 positive cells lacking α and β chains which are so numerous in patients with severe combined deficiency, has it been possible to identify a polypeptide chain gene product. Its close association with T3 strengthens its claim to T-cell receptor status but the nature of the cells they serve is still a mystery. They are not NK-cells but just might be T-suppressors.

THE GENERATION OF DIVERSITY FOR ANTIGEN RECOGNITION

We know that the body produces millions of different antibodies capable as a population of recognizing virtually any pathogen that has arisen or might arise. Since this is probably more than the total number of genes in the body, there must be some clever ways to generate all this diversity. Before examining these mechanisms, we must first look at the genetic building blocks from which the final genes encoding antibody molecules and the T-cell receptor are constructed.

Multiple gene segments code for antibody

These fall into three clusters on three different chromosomes coding for κ, λ and heavy chains respectively. There appears to be only one variable region (V) gene for mouse λ chain and the genetic basis for the synthesis of this peptide is illustrated in figure 3.23. In common with other eukaryotic proteins, the

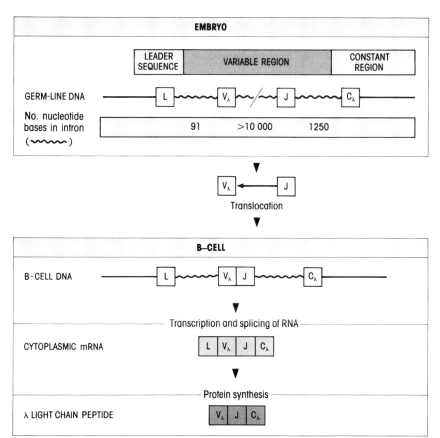

Figure 3.23. *Genetic basis for synthesis of mouse λ chain. As the cell becomes immunocompetent, the variable region is formed by the combination of V_λ with the joining segment J, a process facilitated by base sequences in the intron following the 3' end of the V_λ segment pairing up with sequences in the intron 5' to J. This variable region V_λ J segment is separate from the gene encoding the constant region as originally predicted by Dreyer and Bennett. The final joining occurs when the intervening sequence is spliced out of the mRNA transcript. In the human, the V_λ genes are more complex (cf. V_κ genes below).*

chain is encoded in multiple distinct gene segments separated by intervening nucleotide sequences, *introns*, which are removed either by DNA translocation or by excision of the corresponding mRNA sequence. There is a leader sequence required for passage of the peptide through the endoplasmic reticulum, a V_λ segment coding for amino acid residues 1 to 98, a joining segment (*J*—not to be confused with the J peptide in IgM and IgA) encoding the remaining 11 amino acids of the variable region, and a C_λ gene segment giving rise to the constant region. As a lymphocyte undergoes differentiation to become an immunocompetent cell capable of synthesizing λ chains, there is a rearrangement or translocation of the DNA bringing the L, V_λ and J segments together (figure 3.24) but still separated from the C_λ by an intron of 1250 nucleotides. Splicing of the transcribed RNA in the nucleus produces an mRNA which can now be used for the synthesis of a continuous λ chain peptide.

The same general principles apply to the arrangement of κ and heavy chain genes although they exist in far greater variety (figure 3.25). The 200 or so V_κ genes occur as a series of five families or sets each containing closely related individual genes. Although the genes within a given set show some framework and hypervariable diversity, they resemble each other far more than they do V_κ genes in other sets. There are five different J segments but just a single constant region gene.

The heavy chain constellation shows additional features: the subclass constant region genes form a single cluster and there is a group of 12 highly variable D segments inserted between the V and J regions. The D and J segments together encode almost the entire third hypervariable region, the first two being contributed by the V sequence.

A similar pattern of genes codes for the T-cell receptor

The gene segments encoding the T-cell receptor α and β chains follow a similar arrangement of V, D, J and constant segments to that described for the immunoglobulins (figure 3.26). Similarly, as an immunocompetent T-cell is formed, rearrangement of V, D and J genes occurs to form a continuous *VDJ* sequence and, as in the synthesis of antibody, the intron between *VDJ* and C is spliced out of the mRNA before translation.

The mechanisms which generate tremendous diversity from limited gene pools

Intrachain amplification of diversity

*Simple **VDJ** combinatorial joining increases diversity geometrically*

During the rearrangement of germ-line genes to produce the immunocompetent cell, $V \rightarrow J$, $V \rightarrow D$ and $D \rightarrow J$ joining is random and will produce $V \times J$, or where appropriate, $V \times D \times J$ combinations (see table 3.6).

Variations on the combinatorial theme

Another ploy to squeeze more variation out of the germ-line repertoire involves variable boundary recombinations of V, D and J to produce different junctional sequences (figure 3.27).

Figure 3.24. *Intron sequences facilitating V–J, V–D and D–J recombination. The characteristic sequences forming a base-paired (▬) heptamer, a spacer of 12 or 23 single bases (▬) and then a base-paired nonamer facilitate splicing by enzymes involved in DNA repair.*

Figure 3.25. *Genes coding for κ and heavy chain peptides in the mouse. There are approximately 200 $V_κ$ and 500 V_H genes arranged in a series of families or sets of a closely related sequence. Note the multiple J segments and in the case of heavy chains, the series of D 'minigenes'. Recombination events similar to the rearrangement of $V_λ$ and J in figures 3.23 and 3.24 bring the V, D and J segments together to encode the variable portion of the chosen antibody in an immunocompetent B-cell. The sequence of C_H genes in the human is μ, δ, $γ_1$, $γ_2$, $γ_3$, $γ_4$, ε, $α_1$ and $α_2$.*

51

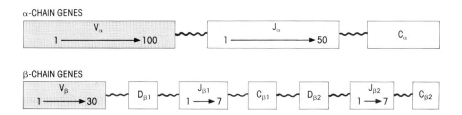

Figure 3.26. *Genes encoding the α and β polypeptides of the T-cell receptor. Note the very large number of α segments. There are approximately 11 $V_α$ and 14 $V_β$ subfamilies of related sequences. In the committed T-cell, one $V_α$ and one $J_α$ segment are combined, while one $V_β$ gene is joined to $D_{β1}$,* plus one of the $J_{β1}$ segments, or to $D_{β2}$ plus a $J_{β2}$ segment. The final peptides would correspond with one $V_αJ_αC_α$ combination together with either a $V_βD_{β1}J_{β1}C_{β1}$ or a $V_βD_{β2}J_{β2}C_{β2}$ combination. The γ chain is made up from one of 12 or so $V_γ$ genes combined with either $J_{γ1}C_{γ1}$ or $J_{γ2}C_{γ2}$.

Table 3.6. *Combinatorial and somatic diversification of mouse V genes.*

The minimum number of specificities generated by straightforward combination of germ-line segments can be calculated. These will be increased by the further mechanisms listed. The calculation for the T-cell receptor β chain requires further explanation. The first of the two D segments, $D_{β1}$ can combine with 30 V genes, can be read in the 3 reading frames and can combine with all 12 $J_{β1}$ and $J_{β2}$ genes (30 × 3 × 12). $D_{β2}$ behaves similarly but can only combine with the 6 downstream $J_{β2}$ genes (30 × 3 × 6). (Reproduced from Goverman J., Hunkappiller T. & Hood L. (1986) Cell 45, 475, with permission. Copyright 1986 by Cell Press.)

	T-CELL RECEPTOR		IMMUNOGLOBULIN	
	ALPHA	BETA	HEAVY	KAPPA
V gene segments	100	30	500	200
D gene segments	—	2	15	—
J gene segments	50	6 + 6	4	4
D's in 3 reading frames	—	+ + +	+	—
N region insertion	+	+ +	+ +	—
Junctional diversity	+ + +	+ + +	+ + +	+
Somatic hypermutation	—	—	+	+
Combinatorial joining	V×J 100×50	V×D×J (30×3×12) +(30×3×6)	V×D×J 500×15×4	V×J 200×4
Total	5000	1620	$3×10^4$	800
Combinatorial association	X $8.1×10^6$		X $2.4×10^7$	

MOLECULES WHICH RECOGNIZE ANTIGEN

Figure 3.27. *Junctional diversity between two germ-line segments producing three variant protein sequences. The nucleotide triplet which is spliced out is coloured blue.*

Further diversity arises from the insertion of nucleotides at the N region of the D and J segments, a process associated with the expression of terminal deoxynucleotidyl transferase. This process greatly increases the repertoire of T-receptor γ genes which are otherwise rather limited in number.

Just to make sure that we are really impressed, it transpires that even after a $V_H D J_H$ rearrangement has occurred, an interchange with a quite different 5′ V_H gene can still take place; since the process is not precise, bases can be lost and/or added at the region joining the new V_H to the N-terminal end of the D sequence. This V_H 'swapping' may prevent bias in the development of the heavy chain V-region repertoire because the earliest differentiating B-cells utilize the V_H segments most proximal to D with high frequency to form their $V_H D J_H$ rearrangements.

Yet additional mechanisms work on the D regions: in some cases the D segment can be read in three different reading frames and in others D−D combinations may be formed.

Interchain amplification

The immune system took an ingenious step forward when two different types of chain were utilized for the recognition molecules because the combinations produce new variability. Thus when one heavy chain is paired with different light chains the specificity of the final antibody is altered; for example, pairing of a heavy chain containing the T15 idiotype with three different light chains produced antibodies with different affinities for phosphorylcholine.

Random association between α and β chains and Ig heavy and light chains yields a geometric in-

crease in diversity. From table 3.6 it can be seen that approximately 200 T-receptor and 700 Ig germ-line segments can give rise to 8 million and 25 million different combinations respectively, by straight-forward associations *without* taking into account all of the fancy additional D/J mechanisms described above. Hats off to evolution!

Somatic hypermutation

There is inescapable evidence that immunoglobulin V region genes can undergo significant somatic mutation. Analysis of 18 murine λ myelomas revealed 12 with identical structure, 4 showing just one amino acid change, 1 with 2 changes and 1 with 4 changes, all within the hypervariable regions and indicative of somatic mutation of the single mouse λ germ-line gene. In another study, following immunization with pneumococcal antigen, a single germ-line T15 V_H gene gave rise by mutation to several different V_H genes all encoding phosphorylcholine antibodies (figure 3.28).

A number of features of this somatic diversification phenomenon deserve mention. The mutations are the result of single nucleotide substitutions, they are restricted to the variable as distinct from the constant region and occur in both framework and hypervariable regions. The mutation rate calculated by dividing the substitutions by the nucleotide bases sequenced is remarkably high, between 2 and 4% for V_H genes as compared with a figure of less than 0.0001% for a non-immunological lymphocyte gene. In addition, the mutational mechanism is bound up in some way with class switch since mutations are more frequent in IgG and IgA than in IgM antibodies, affecting both heavy (figure 3.28) and light chains.

The perceived wisdom at the present time is that somatic mutation does not add to the repertoire available in the early phases of the primary response, but occurs during the generation of memory and is probably responsible for tuning the response towards higher affinity.

T-cell receptor genes, on the other hand, do not appear to undergo somatic mutation. Assuming this result is not biased by the selection of T-cell clones studied, it has been argued that this would be a useful safety measure since T-cells are so close to fully recognizing self, mutations could readily encourage the emergence of high affinity autoreactive receptors and autoimmunity.

One may ask how it is that this array of germ-line genes is protected from genetic drift. With a library

Figure 3.28. *Mutations in a germ-line gene. The amino acid sequences of the V_H regions of five IgM and five IgG monoclonal phosphorylcholine antibodies generated during an anti-pneumococcal response in a single mouse are compared with the primary structure of the T15 germ-line sequence. A line indicates identity with T15 prototype and a blue circle (●) a single amino acid difference. Mutations have only occurred in the IgG molecules and are seen in both hypervariable and framework segments (after Gearhart P.J. (1982)* **Immunol. Today 3,** *107).*

of 800 or so *V* genes, selection would act only weakly on any single gene which had been functionally crippled by mutation and this implies that a major part of the library could be lost before evolutionary forces operated. One idea is that each subfamily of related *V* genes (figure 3.25) contains a prototype coding for an antibody which is indispensable for protection against some common pathogen so that mutation in this gene would put the host at a disadvantage and would therefore be selected against. If any of the other closely related genes in its set become defective through mutation, this indispensable gene could repair them by gene conversion, a mechanism in which it will be remembered that two genes interact in such a way that the nucleotide sequence of part or all of one becomes identical to that of the other. Although gene conversion was invoked earlier (figure 3.19) to account for the diversification of MHC genes, it can also act on families of genes to maintain a degree of sequence homogeneity.

SUMMARY

Immunoglobulins

Immunoglobulins (Ig) have a basic four-peptide structure of two identical heavy and two identical light chains joined by interchain disulphide links. Papain splits the molecule at the exposed flexible hinge region to give two identical univalent antigen binding fragments (Fab) and a further fragment (Fc). Pepsin proteolysis gives a divalent Ag binding fragment F(ab')$_2$ lacking the Fc.

There are perhaps 10^8 or more different Ig mole-

cules in normal serum. Analysis of myeloma proteins which are homogeneous Ig produced by single clones of malignant plasma cells has shown the N-terminal region of heavy and light chains to have a variable amino acid structure and the remainder to be relatively constant in structure. Each chain is folded into globular domains. The variable region domains bind Ag, and three *hypervariable* loops on the heavy and three on the light chain form the Ag binding site. The constant region domains of the heavy chain (particularly the Fc) carry out a secondary biological function after the binding of Ag, e.g. complement fixation and macrophage binding.

In the human there are five major types of heavy chain giving five *classes* of Ig. IgG is the most abundant Ig particularly in the extravascular fluids where it combats micro-organisms and toxins; it fixes complement, binds to phagocytic cells and crosses the placenta. IgA exists mainly as a monomer (basic four-peptide unit) in plasma, but in the sero-mucous secretions where it is the major Ig concerned in the defence of the external body surfaces, it is present as dimer linked to a secretory component. IgM is a pentameric molecule, essentially intravascular, produced early in the immune response. Because of its high valency it is a very effective bacterial agglutinator and mediator of complement-dependent cytolysis and is therefore a powerful first-line defence against bacteraemia. IgD is largely present on the lymphocyte and probably functions as an Ag receptor. IgE binds firmly to mast cells and contact with antigen leads to local recruitment of anti-microbial agents through degranulation of the mast cells and release of inflammatory mediators. IgE is of importance in certain parasitic infections and is responsible for the sympfibrillar protein) do not tend to react well with denatured preparations and this is consistent with the view that the majority recognize topographical (surface) structures (i.e. epitopes) which depend upon the conformation of the native molecule. For this reason, antibodies to native proteins do not usually react as strongly with peptides having the same primary sequence (figure 4.2). When individual epitopes are mapped using homogeneous monoclonal antibodies (cf. p. 107), they are frequently seen to involve amino acid residues far apart in the primary sequence, but brought together by the folding of the peptide chains in the native protein (figures 4.3 and 4.6). It seems reasonable to talk of *discontinuous* or assembled rather than *continuous* or sequential epitopes in these cases.

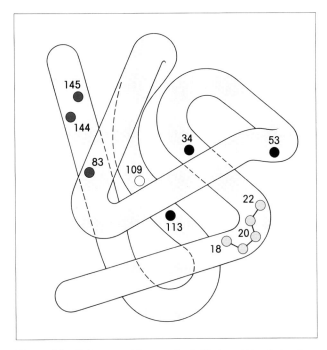

Figure 4.3. *Epitope residues on the folded peptide chain of sperm whale myoglobulin. Amino acid residues 34, 53, and 113 (●) contribute to the epitope recognized by one homogeneous monoclonal antibody, 83, 144 and 145 (●) to another. These are clearly* discontinuous *epitopes. Amino acids 18−22 (○) are postulated to form part of a continuous epitope based on reactions with the isolated peptides. Much of the myoglobin chain is in the α-helical form. Residue 109 (○) is critical for T-cell recognition and so far no antibodies reacting with this site have been demonstrated. (Based on Benjamin et al. (1986)* Ann. Rev. Immunol. **2, 67.)*

	LYSOZYME	ISOLATED LOOP PEPTIDE	REDUCED LOOP PEPTIDE
Anti-lysozyme	+ +	+	−
Anti-loop peptide	+	+ +	−

Figure 4.2. *Specificity and three-dimensional configuration in a globular protein, lysozyme. Antibodies to the whole molecule and to the isolated loop peptide do not react with the peptide after reduction of its disulphide bond, showing that the linear reduced peptide has lost the antigenic configuration it had when held as a loop even though the amino acid sequence was unchanged (from Maron E., Shiowa C., Arnon R. & Sela M. (1971)* Biochemistry 10, 763).*

If one were to take each individual antibody within an antiserum raised to a protein antigen and plot the approximate centre of the corresponding epitope on the antigen surface, one would almost certainly finish up with a 'contour map' of epitope density indicating regions on the antigen surface of *dominant epitope clusters* (figure 4.4a). Each of these clusters is as near as I can get to defining an antigen *determinant*. It is important to be aware that each antigen usually bears several determinants on its surface, which may well be structurally distinct from each other; thus a monoclonal antibody reacting with one determinant will usually not react with any other determinants on the same antigen unless the molecule has axes of symmetry (figure 4.4b).

Antigens and antibodies interact by spatial complementarity not by covalent bonding

Once a method had been found for raising antibodies to small chemically defined haptens (figure 4.1), it then became possible to relate variations in the chemical structure of a hapten to its ability to bind to a given antibody. In one experiment, antibodies raised to *m*-aminobenzene sulphonate were tested for their ability to combine with *ortho, meta* and *para* isomers of the hapten and related molecules in which the sulphonate group was substituted by arsonate or carboxylate (table 4.1). The hapten with the sulphonate group in the *ortho* position combines somewhat less well with the antibody

56

Figure 4.4. *A globular protein antigen usually bears a mosaic of determinants (dominant epitope clusters) on its surface, defined by the heterogeneous population of antibody molecules in a given antiserum. (a) Hypothetical 'contour' map of surface showing how determinants represent regions of clustering but overlapping epitopes whose positions are plotted as the centre of the area making contact with antibody. The actual size of a single epitope may be guaged by looking at figure 4.6. (b) Cross-section of a theoretical antigen with an axis of symmetry displaying six determinants including two pairs which are identical. An antiserum contains clusters of overlapping antibodies to each determinant (one representative of each antibody cluster is shown) which do not react with the other structurally unrelated determinants.*

Table 4.1. *Effect of variations in hapten structure on strength of binding to antibodies raised against **m**-aminobenzene sulphonate.*

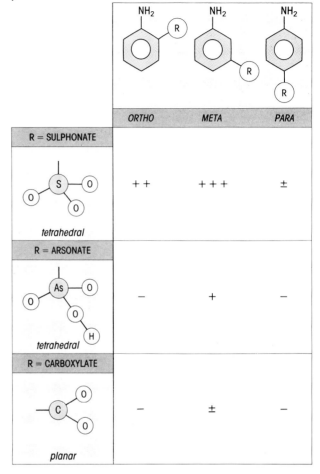

	ORTHO	META	PARA
R = SULPHONATE (tetrahedral)	+ +	+ + +	±
R = ARSONATE (tetrahedral)	−	+	−
R = CARBOXYLATE (planar)	−	±	−

(From Landsteiner K. & van der Scheer J. (1936) J. Exp. Med. 63, 325.)

57

than the original *meta* isomer, but the *para*-substituted compound (chemically similar to the *ortho*) shows very poor reactivity. The substitution of arsonate for sulphonate leads to weaker combination with the antibody; both groups are negatively charged and have a tetrahedral structure but the arsonate group is larger in size and has an extra H atom. The amino benzoates in which the sulphonate is substituted by the negatively charged but planar carboxylate group show even less affinity for the antibody. It would appear that the overall *configuration* of the hapten is even more important than its *chemical* nature, i.e. the hapten is recognized by the overall three-dimensional shape of its outer electron cloud as distinct from its chemical reactivity. The production of antibodies against such strange moieties as benzene sulphonate and arsonate becomes more comprehensible if they are thought to be directed against a particular electron-cloud shape rather than a specific chemical structure. This view is consistent with the nature of antigen–antibody binding which is known not to

involve covalent linkages and, like enzyme–substrate interactions, can be readily reversed. Thus, if one puts a mixture of the hapten with antibody inside a dialysis bag, the hapten will be found to diffuse out into the surrounding fluid until an equilibrium is reached in which some hapten is bound to antibody and some is free; if this exterior fluid is continually renewed, all the hapten will be lost from the bag showing that it can be completely dissociated from the antibody (figure 4.5).

The idea that antibody recognizes antigen through complementariness of shapes on paratope and epitope (simplistically another 'lock and key' arrangement) is beautifully confirmed by the X-ray crystallographic analysis of the interaction of a Fab fragment of monoclonal anti-lysozyme with its antigen where the snugness of fit between the two at their contact region is clearly evident (figure 4.6). Although some of the atomic radii of the contacting

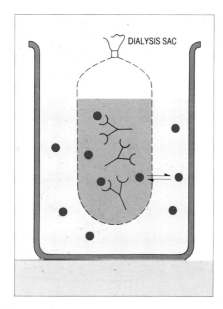

Figure 4.5. *Reversibility of the interaction between antibody (>—c) and hapten (●). Within the dialysis sac the hapten is partly in the free form and partly bound to antibody according to the affinity of the antibody. Only hapten can diffuse through the dialysis membrane and the external concentration then will equal the concentration of unbound hapten within the sac. Measurement of total hapten in the dialysis sac then enables the amount bound to antibody to be calculated. Constant renewal of the external buffer will lead to total dissociation and loss of hapten from inside the dialysis sac showing the reversible nature of the antigen–antibody bond.*

residues are far enough apart to permit the intrusion of water molecules, most exclude water and this has important implications for binding strength as we shall see.

The forces binding antigen to antibody become large as intermolecular distances become small

It should be stressed immediately that the forces which hold antigen and antibody together are in essence no different from the so-called 'non-specific' interactions which occur between any two unrelated proteins (or other macromolecules) as, for example, human serum albumin and human transferrin. These intermolecular forces may be classified under four headings:

(a) Electrostatic

These are due to the attraction between oppositely charged ionic groups on the two protein side-chains

as, for example, an ionized amino group (NH_3^+) on a lysine of one protein and an ionized carboxyl group ($—COO^-$) of, say, glutamate on the other (figure 4.7a). The force of attraction (F) is inversely proportional to the square of the distance (d) between the charges, i.e.

$$F \propto 1/k_D d^2$$

where k_D is the dielectric constant. Thus as the charges come closer together, the attractive force increases considerably: if we halve the distance apart, we quadruple the attraction. Furthermore, since the dielectric constant of water is extremely high, exclusion of water molecules through the contiguity of the interacting residues would greatly increase F.

Dipoles on antigen and antibody can also attract each other. In addition, electrostatic forces may be generated by charge transfer reactions between antibody and antigen; for example, an electron-donating protein residue such as tryptophan could part with an electron to a group such as dinitrophenyl which is electron accepting, thereby creating an effective $+1$ charge on the antibody and -1 on the antigen.

(b) Hydrogen bonding

The formation of reversible hydrogen bridges between hydrophilic groups such as $\cdot OH$, $\cdot NH_2$ and $\cdot COOH$ depends very much upon the close approach of the two molecules carrying these groups (figure 4.7b). Although H-bonds are relatively weak, because they are essentially electrostatic in nature, exclusion of water between the reacting side-chains would greatly enhance the binding energy through the gross reduction in dielectric constant.

(c) Hydrophobic

In the same way that oil droplets in water merge to form a single large drop, so non-polar, hydrophobic groups such as the side-chains of valine, leucine and phenylalanine tend to associate in an aqueous environment. The driving force for this hydrophobic bonding derives from the fact that water in contact with hydrophobic molecules, with which it cannot H-bond, will associate with other water molecules but the number of configurations which allow H-bonds to form will not be as great as that occurring when they are surrounded completely by other water molecules, i.e. the entropy is lower. The greater the area of contact between water and hy-

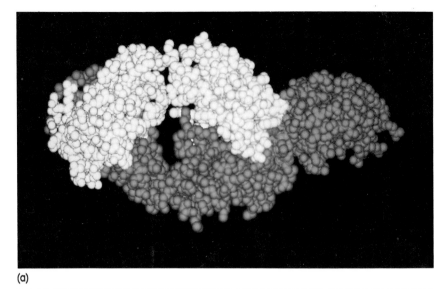

(a)

Figure 4.6. *The structure of the contact regions between a monoclonal Fab anti-lysozyme and lysozyme. (a) Space-filling model showing the Fab and lysozyme molecules fitting together snugly to form the complex. The antibody heavy chain is shown in blue, the light chain in yellow, lysozyme in green with its glutamine 121 in red. (b) Fab and lysozyme models pulled apart to show how the protuberances and depressions of each are complementary to each other. (c) End-on views of antibody combining site (left) and the antigenic region of lysozyme (right) obtained from (b) by rotating each molecule 90° about a vertical axis. Contact residues on both are shown in red except for Gln121 in light purple. The Gln121 fits into an antibody surface cavity surrounded by V_L and V_H residues 2, 5, 6, 7 and 16. The lysozyme epitope contact residues labelled 1−9 lie between residues 18 to 27 and labelled residues 10−16 are contributed by the peptide stretch from 117 to 128, i.e. this is clear evidence for a discontinuous epitope. All the hypervariable (complementarity determining) regions and two framework residues in the Fab make contact with the antigen. Most contacts are made by the heavy chain especially by the 3rd hypervariable region. It is not clear whether all the contacting residues contribute positively to the attractive forces between antigen and antibody; the striking influence of the Gln121 is revealed by the poor binding of lysozymes from other species in which the Gln121 is replaced by histidine. (Reproduced, with permission, from Amit A. et al. (1986)* Science 233, *747−753. Copyright 1986 by the AAAS.)*

(b)

(c)

drophobic surfaces, the lower the entropy and the higher the energy state. Thus if hydrophobic groups on two proteins come together so as to exclude water molecules between them, the net surface in contact with water is reduced (figure 4.7c) and the proteins take up a lower energy state than when they are separated (in other words, there is a force of attraction between them). It has been estimated that hydrophobic forces may contribute up to 50% of the total strength of the antigen–antibody bond.

(d) Van der Waals

These are the forces between molecules which depend upon interaction between the external 'electron clouds'. The deviation of gaseous molecules of say nitrogen or hydrogen from 'ideal' behaviour according to the kinetic theory is attributable to the Van der Waals attractions between them. The nature of this interaction is difficult to describe in non-mathematical terms but it has been likened to a temporary perturbation of electrons in one molecule effectively forming a dipole which induces a dipolar perturbation in the other molecule, the two dipoles then having a force of attraction between them; as the displaced electrons swing back through the equilibrium position and beyond, the dipoles oscillate (figure 4.7d). The force of attraction is inversely proportional to the seventh power of the distance, i.e.

$$F \propto 1/d^7$$

and as a result this rises very rapidly as the interacting molecules come closer together.

This last point underlines one essential feature common to all four types of force—they depend upon the close approach of both molecules before the forces become of significant magnitude, the more so if water molecules are excluded. And this is at the heart of the combination of antigen and antibody. The *complementary* electron-cloud shapes on the combining site of the antibody and the surface determinant of the antigen enable the two molecules to fit snugly together (cf. figure 4.6) so that the intermolecular distance becomes very small and the 'non-specific protein interaction forces' are considerably increased; the greater the areas of antigen and antibody which fit together, the greater the force of attraction, particularly if there is apposition of opposite charges and hydrophobic groupings.

By contrast, when the electron clouds of the two molecules effectively overlap, powerful repulsive forces are generated and energy must be expended

Figure 4.7. *Protein–protein interactions. (a) Coulombic attraction between oppositely charged ionic groupings. (b) Hydrogen bonding between two proteins. (c) Hydrophobic bonding: the region in which the water molecules are in contact with the hydrophobic groups (———) is considerably reduced when the hydrophobic groups on two proteins are in contact with each other (_____) and the lower free-energy of this system makes this a more probable state than separation of the hydrophobic groups. (d) Van der Waals force: the interaction between the electrons in the external orbitals of two different macromolecules may be envisaged (for simplicity!) as the attraction between induced oscillating dipoles in the two electron clouds.*

in displacing the overlapping residues from their normal equilibrium positions.

The affinity or strength of binding of antigen and antibody

We saw from the electron microscope (E.M.) studies on the interaction between bifunctional dinitrophenyl (DNP) conjugates and antibody, that each DNP group fitted into one antibody combining site (figures 3.3 and 3.4). This means that small haptens by themselves are monovalent with respect to reaction with antibody. The experiment on mixing hapten with antibody in a dialysis bag (figure 4.5) showed that the combination with antibody was reversible and that the complex so formed could readily dissociate depending upon the strength of binding. This can be defined through the equilibrium constant (K) of the reaction:

$$Ab + H \rightleftharpoons AbH$$

given by the mass action equation,

$$K = \frac{[AbH]}{[Ab][H]}$$

where [Ab] is the concentration of free antibody combining sites and [H] the concentration of free hapten. If the antibody and hapten fit together very closely, the equilibrium will lie well over to the right; we refer to such antibodies which bind strongly to the hapten as *high affinity antibodies*. At a certain *free* hapten concentration [H_c] where half of the antibody sites are bound,

$$[AbH] = [Ab] \text{ and } K = 1/[H_c]$$

i.e. the affinity constant K is equal to the reciprocal of the concentration of free hapten at the equilibrium point where half the antibody sites are in the bound form. In other words, when an antibody has a high affinity constant and binds hapten strongly, it only needs a low hapten concentration to half-saturate the antibody. It will be appreciated that an individual epitope on the surface of a complex antigen is also (by definition) monovalent and the strength of its combination with a univalent (Fab) antibody would also be defined by an affinity constant.

The value of K is determined by the difference in free energy (ΔG) between the antigen and antibody in the free state on the one hand and in the complexed form on the other, according to the equation

$$\Delta G = -RT \log_e K$$

where R is the universal gas constant and T the absolute temperature. Some energy may be required to alter the conformation of the antigen to allow strongly binding contact residues to interact either because some displacement from the native position is required in order to make the contact, or because a residue has to be displaced ón account of the steric repulsion forces which would be generated if it remained in its normal configuration.

One can study the interaction of hapten and antibody by the dialysis method described in figure 4.5 and use the data to calculate the affinity constant from the mass action equation. K values may sometimes be as high as 10^{11} l/mol.

Analysis of the binding at different hapten concentrations generally shows a heterogeneity (figure 4.8) which indicates that most antisera, even those raised against haptens with a simple structure, contain a variety of different antibodies with a range of binding affinities which depend upon the area of contact between the antibody and the hapten or epitope, the closeness of fit, conformation changes necessitated by electron-cloud overlap and the distribution of charged and hydrophobic groups.

The avidity of antiserum for antigen — the bonus effect of multivalency

While the term affinity describes the binding of antibody to a monovalent hapten or single antigen determinant, in most practical circumstances we are concerned with the interaction of an antiserum (i.e. the serum from an immunized individual) with a multivalent antigen. The term employed to express this binding,

$$nAb + mAg \rightleftharpoons Ab_n Ag_m$$

(Ab = antibody; Ag = antigen) is *avidity*.

The factors which contribute to avidity are complicated, including as they do the heterogeneity of antibodies in a given serum which are directed against each determinant on the antigen, and the heterogeneity of the determinants themselves (figures 4.4 and 4.8). But yet a further factor must be considered. The multivalence of most antigens leads to an interesting 'bonus' effect in which the binding of two antigen molecules by antibody is always greater, usually many-fold greater, than the arithmetic sum of the individual antibody links. This is illustrated in figure 4.9. The binding of the two antibodies to determinants 1 and 2 on the antigen can each be described by the individual change in free energy state on forming the epitope—paratope bond with its corresponding affinity constant, i.e.

$$\Delta G_1 = -RT \log_e k_1 \text{ and } \Delta G_2 = -RT \log_e k_2$$

For both antibodies operating in conjunction, the *overall* free energy change giving the avidity (K_{avid}) would be

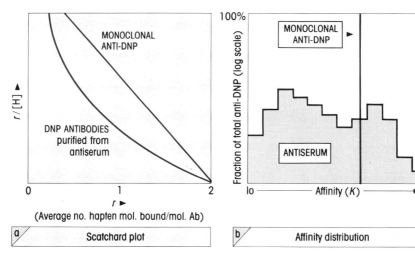

(Average no. hapten mol. bound/mol. Ab)

| a | Scatchard plot |

| b | Affinity distribution |

Figure 4.8. *Heterogeneity of IgG anti-hapten (dinitrophenyl: DNP) antibodies from the serum of an immunized animal contrasting with the homogeneity of a monoclonal IgG anti-DNP. (a) A Scatchard plot of hapten binding to antibodies purified from the serum. If* r *represents the average number of DNP molecules bound to each antibody molecule, of affinity constant* k *and number of binding sites* n, *in the presence of a free hapten concentration [H], then from the mass-action equation of equilibrium relationships (p.61) it can be shown that:*

$$r/[H] = nk - rk$$

Thus, a Scatchard plot of r/[H] *against* r *for a single antibody species will be a straight line of slope* k *as seen for the monoclonal antibody; the deviation from a straight line given*

by anti-DNP from the antiserum clearly indicates the existence of antibodies with different affinities as may be confirmed by the binding of labelled DNP to many different bands after separation of the individual antibodies by isoelectric focusing of the serum. Extrapolation to r/[H] = o *(at infinitely high concentration of antigen) gives the number of binding sites on each IgG molecule as 2 (cf. figure 3.5). For IgM antibodies the value would be 10. (b) Histogram showing a typical distribution of antibody affinities in the anti-DNP serum. Measurable affinities tend to range between* 10^4 *and* 10^{10} *or* 10^{11} *and have skewed and not necessarily unimodal distributions. The monoclonal antibody of course gives a single affinity value.*

62

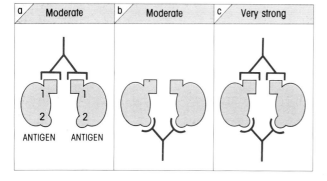

Figure 4.9. *The 'bonus' effect of multivalent attachment on binding strength. The force binding the two antigen molecules in (c) with two antibody bridges is many-fold greater than (a + b). If the affinity for determinant 1 is* k_1 *and for the second determinant* k_2, *the avidity of the mixture of antibodies for the antigen would be* $K_{avid} = k_1 \times k_2$. *To give a concrete example, if* k_1 *is* 10^4 *and* k_2 10^3, K_{avid} *would be* 10^7 *l/mol.*

$$\Delta G = \Delta G_1 + \Delta G_2 = -RT \log_e k_1 - RT \log_e k_2$$
$$= -RT(\log_e k_1 + \log_e k_2) = -RT(\log_e k_1 \times k_2)$$

Since $\Delta G = -RT \log_e K_{avid}$, $K_{avid} = k_1 \times k_2$.

The tremendous increase in equilibrium constant resulting from *multiplying* the contributing affinities (figure 4.9) is responsible for the bonus effect.

For those who prefer a more 'earthy' way of looking at molecular interactions, the mechanism of this effect may be interpreted by considering an analogy. Let us fabricate an unheard-of disease in which we cannot stop our hands opening and closing continuously. If we now try to hold an object in *one* hand it will fall the moment we open that hand. However, if we use *both* hands to hold the object, provided we open and close our hands at different times, there is much less chance of the object falling. The reversible combination of antigen and antibody is like the opening and closing of the hand; the more valencies holding the antigen the less likely it is to be lost when the complex dissociates at any one binding site (figure 4.10).

The same considerations apply to the binding of antibody to a polymeric antigen with repeating determinants such as ovalbumin substituted by several DNP groups, or most bacterial polysaccharides or red cells with repeating blood-group determinants. As one moves from a univalent Fab fragment to a divalent IgG to a pentameric IgM, the bonus effect of multivalency produces striking increases in the strength of antigen−antibody complex formation.

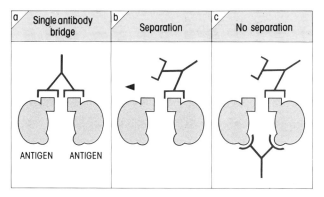

a. Single antibody bridge	b. Separation	c. No separation
ANTIGEN ANTIGEN		

Figure 4.10. *The mechanism of the bonus effect. Each antigen–antibody bond is reversible and with a single antibody bridge between two antigen molecules (a), dissociation of either bond could enable an antigen molecule to 'escape' as in (b). If there are two antibody bridges, even when one dissociates the other prevents the antigen molecule from escaping and holds it in position ready to reform the broken bond. In effect, the orientation of the broken bond greatly increases the effective* **combining** *concentration of antibody and thereby speeds up the velocity of the association reaction:* $V_a = k_a[Ag][Ab\uparrow]$.

Avidity being a measure of the functional affinity of an antiserum for the whole antigen is of obvious relevance to the reaction with antigen in the body. High avidity is superior to low for a wide variety of functions *in vivo*, immune elimination of antigen, virus neutralization, protective role against bacteria and so on.

The specificity of antigen recognition by antibody is not absolute

The ability of antibodies to discriminate between different antigens was well illustrated by the range of reactivity of an anti-hapten for a series of structurally related molecules as described in table 4.1. Since the strength of the reaction can be quantified by the affinity or avidity, we would relate the *specificity* of an antiserum to its relative avidity for the antigens which are being discriminated.

In so far as we recognize that an antiserum may have a relatively greater avidity for one antigen rather than another, by the same token we are saying that the antiserum is displaying relative rather than absolute specificity; in practice we speak of degrees of *cross-reactivity*. An antiserum raised against a given antigen can cross-react with a partially related antigen which bears one or more identical or similar determinants. In figure 4.11 it can be seen that an antiserum to antigen₁ (Ag₁) will react

less strongly with Ag₂ which bears just one identical determinant because only certain of the antibodies in the serum can bind. Ag₃ which possesses a similar but not identical determinant will not fit as well with the antibody and the binding is even weaker. Ag₄, which has no structural similarity at all, will not react significantly with the antibody. Thus, based upon stereochemical considerations, we can see why the avidity of the antiserum for Ag₂ and Ag₃ is less than for the homologous antigen, while for the unrelated Ag₄ it is negligible. It would be customary to describe the antiserum as being highly specific for Ag₁ in relation to Ag₄ but cross-reacting with Ag₂ and Ag₃ to different extents.

Original antigen	One identical determinant	Similar determinant	No structural similarity
Ag₁	Ag₂	Ag₃	Ag₄
	CROSS-REACTION		NO REACTION

Figure 4.11. *Specificity and cross-reaction. The avidity of the serum antibodies (and) for Ag₁ > Ag₂ > Ag₃ ≫ Ag₄.*

By being directed towards single epitopes on the antigen, monoclonal antibodies frequently show high specificity in terms of their low cross-reactivity with other antigens. Occasionally, however, one sees quite unexpected binding to antigens which react poorly, if at all, with a specific antiserum. It is an instructive exercise to see how it is that a polyclonal antiserum containing a heterogeneous collection of antibodies can be more specific in discriminating between two antigens than a monoclonal antibody. The six hypervariable regions of an antibody encompass a relatively large molecular area composed of highly diverse amino acid side-chains and it is self-evident that a number of different epitopic structures could fit into different parts of this hypervariable 'terrain', albeit with a spectrum of combining affinities.

Thus, each antibody will react not only with the antigen which stimulated its production, but also with some possibly quite unrelated molecules. Figure 4.12 explains (I hope) how this may translate into a higher specificity for the polyclonal serum.

63

ANTIGEN RECOGNITION – PRIMARY INTERACTION

Specificity of antiserum	Specificity of a monoclonal antibody
A	A
a	
b	
c	a
d	
etc.	

Figure 4.12. *Antigen A stimulates lymphocytes whose polyfunctional receptors bind A but could also bind other determinants as indicated (small letters). All antibodies in the resulting antiserum will have anti-A as a common specificity but the other specificities will be so diverse, none of them will reach appreciable concentrations to cross-react* *significantly with another antigen bearing a or b etc., i.e. the antiserum shows specificity for A. A monoclonal antibody on the other hand cannot dilute out its alternative specificity so in the example shown there would be strong cross-reaction with an unrelated antigen a. (With acknowledgement to Talmage D.W. (1959)* Science 129, 1643.*)*

What the T-cell sees

We have on several occasions alluded to the fact that the T-cell receptor sees antigen on the surface of cells associated with an MHC class I or II molecule. Now is the time for us to go into the nuts and bolts of this relationship.

Haplotype restriction reveals the need for MHC participation

Of dramatic significance has been the revelation that cytotoxic T-cells taken from an individual recovering from a viral infection will only kill virally infected cells which share an MHC haplotype. In the original experiments of Doherty and Zinkernagel, cytotoxic T-cells from mice of the H-2^d haplotype infected with lymphocytic choriomeningitis virus could kill virally infected cells derived from any H-2^d strain but not cells of H-2^k or other H-2 haplotype. The reciprocal experiment with H-2^k mice shows that this is not just a special property associated with H-2^d (figure 4.13). Studies with recombinant strains (cf. table 3.5) pin-pointed class I MHC as the restricting element and this was confirmed by showing that antibodies to class I MHC block this killing reaction. The same phenomenon has been repeatedly observed in the human. HLA-A2 individuals recovering from influenza have cytolytic T-cells which kill HLA-A2 target cells infected with influenza virus but not cells of a different HLA-A tissue-type specificity.

An entirely comparable series of experiments has established the role of MHC class II molecules in antigen presentation to helper T-cells. For example, a T-cell clone proliferating in response to ovalbumin on antigen-presenting cells with the I-A^b phenotype will fail to respond if antigen is presented in the context of I-A^k.

Finally, transfection of the appropriate MHC genes endows cells of the wrong haplotype with the ability to present antigen to T-effector cells restricted to the haplotype of the transfected genes. Taken together, these findings unequivocally establish the participation of MHC molecules in T-cell recognition. What then of the antigen?

Do T-cells see 'processed' antigen?

It has long been known that denatured antigens tend to be better at eliciting T-cell-mediated skin reactions (delayed-type hypersensitivity) than native protein. There is now good evidence that soluble proteins, at least, need to be metabolically processed in some way by antigen-presenting cells before they can be recognized by T-helper cells. Consider the following experiment: if macrophages are pulsed with ovalbumin at 0°C, washed and then allowed to warm up to 37°C, they will induce a proliferative response in a T-cell clone specific for ovalbumin and the H-2 haplotype of the antigen-presenting macrophage. If the pulsed macrophages are fixed with glutaraldehyde within a few minutes of reaching 37°C, they are unable to stimulate the T-cells, but if one waits for 1 hour at 37°C before fixation, a full-blooded T-cell proliferation can be induced (figure 4.14a). Clearly the antigen-presenting cell has to act on the ovalbumin in some way for it to be

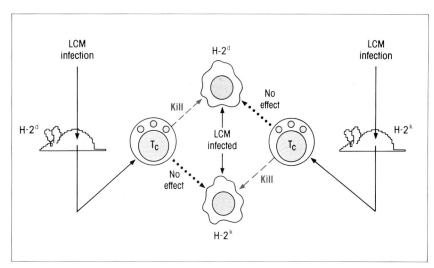

Figure 4.13. *Haplotype restricted killing of lymphocytic choriomeningitis (LCM) virus infected target cells by cytotoxic T-cells. Killer cells from H-2ᵈ hosts only killed H-2ᵈ infected targets, not those of H-2ᵏ haplotype and vice versa.*

recognized by the T-cell and this processing takes around 1 hour. It is also inhibited by chloroquine (figure 4.14b) which prevents the development of low pH in lysosomes and endosomes and there is a current view that native antigen loosely bound to the surface of the antigen-presenting cell is taken into endosomes where the relatively low pH allows limited denaturation or breakdown of antigen before it is returned to the surface of the cell for presentation. Speculatively, it is also suggested that endosomes which have incorporated class II MHC molecules are geared to return to the surface and those which have not are destroyed without trace by lysosomal fusion.

Whether the viral glycoproteins on virally infected cells which are thought to be the target for cytolytic T-cells are processed in a similar fashion is still debatable. However, recent studies with human T-cell clones cytolytic for influenza-infected target cells are consistent with some processing step in that simple addition of certain 16 amino acid peptides from influenza nucleoprotein to uninfected cells conferred susceptibility to T-cell lysis whereas addition of the whole nucleoprotein did not (figure 4.15).

Since T-cells have to recognize MHC together with some surface membrane form of the antigen (often referred to as 'nominal' antigen), it seems likely that a type of 'processing' which reveals hydrophobic segments of the antigen for membrane insertion will be necessary. It may be of relevance to call attention to the observation that a relatively

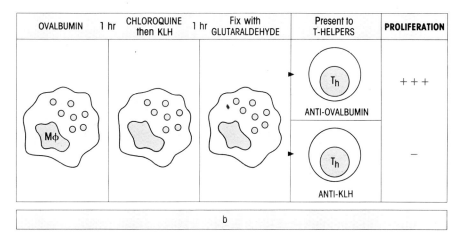

OVALBUMIN	1 hr	CHLOROQUINE then KLH	1 hr	Fix with GLUTARALDEHYDE	Present to T-HELPERS	PROLIFERATION
					Tₕ ANTI-OVALBUMIN	+ + +
					Tₕ ANTI-KLH	−

Figure 4.14. *Evidence of processing of soluble protein by antigen-presenting cell. (a) Antigen-presenting cells are kept at 37°C after pulsing with antigen before fixation with glutaraldehyde; the ability to cause proliferation of specific T-cells does not appear until after 45 min. (b) Chloroquine, an agent which prevents low pH in lysosomes and endosomes*

blocks the processing of keyhole limpet haemocyanin (KLH) but has no effect on previously processed ovalbumin. (Based on Grey H.M. & Chesnut R. (1985) Immunology Today 6, 101; *Ziegler K. & Unanue E. (1982)* Proc. Nat. Acad. Sci. 79, 175.)

65

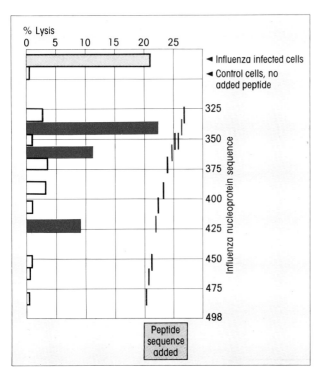

Figure 4.15. *Cytotoxic T-cells, from a human donor, kill uninfected target cells in the presence of short influenza nucleoprotein peptides. The peptides indicated were added to ^{51}Cr-labelled syngeneic (i.e. same as T-cell donor) mitogen-activated lymphoblasts and cytotoxicity assessed by ^{51}Cr release with a killer : target ratio of 50:1. The three peptides indicated in dark blue induced good killing. Blasts infected with influenza virus of a different strain served as a positive control. (Reproduced from Townsend A.R.M. et al. (1986) Cell 44, 959, with permission. Copyright 1986 by Cell Press.)*

weak-kneed antigen can be made strongly immunogenic by using recombinant DNA technology to attach the hydrophobic C-terminal peptide of the lymphocyte receptor form of IgM which anchors it to the surface membrane.

Does specificity imply dual T-cell receptors?

Transfection of α and β T-cell receptor genes shows that these carry the information to recognize both antigen and MHC and models of this relationship have fallen into two main types in which the ligands are recognized separately by α and β chains (figure 4.16a) or as a complex (figure 4.16b or c). However, if a T-cell hybridoma which recognizes antigen A in the context of H-2^d is fused with one recognizing antigen B in association with haplotype H-2^k, the resulting cell retains the original haplotype restriction for the recognition of each antigen and cannot respond to antigen A/H-2^k or antigen B/H-2^d; this is not the result to be expected if there are separate

receptors for antigen and H-2 unless there is some, as yet unrecognized, restriction in their association with each other.

On the other hand, photo-affinity reagents show that MHC and antigen become closely associated on the membrane. Assuming then that the two are seen as a complex, the receptor may recognize both components (figure 4.16b) or just the MHC alone, specifically altered in conformation by instruction from the nominal antigen (figure 4.16c). The latter is a slightly indirect way of generating the large number of specificities which T-cells can perceive and one guesses that both MHC and antigen will prove to be involved in the contact with T-cell receptor, not excluding the possibility of some concomitant alteration in the MHC. The ability of avidin to block the presentation of a biotinylated peptide to T-cells would seem to be strong evidence for a direct contribution from nominal antigen to the complex recognized by the T-cell receptor.

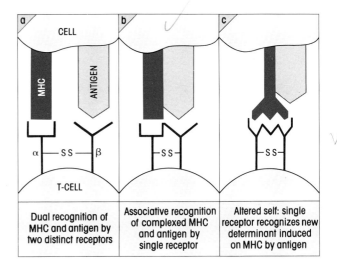

Figure 4.16. *Models for recognition of cell-surface antigen plus MHC by the T-cell receptor.*

Do MHC and nominal antigen interact positively to form a complex?

At the time of writing, this is still a vexed question and difficult to resolve unequivocally. Mice of H-2^d but not H-2^k haplotype give good T-cell responses to the 323–339 17 amino acid peptide from ovalbumin which are restricted to I-A. Equilibrium dialysis experiments between I-A^d and labelled peptide indicate a weak interaction which is not seen with I-A^k or I-E^d or I-E^k. More indirectly, the response of a T-cell hybridoma to pigeon and moth cytochrome *c* peptides on two different but related

Table 4.2. *Evidence for interaction between MHC class II I-E molecules and the cytochrome c peptide 81–103.*

Expt	Peptide origin	Antigen-presenting cell		Proliferation of specific T-cell hybridoma
1	Pigeon	B 10.A	I-E$_\alpha^k$ E$_\beta^k$	+ +
2	Pigeon	B 10.A(5R)	I-E$_\alpha^k$ E$_\beta^b$	–
3	Moth	B 10.A	I-E$_\alpha^k$ E$_\beta^k$	+ +
4	Moth	B 10.A(5R)	I-E$_\alpha^k$ E$_\beta^b$	+ +

(From Heber-Katz E., Hansburg D. & Schwartz R. (1983) J. Mol. Cell. Immunol. 1, 3.)

antigen-presenting cells, were studied. From the data in table 4.2, experiment 1 shows that the T-cell hybridoma recognizes pigeon cytochrome *c* while experiment 4 shows that it responds to the I-E restriction element on BI0.A(5R). The failure to be stimulated by the pigeon peptide in association with BI0.A(5R) (expt 2) seems therefore to be due to an inability of the antigen to complex with the I-E of BI0.A(5R).

Energy transfer studies show that class II molecules and nominal antigen do not come close to each other until the recognition by the T-cell receptor occurs. Thus, if there is a positive interaction between MHC and antigen, it is probably relatively feeble and only achieves significance when the ternary complex with the T-cell receptor is formed (figure 4.17).

Features associated with antigenicity

This is a subject of particular interest to those wishing to make simple peptide substitutes for complex protein antigens. In general, large proteins, because they have more potential determinants, are better antigens than small ones. The more foreign an antigen, that is the less similar to self-configurations which induce tolerance, the more effective it is in provoking an immune response.

Parts of the peptide chains which protrude significantly from the globular surface tend to be sites of high epitope density. The least antigenic segments of the surface are associated with neighbouring concave regions containing water molecules which may be more difficult to displace, and we have noted earlier the importance attached to driving out the water molecules between antigen and antibody to achieve high binding forces. Much attention has been focused on the association between dominant

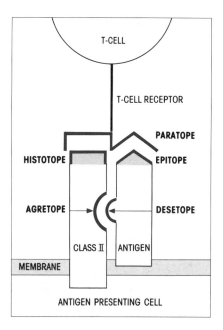

Figure 4.17. *Ternary complex between T-cell receptor, MHC class II and nominal antigen. The model assumes a strengthening of complex formation through positive interaction between class II and antigen through hypothetical structures, the agretope (antigen recognizing) and the desetope (determinant selecting). Note that giving them names does not of itself strengthen the case for their existence!*

antigenic regions and flexibility in the peptide chains as measured by the temperature factors derived from X-ray crystallography. If one considers the large area of potential contact between antigen and antibody, it is likely to be of value to have some flexibility in the shape of the antigen to allow it to take up a conformation which maximizes antibody contact; the assumption is that the energy expended in inducing this conformational change is more than compensated by the intrinsic free energy change associated with formation of the new binding sites. This input of energy to produce conformational change leading to strong binding appears to be the factor behind the frequent occurrence of normally 'buried' hydrophobic side-chains as contact residues for antibody.

T-cell epitopes are less well defined. They may well involve parts of the antigen which are not concerned in the stimulation of antibodies (figure 4.3) which is not surprising if one thinks of a possible requirement for hydrophobic insertion into the antigen-presenting cell membrane. The Berzofsky model for predicting potential T-cell-reacting epitopes looks for amphipathic sequences forming a helix with hydrophilic residues on one side and hydrophobic on the other. Because B-cells

67

tend to react with the natively folded protein antigen while T-cells recognize somewhat unfolded peptide chains, linear peptides mimic the potency of the parent antigen for stimulation of T-cells much more readily than they do for reaction with antibody.

SUMMARY

An antigen is defined by its antibody. The contact area with an antibody is called an *epitope* and the corresponding area on an antibody, a *paratope*. Antisera recognize a series of dominant epitope clusters on the surface of an antigen; each cluster is called a determinant. Antigens and antibodies interact by spatial complementarity, not by covalent binding, and the forces of interaction include electrostatic, hydrogen-bonding, hydrophobic and Van der Waals; the forces become large as separation of antigen and antibody diminishes, especially when water molecules are excluded.

The strength of binding to a single antibody combining site is measured by the affinity. The reaction of multivalent antigens with the heterogeneous mixture of antibodies in an antiserum is defined by avidity and is usually much greater than affinity due to the 'bonus effect of multivalency'.

Specificity of antibodies is not absolute and they may cross-react with other antigens to different extents measured by their relative avidities.

T-cells see antigen in association with MHC molecules. They are restricted to the haplotype of the cell which first primed the T-cell. Antigens, certainly soluble antigens, appear to be 'processed' by antigen-presenting cells and T-cells do not necessarily react with conformations of antigen identical to those of the native state. There is some evidence for a weak interaction between class II MHC and the nominal antigen which may contribute to the final strength of the termolecular complex formed between T-cell receptor, antigen and MHC.

The larger and more foreign a protein, the more likely it is to provoke antibody production; the protruding regions and probably the 'flexible' segments of globular proteins tend to be associated with higher epitope densities.

Further reading

Cresswell P. (1987) Antigen recognition by T-lymphocytes. *Immunology Today*, **8**, 67.

Geysen H.M. *et al.* (1987) Chemistry (and mechanisms) of antibody binding to a protein. *Science*. In press.

Glynn L.E. & Steward M.W. (eds) (1977) *Immunochemistry: an Advanced Textbook*. John Wiley & Sons, Chichester, UK.

Karush F. (1976) Multivalent binding and functional affinity. In *Contemporary Topics in Molecular Immunology*. F.P. Inman (ed.). Vol. 5, p. 217. Plenum Press, New York. (Bonus effect of multivalency.)

Nisonoff A. & Pressman D. (1957) Closeness of fit and forces involved in the reactions of antibody homologous to the p-(p'azophenylazo)-benzoate ion group. *J. Amer. Chem. Soc.*, **79**, 1616.

Novotny J. Handschumacher M. & Bruccoleri R.E. (1987) Protein antigenicity: a static surface property. *Immunology Today*, **8**, 26.

THE RECOGNITION OF ANTIGEN

II – Detection and Application

After exploring the intimacy of antigen−antibody interactions at the molecular level, this chapter will be more concerned with the practical aspects of methods used to detect and exploit antigen recognition.

Precipitation

The classical precipitin reaction

When an antigen solution is mixed in correct proportions with a potent antiserum, a precipitate is formed. Quantitative analysis of this interaction by the method shown in figure 5.1 gives both the antibody content of the immune serum and also an indication of the valency of the antigen, i.e. the effective number of dominant combining sites (determinants). This can vary enormously depending on the antigen, its size, and the species making the antibody. With hyperimmune rabbit antisera containing predominantly IgG antibodies, ovalbumin may have a valency of 10 and human thyroglobulin as many as 40 determinants on its surface.

It will be noted from the precipitin curve in figure 5.1 that as more and more antigen is added, an optimum is reached after which consistently less precipitate is formed. At this stage the supernatant can be shown to contain soluble complexes of antigen (Ag) and antibody (Ab), many of composition Ag_4Ab_3, Ag_3Ab_2 and Ag_2Ab (figure 5.2). In extreme antigen excess (AgXS; figure 5.1) ultracentrifugal analysis reveals the complexes to be mainly of the form Ag_2Ab, a result directly attributable to the two combining sites or divalence of the IgG antibody molecule (cf. E.M. study, figure 3.4 and Scatchard analysis, figure 4.8). Between these extremes the cross-linking of antigen and antibody will generally give rise to three-dimensional lattice structures, as suggested by Marrack, which coalesce, largely through Fc−Fc interaction, to form large precipitating aggregates.

Quantification by nephelometry

The small aggregates formed when dilute solutions of antigen and antibody are mixed creates a cloudiness or turbidity which can be measured by the scattering of an incident light source (nephelometry). Greater sensitivity can be obtained by using monochromatic light from a laser and by adding polyethylene glycol to the solution so that aggregate size is increased. In favoured laboratories which can sport the appropriate equipment, this method is replacing single radial immunodiffusion for the estimation of immunoglobulins, C3, C-reactive protein, etc.

Visualization of the precipitation reaction in gels

Ouchterlony double diffusion

In this method, antigen and antibody placed in wells cut in agar gel diffuse towards each other and precipitate to form an opaque line in the region

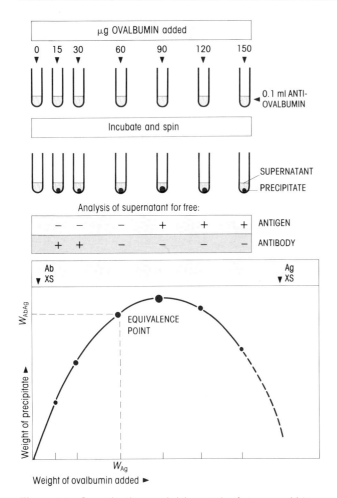

Figure 5.1. *Quantitative precipitin reaction between rabbit anti-ovalbumin and ovalbumin (after Heidelberger & Kendall). The antibodies are predominantly IgG. Increasing amounts of ovalbumin are added to a constant volume of the antiserum placed in a number of tubes. After incubation the precipitates formed are spun down and weighed. Each supernatant is split into two halves: by adding antigen to one and antibody to the other, the presence of reactive antibody or antigen respectively can be demonstrated. The antibody content of the serum can be calculated from the equivalent point where virtually no antigen or antibody is present in the supernatant. All the antigen added is therefore complexed in the precipitate with all the antibody available and the antibody content in 0.1 ml of serum would therefore be given by ($W_{AgAb} - W_{Ag}$). Analysis of the precipitate formed in antibody excess (AbXS), where the antigen-combining sites are largely saturated, gives a measure of the molar ratio of antibody to antigen in the complex and hence an estimate of the effective antigen valency.*

where they meet in optimal proportions. A preparation containing several antigens will give rise to multiple lines. The immunological relationship between two antigens can be assessed by setting up the precipitation reactions in adjacent wells; the lines formed by each antigen may be completely

confluent indicating immunological identity, they may show a 'spur' as in the case of partially related antigens, or they may cross, indicative of unrelated antigens (figure 5.3). The origins of these patterns are explained in figure 5.4. It should be emphasized that even in the case of confluent lines this can only indicate immunological identity in terms of the antiserum used, not necessarily molecular identity. For example, purified antibodies to the dinitrobenzene hapten would give a line of confluence when set up against dinitrophenyl (DNP)—ovalbumin and DNP—serum albumin conjugates placed in adjacent wells.

Where reagents are present in balanced proportions, the line formed will generally be concave to the well containing the reactant of higher molecular weight, be it antigen or antibody. This is a consequence of the usually slower diffusion rate of larger sized molecules.

The gel precipitation method can be made more sensitive by incorporating the antiserum in the agar and allowing the antigen to diffuse into it; up to 90% serum in agar may be employed (Feinberg). This method of single radial immunodiffusion is used for the quantitative estimation of antigens.

Single radial immunodiffusion (SRID)

When antigen diffuses from a well into agar containing suitably diluted antiserum, initially it is present in a relatively high concentration and forms soluble complexes; as the antigen diffuses further the concentration continuously falls until the point is reached at which the reactants are nearer optimal proportions and a ring of precipitate is formed. The higher the concentration of antigen, the greater the diameter of this ring (figure 5.5). By incorporating, say, three standards of known antigen concentration in the plate, a calibration curve can be obtained and used to determine the amount of antigen in the unknown samples tested (figure 5.6). The method is used routinely in clinical immunology, particularly for immunoglobulin determinations, and also for substances such as the third component of complement, transferrin, C-reactive protein and the embryonic protein, α-fetoprotein, which is associated with certain liver tumours.

Immunoelectrophoresis

The principle of this is described in figure 5.7. The method is of value for the identification of antigens by their electrophoretic mobility, particularly when

71

Figure 5.2. *Diagrammatic representation of complexes formed between a hypothetical tetravalent antigen (●┼●) and bivalent antibody (○—○) mixed in different proportions. In practice, the antigen valencies are unlikely to lie in the same plane or to be formed by identical determinants as suggested in the figure. (a) In extreme antibody excess, the antigen valencies are saturated and the molar ratio Ab:Ag approximates to the valency of the antigen. (b) At equivalence, large lattices are formed which aggregate to form a typical immune precipitate. This secondary aggregation, and hence precipitation tends to be inhibited by high salt concentration. (c) In extreme antigen excess where the two valencies of each antibody molecule become rapidly saturated, the complex Ag_2Ab tends to predominate. (d) A monovalent hapten binds but is unable to cross-link antibody molecules.*

Figure 5.3. *Multiple lines formed in the Ouchterlony test (double-diffusion precipitation) when rabbit antiserum (centre well) reacts in agar gel with four different antigen preparations (peripheral wells). Non-identity and partial identity of antigens are shown respectively by crossing over and spur formation between precipitin lines.*

ANTIGEN RECOGNITION — DETECTION

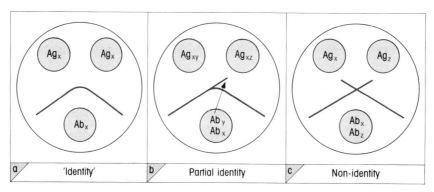

Figure 5.4. *(a) Line of confluence obtained with two antigens which cannot be distinguished by the antiserum used. (b) Spur formation by partially related antigens having a common determinant x but individual determinants y and z reacting with a mixture of antibodies directed against x and y. The antigen with determinants x and z can only* precipitate antibodies directed to x. The remaining antibodies (Ab$_y$) cross the precipitin line to react with the antigen from the adjacent well which has determinant y giving rise to a 'spur' over the precipitin line. (c) Crossing over of lines formed with unrelated antigens.

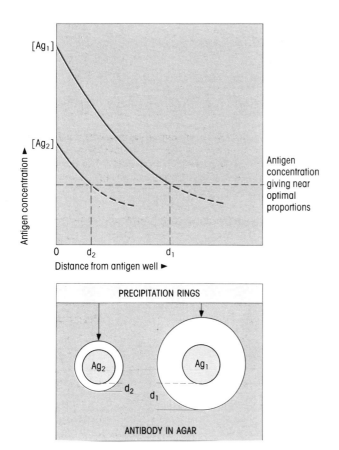

Figure 5.5. *Single radial immunodiffusion: relation of antigen concentration to size of precipitation ring formed. Antigen at the higher concentration [Ag$_1$] diffuses further from the well before it falls to the level giving precipitation with antibody near optimal proportions.*

Figure 5.6. *Measurement of IgG concentration in serum by single radial immunodiffusion. The diameter of the standards (●) enables a calibration curve to be drawn and the concentration of IgG in the sera under test can be read off:*
T$_1$—serum from patient with IgG myeloma; 15 mg/ml
T$_2$—serum from patient with hypogammaglobulinaemia; 2.6 mg/ml
T$_3$—normal serum; 9.6 mg/ml.
(Courtesy of Dr F.C. Hay.)

other antigens are also present. In clinical immunology, semi-quantitative information regarding immunoglobulin concentrations and identification of myeloma proteins is provided by this technique (figure 5.8).

There have been some felicitous developments of

ANTIGEN	ANTIBODY	ANTIGEN
Stage 1	Stage 2	

Figure 5.7. *The principle of immunoelectrophoresis.* **Stage 1:** *Electrophoresis of antigen in agar gel. Antigen migrates to hypothetical position shown.* **Stage 2:** *Current stopped. Trough cut in agar and filled with antibody. Precipitin arc formed. Because antigen theoretically at a point source diffuses radially and antibody from the trough diffuses with a plane front, they meet in optimal proportions for precipitation along an arc. The arc is closest to the trough at the point where antigen is in highest concentration.*

Figure 5.8. *Major human immunoglobulin classes demonstrated by immunoelectrophoretic analysis of human serum using a rabbit antiserum in the trough. The position of the main electrophoretic globulin fractions is indicated. Three of the five major immunoglobulin classes can be recognized: immunoglobulin G (IgG), immunoglobulin A (IgA) and immunoglobulin M (IgM). The IgG precipitin arc extends from the γ region well into the α₂-globulin mobility range reflecting the tremendous heterogeneity of the antibody population with respect to amino acid composition and net charge.*

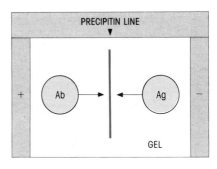

Figure 5.9. *Countercurrent immunoelectrophoresis. Antibody moves 'backwards' in the gel on electrophoresis due to endosmosis; an antigen which is negatively charged at the pH employed will move towards the positive pole and precipitate on contact with antibody.*

the principle combining electrophoresis with immunoprecipitation in which movement in an electric field drives the antigen directly into contact with antibody. *Countercurrent immunoelectrophoresis* may be applied to antigens which migrate towards the positive pole in agar (see figure 5.9). This qualitative technique is much faster and considerably more sensitive than double diffusion (Ouchterlony) and is used for the detection of hepatitis B antigen or antibody, DNA antibodies in SLE (p. 240), autoantibodies to soluble nuclear antigens in mixed connective tissue disease, and *Aspergillus* precipitins in cases with allergic bronchopulmonary aspergillosis. *Rocket electrophoresis* is a quantitative method which involves electrophoresis of antigen into a gel containing antibody. The precipitation arc has the appearance of a rocket, the length of which is related to antigen concentration (figure 5.10). Like countercurrent electrophoresis this is a rapid method but again the antigen must move to

the positive pole on electrophoresis; it is therefore suitable for proteins such as albumin, transferrin and caeruloplasmin but immunoglobulins are more conveniently quantitated by single radial immunodiffusion. One powerful variant of the rocket system, Laurell's *two-dimensional* or *crossed immunoelectrophoresis*, involves a preliminary electrophoretic separation of an antigen mixture in a direction perpendicular to that of the final 'rocket-stage' (figure 5.11). In this way one can quantitate each of several antigens in a mixture. One straightforward example is the estimation of the degree of conversion of the third component of complement (C3) to the inactive form C3c (cf. figure 1.10) which may occur in the serum of patients with active SLE or the synovial fluid of affected joints in active rheumatoid arthritis, to give but two examples (figure 5.11b). The remarkable ability of the technique to resolve a highly complex mixture of antigens is clearly seen in figure 5.11c.

Indirect precipitation of complexes

For a variety of reasons, addition of antibody to an

73

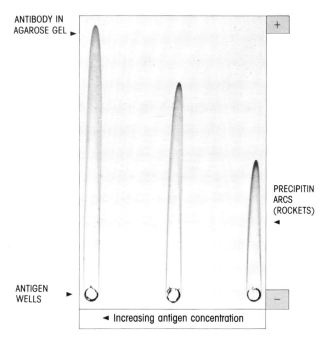

ANTIBODY IN AGAROSE GEL

PRECIPITIN ARCS (ROCKETS)

ANTIGEN WELLS

◄ Increasing antigen concentration

Figure 5.10. *Rocket electrophoresis. Antigen, in this case human serum albumin, is electrophoresed into gel containing antibody. The distance from the starting well to the front of the rocket-shaped arc is related to antigen concentration. In the example shown, human serum albumin is present at relative concentrations from left to right: 3, 2 and 1. (Reproduced from Weir et al. (eds) (1986)* **Handbook of Experimental Immunology 1,** *figure 32.42, with permission.)*

antigen may give rise to a soluble complex. If one wishes to analyse the complex for its antibody content or to identify the antigens within it, the complex can be brought out of solution either by changing its solubility or by adding an anti-immunoglobulin precipitating reagent as in figure 5.12. An example of how this technique was used to characterize the main chain of human class I MHC molecules is given in figure 5.13.

Figure 5.11. *Crossed immunoelectrophoresis. (a) Antigens are separated on the basis of electrophoretic mobility in agar gel. A narrow longitudinal strip (dotted) containing the separated antigens is cut out as shown, laid over another gel which contains antiserum, and electrophoresis carried out in a direction at right angles to the first to drive the antigens through the antiserum in the gel, so forming precipitin peaks; the area under the peak is related to the concentration of antigen. (b) Actual run showing C3 conversion (C3→C3c) in serum after staining of the gel. In this case the arcs interact because of common antigenic determinants. (Courtesy of Dr C. Loveday.) (c) 'Himalayan fantasy' showing the analysis of a highly complex mixture of antigens from* **Mycobacterium intracellulare.** *(Reproduced from Weir et al. (eds) (1986)* **Handbook of Experimental Immunology 1,** *figure 32.44, with permission.)*

Agglutination by antibody

Whereas the cross-linking of multivalent protein antigens by antibody leads to precipitation, cross-linking of cells or large particles by antibody directed against surface antigens leads to agglutination. Since most cells are electrically charged, a reasonable number of antibody links between two cells is required before the mutual repulsion is overcome. Thus agglutination of cells bearing only a small

a

Ag_2 Ag_1 STARTING WELL

PRECIPITIN PEAKS

Ag_2

Ag_1

AGAR GEL

ANTIBODY IN GEL

First run

Second run

b

C3c C3

◄ Direction of first run

c

Figure 5.12. *Precipitation of soluble complexes either (i) by changing the solubility so that the complexes are precipitated while the uncombined Ag and Ab remain in solution, or (ii) by adding a precipitating anti-immunoglobulin antibody or staphylococcal organisms which bind immunoglobulin Fc to the protein A on their surface and can then be spun down.*

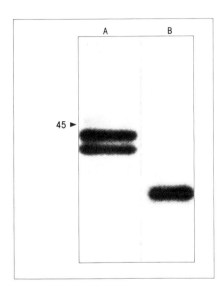

Figure 5.13. *Analysis of membrane-bound class I MHC antigens (cf. p. 45). The membranes from human cells pulsed with ^{35}S-methionine were solubilized in a detergent, mixed with a monoclonal antibody to HLA-A and B molecules and immunoprecipitated with staphylococci. An autoradiograph (A) of the precipitate run in SDS-polyacrylamide gel electrophoresis shows the HLA-A and B chains as a 43 000 molecular weight doublet (the position of a 45 000 marker is arrowed). If membrane vesicles were first digested with Proteinase K before solubilization, a labelled band of molecular weight 39 000 can be detected (B) consistent with a transmembrane orientation of the HLA chain: the 4000 hydrophilic C-terminal fragment extends into the cytoplasm and the major portion, recognized by the monoclonal antibody and by tissue typing reagents, is present on the cell surface (cf. figure 3.16). (From data and autoradiographs kindly supplied by Dr M.J. Owen.)*

Figure 5.14. *Mechanism of agglutination of antigen-coated particles by antibody cross-linking to form large macroscopic aggregates. If red cells are used, several cross-links are needed to overcome the electrical charge at the cell surface. IgM is superior to IgG as an agglutinator because of its multivalent binding and because the charged cells are further apart.*

Agglutination reactions are used to identify bacteria and to type red cells; they have been observed with leucocytes and platelets and even with spermatozoa in certain cases of male infertility due to sperm agglutinins. Because of its sensitivity and convenience, the test has been extended to the identification of antibodies to soluble antigens which have been artificially coated on to various types of particle. Red cells have been popular and they can be coated with proteins after first modifying their surface with tannic acid or chromium chloride, or by direct use of bifunctional cross-linking agents such as bisdiazobenzidine. The large, rapidly sedimenting red cells of the turkey are finding increasing favour for this purpose. The tests are usually carried out in the wells of plastic agglutination trays where the settling pattern of the cells on the bottom of the cup may be observed (figure 5.15); this provides a more sensitive indicator than macroscopic clumping. Inert particles such as bentonite and polystyrene latex have also been coated with antigens for agglutination reactions, particularly those used to detect the rheumatoid factors (figure 5.16).

number of determinants may be difficult to achieve unless special methods such as further treatment with an antiglobulin reagent are used. Similarly, the higher avidity of multivalent IgM antibody relative to IgG (cf. p. 61) makes the former more effective as an agglutinating agent, molecule for molecule (figure 5.14).

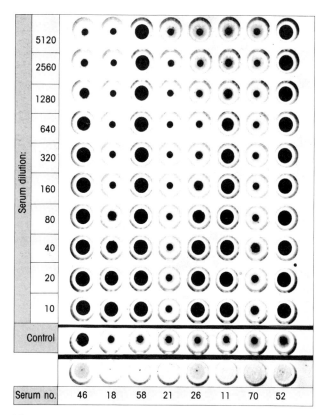

Serum dilution: 5120, 2560, 1280, 640, 320, 160, 80, 40, 20, 10, Control

Serum no. 46 18 58 21 26 11 70 52

Figure 5.15. *Tanned red cell haemagglutination test for thyroglobulin autoantibodies. Thyroglobulin-coated cells were added to dilutions of patients' sera. Uncoated cells were added to a 1:10 dilution of serum as a control. In a positive reaction, the cells settle as a carpet over the bottom of the cup. Because of the 'V'-shaped cross-section of these cups, in negative reactions the cells fall into the base of the 'V' forming a small easily recognizable button. The reciprocal of the highest serum dilution giving an unequivocally positive reaction is termed the* **titre**. *The titres reading from left to right are: 640, 20, >5120, neg, 40, 320, neg, > 5120. The control for serum No. 46 was slightly positive and this serum should be tested again after absorption with uncoated cells.*

Purification of antigens and antibodies by affinity chromatography

The principle is simple and *very* widely applied. Antigen or antibody is bound through its free amino groups to cyanogen-bromide-activated Sepharose particles. Insolubilized antibody, for example, can be used to pull the corresponding antigen out of solution in which it is present as one component of a complex mixture, by absorption to its surface. The uninteresting garbage is washed away and the required ligand released from the affinity absorbent by disruption of the antigen−antibody bonds by changing the pH or adding chaotropic ions such as thiocyanate (figure 5.17). Likewise, an antigen immunosorbent can be used to absorb out an antibody from a mixture whence it can be purified by elution.

Immunoassay of antigen and antibody with labelled reagents

Antigen and antibody can be used for the detection of each other and an ingenious plethora of immunoassay techniques have been developed in which the final read-out of the reaction involves a reagent conjugated with an appropriate label.

A wide variety of labels is available

Radiolabelling with ^{131}I, or now more usually ^{125}I, is a tried and trusted technique with a very long history. Because of health hazards and the deterioration of reagents through radiation damage, other types of label have been sought. Enzymes such as peroxidase and phosphatase which give a coloured reaction product have been successfully employed particularly in the ELISA (enzyme-linked immunosorbent assay), an immunoradiometric assay for antibody and sometimes for antigen. One clever ploy for amplifying the phosphatase reaction is to use NADP as a substrate to generate NAD which now acts as a co-enzyme for a second enzyme system. Conjugation with the vitamin biotin is finding increasing favour since this can be readily detected by its reaction with enzyme-linked avidin to which it binds with ferocious specificity and affinity ($K = 10^{15}M^{-1}$). Other active approaches utilize chemiluminescent and new-style fluorescent tags.

Soluble phase immunoassays

For antibody

If a reasonable excess of labelled antigen is added to an antiserum, most of the antibodies of moderate affinity will be complexed and precipitation of the complexes followed by measurement of the label will give an estimate of the antigen binding capacity of the serum (figure 5.18). By using antibodies to different immunoglobulin classes and subclasses as the antiglobulin reagent, it is possible to determine the distribution of antibody activity among the classes. For example, addition of a radioactive antigen to human serum followed by a precipitating

CHAPTER 5

Figure 5.16. *Macroscopic agglutination of latex coated with human IgG by serum from a patient with rheumatoid arthritis. This contains rheumatoid factor, an autoantibody directed against determinants on IgG. (a) Normal serum, (b) patient's serum.*

(a)   (b)

ACTIVATED SEPHAROSE	MONOCLONAL ANTIBODY	AFFINITY ABSORBENT	ANTIGEN MIXTURE			PURIFIED ANTIGEN
▷	+	Conjugate	+	Absorb antigen	Wash Elute	

Figure 5.17. *Affinity chromatography. A column is filled with Sepharose-linked antibody. The antigen mixture is poured down the column. Only the antigen binds and is released by* change in pH for example. An antigen-linked affinity column will purify antibody obviously.

Figure 5.18. *Determination of antigen-combining capacity of an antiserum using antigen coupled to ^{125}I or some other label (cf. figure 5.12). The radioactivity of the precipitate provides a measure of the antigen-combining capacity.*

rabbit anti-human IgA would indicate how much antigen had been bound to the serum IgA.

Classical radioimmunoassay (RIA) for antigen

The binding of radioactively labelled antigen to a limited fixed amount of antibody can be partially inhibited by addition of unlabelled antigen and the extent of this inhibition can be used as a measure of the unlabelled material added. The principle of this form of saturation analysis is explained in figure 5.19. Methods vary in the means used to separate free antigen from that bound to antibody and we have discussed the main ones already.

With the development of methods for labelling antigens to a high specific activity, very low concentrations down to the 10^{-12} g/ml level can be detected and most of the protein hormones can now be assayed with this technique. One disadvantage is that these methods cannot distinguish active protein molecules from biologically inactive fragments which still retain antigenic determinants. Other applications include the assay of carcinoembryonic antigen, hepatitis B (Australia) antigen and smaller molecules such as steroids, prostaglandins and morphine-related drugs (appropriate antibodies are raised by coupling to an immunogenic carrier).

ANTIGEN RECOGNITION – DETECTION

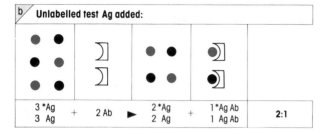

*Ag = radioactive antigen Ag = unlabelled antigen	FREE ANTIGEN	BOUND ANTIGEN	RATIO FREE:BOUND RADIOACTIVITY
a BASELINE:			
3 *Ag + 2 Ab ▶	1 *Ag +	2 *Ag Ab	**1:2**
b Unlabelled test Ag added:			
3 *Ag 3 Ag + 2 Ab ▶	2 *Ag 2 Ag +	1 *Ag Ab 1 Ag Ab	**2:1**

Calibration curve

Figure 5.19. *Principle of radioimmunoassay (simplified by assuming a very highly avid antibody and one combining site per antibody molecule). (a) If we add 3 mol of radio-labelled Ag (●) to 2 mol of Ab, 1 mol of Ag will be free and 2 bound to Ab. The ratio of the counts of free to bound will be 1:2. (b) If we now add 3 mol of unlabelled Ag (●) plus 3 mol radio Ag to the Ab, again only 2 mol of total Ag will be bound, but since the Ab cannot distinguish labelled from unlabelled Ag, half will be radioactive. The remaining antigen will be free and the ratio free: bound radioactivity changes to 2:1. This ratio will vary with the amount of unlabelled Ag added and this enables a calibration curve to be constructed.*

Solid phase immunoassays

For antibody

The antibody content of a serum can be assessed by the ability to bind to antigen which has been insolubilized by physical adsorption to a plastic tube or micro-agglutination tray with multiple wells; the bound immunoglobulin may then be estimated by addition of a labelled anti-Ig raised in another species. Consider, for example, the determination of DNA autoantibodies in systemic lupus erythematosus (cf. p. 240). When a patient's serum is added to a microwell coated with antigen (in this case DNA), the autoantibodies will bind to the plastic and remaining serum proteins can be readily washed away. Bound antibody can now be estimated by addition of ^{125}I-labelled purified rabbit anti-human IgG; after rinsing out excess unbound reagent, the radioactivity of the tube will clearly be a measure of the autoantibody content of the patient's serum. The distribution of antibody in different classes can obviously be determined by using specific antisera. Take the radioallergosorbent test (RAST) for IgE antibodies in allergic patients. The allergen (e.g. pollen extract) is covalently coupled to an immunoabsorbent, in this case a paper disc, which is then treated with patient's serum. The amount of specific IgE bound to the paper can now be estimated by addition of labelled anti-IgE.

Immunoradiometric assay for antigen

This differs from radioimmunoassay in the sense

that the labelled reagent is used in excess. For the estimation of antigen, antibodies are coated on to a solid surface such as plastic and the test antigen solution added; after washing, the amount of antigen bound to the plastic can be estimated by adding an excess of radio-labelled antibody. The specificity of the method can be improved by using solid phase and labelled antibodies with specificities for different parts of the antigen:

One widely used application is the radioimmunosorbent test (RIST) for IgE. Rabbit anti-IgE is coupled by cyanogen bromide to microcrystalline cellulose and reacted with dilutions of an IgE-containing standard serum or the patient's serum under test. Bound IgE is then measured by addition of labelled anti-IgE.

Immunoblotting (Western blots)

After separation from a complex mixture by electrophoresis in a solid phase such as polyacrylamide or agar gel, antigens can be 'blotted' by transverse electrophoresis on to nitrocellulose sheets where they bind non-specifically and can be identified by staining with appropriately labelled antibodies. This technique has been used widely, as for example in the identification of components of neurofilaments which have been separated in sodium dodecyl sulphate (SDS)-polyacrylamide gels; obviously, such a procedure will not work with antigens which are irreversibly denatured by this detergent. Conversely, the spectrotype of an antiserum can be revealed by isoelectric focusing, blotting and then staining with labelled antigen.

Immunohistochemistry—localization of antigens in cells and tissues

Immunofluorescence

Fluorescent dyes such as fluorescein and rhodamine can be coupled to antibodies without destroying their specificity. Coons showed that such conjugates would combine with antigen present in a tissue section and that the bound antibody could be visualized in the fluorescence microscope. In this way the distribution of antigen throughout a tissue and within cells can be demonstrated. Looked at another way, the method can also be used for the detection of antibodies directed against antigens already known to be present in a given tissue section or cell preparation. There are three general ways in which the test is carried out.

1. Direct test

The antibody to the tissue substrate is itself conjugated with the fluorochrome and applied directly (figure 5.20a). For example, suppose we wished to show the tissue distribution of a gastric autoantigen reacting with the autoantibodies present in the serum of a patient with pernicious anaemia. We would isolate IgG from the patient's serum, conjugate it with fluorescein, and apply it to a section of human gastric mucosa on a slide. When viewed in the fluorescence microscope we would see that the cytoplasm of the parietal cells was brightly stained. By using antisera conjugated to dyes which emit fluorescence at different wavelengths, two different antigens can be identified simultaneously in the same preparation. In figure 2.5h (p. 18), direct staining of fixed plasma cells with a mixture of rhodamine-labelled anti-IgG and fluorescein-conjugated anti-IgM craftily demonstrates that these two classes of antibody are produced by different cells. The technique of coupling biotin to the antiserum and then finally staining with fluorescent avidin is finding increasing favour.

2. Indirect test

In this double-layer technique, the unlabelled antibody is applied directly to the tissue substrate and visualized by treatment with a fluorochrome-conjugated anti-immunoglobulin serum (figure 5.20b). In this case, in order to find out whether or not the serum of a patient has antibodies to gastric parietal cells, we would first treat a gastric section with the serum, wash well and then apply a fluorescein-labelled rabbit anti-human immunoglobulin; if antibodies were present, there would be staining of the parietal cells (figure 5.21).

This technique has several advantages. In the first place the fluorescence is brighter than with the direct test since several fluorescent anti-immunoglobulins bind on to each of the antibody molecules present in the first layer (figure 5.20b). Secondly, since the conjugation process is lengthy, much time

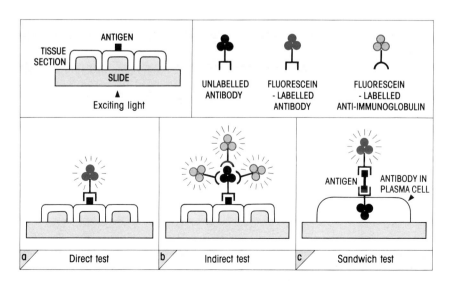

Figure 5.20. *The basis of fluorescence antibody tests for identification of tissue antigens or their antibodies.*
● = *fluorescein labelled.*

(a)

(b)

Figure 5.21. *Staining of gastric parietal cells by (a) fluorescein and (b) peroxidase-linked antibody. The sections were sequentially treated with human parietal cell autoantibodies and then with the conjugated rabbit anti-human IgG. The enzyme was visualized by the peroxidase reaction. (Courtesy of Miss V. Petts.)*

can be saved when many sera have to be screened for antibody because it is only necessary to prepare a single labelled reagent, viz. the anti-immunoglobulin. Furthermore, the method has great flexibility. For example, by using conjugates of antisera to individual immunoglobulin heavy chains, the distribution of antibodies among the various classes and subclasses can be assessed at least semi-quantitatively. One can also test for complement fixation on the tissue section by adding a mixture of the first antibody plus a source of complement, followed by a fluorescent anti-complement reagent as the second layer. Even greater sensitivity can be attained by using a third layer. Thus, in the example quoted of antibodies to parietal cells, we could treat the stomach section sequentially with the following: patient's serum containing antibodies to parietal cells, then a rabbit anti-human IgG, and finally a fluorescein-conjugated goat anti-rabbit IgG. However, as with most immunological techniques as *sensitivity* is increased, *specificity* becomes progressively reduced and careful controls are essential.

Applications of the indirect test may be seen in figure 5.21a and in Chapter 14 (e.g. figure 14.2, p. 242).

3. Sandwich test

This is a double-layer procedure designed to visualize specific antibody. If, for example, we wished to see how many cells in a preparation of lymphoid tissue were synthesizing antibody to pneumococcus polysaccharide, we would first fix the cells with ethanol to prevent the antibody being washed away during the test, and then treat with a solution of the polysaccharide antigen. After washing, a fluorescein-labelled antibody to the polysaccharide would then be added to locate those cells which had specifically bound the antigen (figure 5.20c). The name of the test derives from the fact that antigen is sandwiched between the antibody present in the cell substrate and that added as the second layer.

Reaction with cell surface antigens

Surface antigens can be detected and localized by the use of labelled antibodies. Because antibodies cannot readily penetrate living cells except by endocytosis, treatment of cells with labelled antibody in the cold (to minimize endocytosis) leads to staining only of antigens on the surface. We have previously seen the example of fluorescent staining of the surface of B-lymphocytes with anti-immunoglobulin, and figure 2.5f in Chapter 2 shows the distribution of antigens on the surface of viable human thyroid cells demonstrated with thyroid autoantibodies by the indirect test.

A close look at these examples reveals the patchy distribution of these surface antigens seen when they are visualized with conventional divalent antibodies. However, when B-cells are stained directly with a fluorescein-tagged *uni*valent Fab anti-immunoglobulin, the resulting fluorescence is seen as a smooth ring. This implies that the patchy fluorescence is the result of micro-agglutination through cross-linking of the antigens and, further, that the antigens are freely mobile in the plane of the surface membrane; this becomes quite striking as the cells are warmed up to 37°C when the patches coalesce into caps at one pole of the cell (figure 2.5f) before being taken into the cytoplasm by endocytosis. In fact, after combination with antibody, many antigens are removed from the cell surface either through capping and endocytosis, or shedding into the extracellular medium as complexes. This 'stripping' process may have deleterious consequences for the host if it makes virally infected cells or tumours refractory to immunological attack.

Measurement of cell surface fluorescence by flow cytofluorography

The amount of fluorescent antibody bound to each cell can be quantified by a technique known as flow cytofluorography. Suppose we have stained a subpopulation of lymphocytes with a specific antibody; it is now possible to make the cells flow obediently in a single stream past a laser beam. A light detector at right angles to the beam can be used to record the strength of the fluorescent signal while another detector gives information about cell size by forward light scatter (figure 5.22). An example of the quantitative data which can be generated by these machines is given in figure 5.23.

Other labelled antibody methods

In place of fluorescent markers, other workers have evolved methods in which enzymes such as peroxidase or phosphatase are coupled to antibodies and these can be visualized by conventional histochemical methods at both light microscope (figure 5.21b) and electron microscope (figure 5.24) level. Intracytoplasmic antigens pose certain problems for the latter since the cells must be damaged to allow penetration by the labelled antibody, and in order to avoid morphological degeneration of cellular structures it is necessary to fix the tissue; however, the greater the degree of fixation, the more difficult it is for the antibody to diffuse through the cytoplasm. Technological improvements in this area would not be amiss.

Cell separation techniques

Certain useful gross separations of immunological cells can be achieved by physical means. Adherence to plastic surfaces largely removes phagocytic cells while passage down nylon-wool columns greatly enriches lymphocyte populations for T- at the expense of B-cells. Lymphocyte preparations are customarily made by centrifugation over a Ficoll density

Figure 5.22. *The principle of the fluorescence activated cell sorter (FACS), designed by the Herzenbergs and colleagues, for flow cytofluorographic measurement of the fluorescence on stained cells (blue rimmed circles) and physical separation from unstained cells (grey circles). The charge signal can be activated to separate cells of high from low fluorescence or of large from small size.*

Figure 5.23. *Flow cytofluorographic analysis in a fluorescence activated cell sorter (FACS) of spleen cells from (a) CBA/J and (b) CBA/N mice stained with both fluorescein-labelled anti-IgM and Texas Red conjugated anti-IgD. The axes represent relative fluorescence while the contours give an indication of cell numbers. The CBA/N strain which is defective in its response to type II thymus independent antigens like pneumococcus polysaccharide (cf. p. 96) lacks the population with low surface IgM and high IgD seen in the normally responding strain CBA/J (Parks D.R., Hardy R.R. & Herzenberg L.A. (1983)* **Immunol. Today 4, 145).** *Since Texas*

Red is excited at a different wavelength from fluorescein, the FACS had to be fitted with two lasers to acquire this data; with the advent of newer dyes such as the algal photosynthetic pigment, phycoerythrin, which have fluorescence emission peaks well separated from fluorescein yet can be excited at the same wavelength, comparable results should be obtainable with a single laser. Light scatter measurements in the FACS also provide information on cell size and viability which allows discrimination against dead cells and analysis of fluorescence in relation to cell size.

Figure 5.24. *Electron microscopic visualization of human IgG on the surface of a B-lymphocyte by treatment of viable cell suspensions with peroxidase-coupled anti-IgG. Note the adjacent unstained lymphocyte. (Courtesy of Miss V. Petts.)*

step which separates them from other peripheral blood white cells of higher buoyant density.

However, the development of a wide range of monoclonal antibodies directed to specific differentiation antigens on the surface of different cellular subpopulations can be exploited by a variety of techniques to achieve more effective fractionation (summarized in figure 5.25).

We have already looked at the manner in which cells stained by fluorescent antibodies can be analysed one at a time in a flow cytofluorimeter. After flowing past the laser, the liquid stream is broken up into droplets each containing a single cell and if one wishes to separate the stained cell population, the droplet containing a cell giving a fluorescent signal is charged and deviated from the stream by an electric field into a suitable collector—hence the name *fluorescence activated cell sorter* (FACS; cf.

CYTOTOXICITY	ROSETTING

ANTI-Ig-RICIN CONJUGATE or COMPLEMENT

ANTI-Ig COATED RED CELLS

ANTIBODY-COATED CELL

FLUORESCENT ANTI-Ig

ANTI-Ig COATED DISHES

FLUORESCENCE ACTIVATED CELL SORTING	PANNING

Figure 5.25. *Major methods for separating cells coated with a specific antibody.*

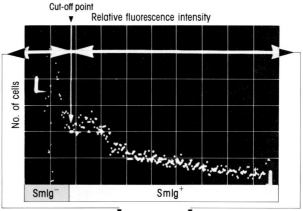

Cut-off point

Relative fluorescence intensity

No. of cells

SmIg⁻   SmIg⁺

Markers	SmIg⁻	SmIg⁺	Unseparated
Sheep cell rosettes	95	2	56
C3 rosettes	13	94	46
SmIg⁺/anti T⁺	<1	8	9
SmIg⁺/anti T⁻	<1	80	38
SmIg⁻/anti T⁺	94	8	51
'null'	6	4	2

Figure 5.26. *Separation of B- and T-cells from human tonsil lymphocytes by the fluorescence activated cell sorter. After staining with fluorescein-conjugated anti-Ig, the viable cells were analysed by flow cytofluorimetry to give the histogram shown. The lymphocytes were separated into a surface membrane Ig positive (SmIg⁺) and a negative (SmIg⁻) population depending upon the fluorescence intensity being either above or below the arbitrary cut-off point. Analysis of the % of cells positive for each marker is shown. 'Null' cells were negative with both anti-Ig and anti-T reagents. (Data kindly provided by Dr M.F. Greaves.)*

figure 5.22). An experiment in which cells were sorted on the basis of surface immunoglobulin in one of these elegant but expensive machines is documented in figure 5.26.

Cells bearing antibody can also be selected by *panning* to dishes coated with an anti-immunoglobulin (figure 5.25). Alternatively, they can form *rosettes* with anti-immunoglobulin-coated erythrocytes and these can readily be separated from un-rosetted cells by centrifugation. Such techniques have frequently been employed to fractionate T4 (helper) from T8 (cytotoxic/suppressor) human lymphocytes (cf. table 6.2) or the corresponding L3T4 and Ly2 mouse populations.

Sometimes one wishes to deplete certain populations such as mature T-lymphocytes in bone marrow cell suspension to limit graft-versus-host reactions (cf. p. 217). For this, cells labelled with anti-T can be killed by addition of complement or of an antibody conjugated to a highly toxic molecule such as ricin-A chain (figure 5.25).

Neutralization of biological activity

To continue our discussion on the interaction of antigen and antibody we may focus attention on a

number of biological reactions which can be inhibited by addition of specific antibody. Thus the agglutination of red cells by interaction of influenza virus with receptors on the erythrocyte surface can be blocked by anti-viral antibodies and this forms the basis for their serological detection. Neutralization of the growth of hapten-conjugated bacteriophage provides an exquisitely sensitive assay for anti-hapten antibodies. A test for antibodies to salmonella H antigen present on the flagella depends upon their ability to inhibit the motility of the bacteria *in vitro*. Likewise, mycoplasma antibodies can be demonstrated by their inhibitory effect on the metabolism of the organisms in culture. The successful treatment of cases of drug overdose with the Fab fragment of specific antibodies has been described and may become a practical proposition if a range of hybridomas can be assembled. Antibodies to hormones such as insulin and thyroid stimulating hormone (TSH) can be used to probe the specificity of biological reactions *in vitro*; for example, the specificity of the insulin-like activity of a serum sample on rat epididymal fat pad can be checked by the neutralizing effect of an antiserum. Such antibodies can be effective *in vivo* and, as part of the world-wide effort to prevent disastrous over-population, attempts are in progress to immunize against chorionic gonadotropin using fragments of the β chain coupled to appropriate carriers, since this hormone is needed to sustain the implanted ovum.

SUMMARY

The formation of single bands of precipitate when antigen and antibody react in gels can be used qualitatively to study the number of reacting components and the immunological relationship between different antigens (Ouchterlony double-diffusion system) and the electrophoretic mobility of the antigens (immunoelectrophoresis). Quantitative measurement of antigen concentration is made by single radial immunodiffusion, 'rocket' electrophoresis and two-dimensional electrophoresis. Laser nephelometry provides a sensitive method for the quantification of antigens in solution.

Antibodies can also be detected by macroscopic agglutination of particles coated with antigen. Insoluble immunoabsorbents prepared by coupling antibody to Sepharose can be used to affinity-purify antigens from complex mixtures and reciprocally to purify antibodies.

Many immunoassay techniques which exploit the mutual interaction of antigens and antibodies using labelled reagents have been devised. Labels include radioactivity and enzymes. In soluble phase systems, antibody can be estimated by addition of excess labelled antigen followed by precipitation of the complex. Radioimmunoassay of antigen is a form of saturation analysis in which the test material competes with labelled antigen for a limited amount of antibody, the amount of label displaced being a measure of the antigen in the test sample.

Immunoradiometric tests involve the binding of antigen to solid phase antibody and of antibody to solid phase antigen followed by estimation of ligand by excess of an appropriate labelled antibody. Antigens in mixtures can be identified by 'immunoblotting'.

The localization of antigens in tissues, within cells or on the cell surface can be achieved microscopically using antibodies tagged with fluorescent dyes or enzymes such as peroxidase whose reaction product can be readily visualized. In the direct test, the labelled antibody is applied directly to the tissue; in the indirect test the label is conjugated to an anti-Ig used as a second amplifying antibody. Fluorescent antibody bound to the surface of single cells, e.g. lymphocytes, can be quantified by flow cytofluorography. For ultrastructural studies, antibodies are usually tagged with peroxidase.

Cells labelled on their surface by a specific antibody can be selectively fractionated by the fluorescence activated cell sorter, by panning or rosette formation, or killed by complement-mediated cytotoxicity or by an anti-immunoglobulin conjugated to a toxin.

Antigens with biological activity, e.g. bacterial toxins or hormones such as human chorionic gonadotropin, may be neutralized *in vivo* by antibody.

Further reading

Beverley P.C.L. (ed.) (1986) Monoclonal antibodies. *Methods in Hematology*, **13**. Churchill Livingstone, Edinburgh, UK.

Cuello A.C. (ed.) (1983) *Immunohistochemistry*. Wiley, Chichester, UK.

Edwards R. (1985) *Immunoassay: an Introduction*. Heinemann Medical Books, London.

Hudson L. & Hay F.C. (1980) *Practical Immunology*, 2nd edn. Blackwell Scientific Publications, Oxford.

Polak J.M. & Noorden S. van (1987) *An Introduction to Immunocytochemistry: Current Techniques and Problems*. Oxford Science Publishers, Oxford.

Thompson R.A. (1981) *Techniques in Clinical Immunology*, 2nd edn. Blackwell Scientific Publications, Oxford.

Weir D.M. (ed.) (1986) *Handbook of Experimental Immunology*, **1–4**, 4th edn. Blackwell Scientific Publications, Oxford.

CHAPTER 6

THE ACQUIRED IMMUNE RESPONSE

I – Consequences of Antigen Recognition

WHERE DOES IT ALL HAPPEN?—THE ANATOMY OF THE IMMUNE RESPONSE

For an effective immune response an intricate series of cellular events must occur. Antigen must bind and if necessary be processed by antigen-presenting cells which must then make contact with and activate T- and B-cells; T-helpers must assist certain B-cells and cytotoxic T-cell precursors and there have to be mechanisms which amplify the numbers of potential effector cells by proliferation and then bring about differentiation to generate the mediators of humoral and cellular immunity. In addition, memory cells for secondary responses must be formed and the whole response controlled so that it is adequate but not excessive and is appropriate to the type of infection being dealt with. By working hard, we can isolate component cells of the immune system and persuade them to carry out a number of responses to antigen in the test tube, but compared with the efficacy of the overall development of immunity in the body, our efforts still leave much to be desired. *In vivo* the integration of the complex cellular interactions which form the basis of the immune response takes place within the organized architecture of peripheral, or secondary, lymphoid tissue which includes the lymph glands, spleen and unencapsulated tissue lining the respiratory, alimentary and genito-urinary tracts.

These tissues become populated by cells of reticular origin and by macrophages and lymphocytes derived from bone marrow stem cells, the T-cells first differentiating into immunocompetent cells by a high pressure training period in the thymus, the B-cells undergoing their education in the bone marrow itself (figure 6.1). In essence, the lymph nodes filter off and if necessary respond to foreign material draining body tissues, the spleen monitors the blood and the unencapsulated lymphoid tissue is strategically integrated into mucosal surfaces of the body as a forward defensive system based on IgA secretion.

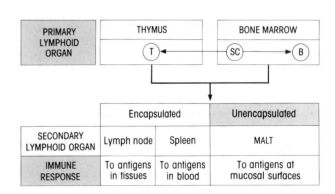

Figure 6.1. *Organized lymphoid tissue. Stem cells (SC) arising in the bone marrow differentiate into immunocompetent T- and B-cells in the primary lymphoid organs and then colonize the secondary lymphoid tissues where immune responses are organized. The mucosal-associated lymphoid tissue which produces the antibodies for mucosal secretions is often referred to as the MALT system.*

Communication between these tissues and the rest of the body is maintained by a pool of recirculating lymphocytes which pass from the blood into the lymph nodes, spleen and other tissues and back to the blood by the major lymphatic channels such as the thoracic duct (figures 6.2 and 6.6).

Lymph node

The encapsulated tissue of the lymph node contains a meshwork of reticular cells and their fibres organized into sinuses. These act as a filter for lymph draining the body tissues and possibly bearing foreign antigens which enters the subcapsular sinus by the afferent vessels and diffuses past the lymphocytes in the cortex to reach the macrophages of the medullary sinuses (figure 6.3e) and thence the efferent lymphatics (figures 6.2 and 6.3a). What is so striking about the organization of the lymph node is that the T- and B-lymphocytes are very largely separated into different anatomical compartments.

B-cell areas

The follicular aggregations of B-lymphocytes are a prominent feature of the outer cortex. In the unstimulated node they are present as spherical collections of cells termed *primary nodules* but after antigenic challenge they form *secondary follicles* (figure 6.3c) which consist of a corona or mantle of concentrically packed resting small B-lymphocytes surrounding a pale-staining *germinal centre* which contains large, often proliferating, B-blasts, scattered conventional reticular macrophages and the specialized dendritic macrophages with elongated cytoplasmic processes and few, if any, lysosomes. Germinal centres are greatly enlarged in secondary antibody responses and it is reasonable to regard them as important sites of B-cell memory. Following antigenic stimulation, differentiating plasmablasts appear and become plasma cells in the medullary cords of lymphoid cells which project between the medullary sinuses (figure 6.3d). This maturation of antibody-forming cells at a site distant from that at which antigen triggering has occurred is also seen in the spleen where plasma cells are found predominantly in the marginal zone. My guess is that this movement of cells acts to prevent the generation of high local concentrations of antibody in the region of the macrophage-processed antigen to avoiding neutralization of the antigen and premature shutting off of the immune response.

The remainder of the outer cortex is also essentially a B-cell area with scattered T-cells.

T-cell areas

T-cells are largely confined to a region of the node referred to as the paracortical (or thymus-dependent) area (figure 6.3a); if one looks at nodes taken from children with selective T-cell deficiency (figure 11.11) or neonatally thymectomized mice (figure 6.3h), the paracortical region is seen to be virtually devoid of lymphocytes. Furthermore, when a T-cell-mediated response is elicited in a normal animal, say by a skin graft or by painting chemicals such as

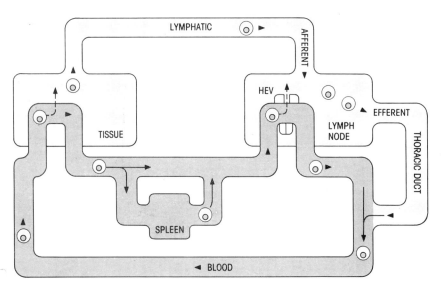

Figure 6.2. *Traffic and recirculation of lymphocytes through encapsulated lymphoid tissue. Blood-borne lymphocytes enter the tissues and lymph nodes passing through the high-walled endothelium of the post-capillary venules (HEV) and leave via the draining lymphatics. The efferent lymphatics finally emerging from the last node in each chain join to form the thoracic duct which returns the lymphocytes to the bloodstream where it empties into the left subclavian vein (in the human). In the spleen, lymphocytes enter the lymphoid area (white pulp) from the arterioles, pass to the sinusoids of the erythroid area (red pulp) and leave by the splenic vein.*

86

picryl chloride on the skin to induce contact hypersensitivity, there is a marked proliferation of cells in the thymus-dependent area and typical lymphoblasts are evident (figure 6.3g). In contrast, stimulation of antibody formation by the thymus-independent antigen, pneumococcus polysaccharide SIII, leads to proliferation in the cortical lymphoid follicles with development of germinal centres while the paracortical region remains inactive reflecting the inability to develop cellular hypersensitivity to the polysaccharide (figure 6.3f). As would be expected, nodes taken from children with congenital hypogammaglobulinaemia associated with failure of B-cell development are conspicuously lacking in primary and secondary follicular structures.

Lymphocyte traffic

Lymphocytes enter the node through the afferent lymphatics and by passage across the specialized high-walled endothelium of the postcapillary venules (HEV) (cf. figure 6.2). A highly specialized polyubiquinated receptor on the HEV defined by the monoclonal antibody MEL-14, acts as a lectin which recognizes a mannose-6-phosphate-containing molecule on the lymphocyte surface and presumably guides the relevant lymphocyte subset into the lymph node. This interaction can be demonstrated *in vitro* by the adherence of lymphocytes to the HEV of thin lymph node sections and the technique has revealed a quite distinct homing receptor on Peyer's patch HEV.

This traffic of lymphocytes between the tissues, the bloodstream and the lymph glands enables antigen-sensitive cells to seek the antigen and to be recruited to sites at which a response is occurring, while the dissemination of memory cells and their progeny enables a more widespread response to be organized throughout the lymphoid system. Thus, antigen-reactive cells are depleted from the circulating pool of lymphocytes within 24 hours of antigen first localizing in the lymph nodes or spleen; several days later, after proliferation at the site of antigen localization, a peak of activated cells appears in the thoracic duct. When antigen reaches a node in a primed animal, there is a dramatic fall in the output of cells in the efferent lymphatics, a phenomenon described variously as 'cell shutdown' or 'lymphocyte trapping' and which probably results from the antigen-induced release of a T-cell soluble factor (cf. the lymphokines, p. 25); this is followed by an output of activated blast cells which peaks at around 80 hours.

Spleen

On a fresh section of spleen, the lymphoid tissue forming the white pulp is seen as circular or elongated grey areas within the erythrocyte-filled red pulp consisting of splenic cords lined with macrophages and venous sinusoids. As in the lymph node, T- and B-cell areas are segregated (figure 6.4). The spleen is a very effective blood filter removing effete red and white cells and responding actively to blood-borne antigens, the more so if particulate. Plasmablasts and mature plasma cells are present in the marginal zone extending into the red pulp.

Mucosal-associated lymphoid tissue

The respiratory, alimentary and genito-urinary tracts are guarded immunologically by subepithelial accumulations of lymphoid tissue which are not constrained by a connective tissue capsule (figure 6.5). These may occur as diffuse collections of lymphocytes, plasma cells and phagocytes throughout the lung and the lamina propria of the intestinal wall (figure 6.5a and b) or as more clearly organized tissue with well-formed follicles. In man, the latter includes the lingual, palatine and pharyngeal tonsils (figure 6.5c), the small intestinal Peyer's patches (figure 6.5d) and the appendix. It has been suggested that this mucosal-associated lymphoid tissue (MALT) forms a separate interconnected secretory system within which cells committed to IgA or IgE synthesis may circulate.

In the gut, antigen enters the Peyer's patches (figure 6.5d) across specialized epithelial cells and stimulates the antigen-sensitive lymphocytes; after activation these drain into the lymph and after a journey through the mesenteric lymph nodes and the thoracic duct, they pass from the bloodstream into the lamina propria (figure 6.6) where they become IgA-forming cells which, because they are now widely distributed, protect a wide area of the bowel with protective antibody. The cells also appear in the lymphoid tissue of the lung and in other mucosal sites presumably using homing receptors analogous to the MEL-14 positive sites on the HEV of lymph nodes.

Bone marrow can be a major site of antibody synthesis

A few days after a secondary response, activated

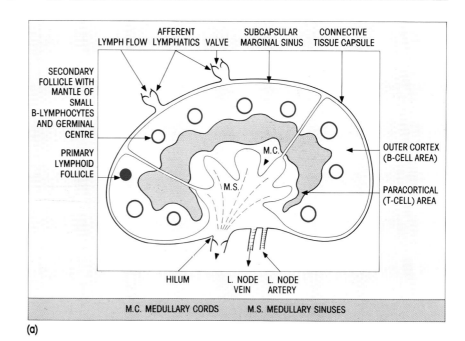

Figure 6.3 above and facing page. *Lymph node.*
(a) Diagrammatic representation. (b) Human lymph node,
low power view. (c) Secondary lymphoid follicle showing
germinal centre surrounded by a mantle of small
B-lymphocytes stained by anti-human IgD labelled with
horse-radish peroxidase (brown colour). There are few IgD
positive cells in the centre but both areas contain IgM
positive B-lymphocytes. (d) Medulla stained with methyl
green pyronin to show the basophilic (pink) cytoplasm of the
plasma cells with their abundant ribosomes. (e) Medullary
sinus of lymph node draining site of lithium carmine injection
showing macrophages which have phagocytosed the colloidal
dye. (f) Node from mouse immunized with the thymus-
independent antigen, pneumococcus polysaccharide SIII,
revealing prominent stimulation of secondary follicles with
germinal centres. (g) Methyl green pyronin stain of lymph

node draining site of skin painted with the contact sensitizer
oxazolone, highlighting the generalized expansion and
activation of the paracortical (T-cell), the T-blasts being
strongly basophilic. (h) The same study in a neonatally
thymectomized mouse shows a lonely primary nodule
(follicle) with complete lack of cellular response in the
paracortical area.

SS, subcapsular sinus; PN, primary nodule; SF, secondary
follicle; LM, lymphocyte mantle of SF; GC, germinal centre;
PA, paracortical area; MC, medullary cords; MS, medullary
sinus; PC, plasma cell; SM, sinusoidal macrophage. ((b)
photographed by Dr P.M. Lydyard, (c) and (d) photographed
by Dr K.A. MacLennan, (e) courtesy of Anatomy Dept.,
Middlesex Hospital Medical School, (f), (g) and (h) courtesy
of Dr M. de Sousa and Prof. D.M.V. Parrott.)

memory B-cells can be shown to migrate to the bone marrow where they mature into plasma cells. Bone marrow is a much neglected site of antibody synthesis which proves to be a major source of serum Ig, contributing up to 80% of the total Ig-secreting cells in the 100-week-old mouse. The peripheral lymphoid tissue responds rapidly to antigen, but only for a relatively short time, whereas bone marrow starts slowly and gives a long-lasting massive production of antibody to antigens which repeatedly challenge the host.

Where does antigen go?

It depends where it enters the body. If it penetrates the tissues it will tend to finish up in the draining lymph nodes. Antigens which are encountered in the upper respiratory tract or intestine are trapped by local mucosal-associated lymphoid tissue, whereas antigen in the blood provokes a reaction in the spleen. Macrophages in the liver and lung will filter blood-borne antigens but do not produce an immune response.

Within lymphoid tissue, large particulate antigens are taken up by macrophages and partly degraded; a fraction may reappear on the surface and soluble fragments may be released. There is general agreement that the antigen-presenting cell must bear antigen on its surface for effective activation of lymphocytes; macrophages which handle antigen in this way can switch on B-cells and, provided they express MHC class II, T-cells as well. Macrophages in the marginal zone of the spleen or the lymph node subcapsular sinus specialize in trapping and presenting polymeric T-independent antigens such

(b)

(c)

(d)

(e)

(f)

(g)

(h)

(a)

(b)

(c)

(d)

(e)

CHAPTER 6

(a)

(b)

(c)

(d)

Figure 6.5. *The IgA secretory immune system (MALT).*
(a) Section of lung showing a diffuse accumulation of
lymphocytes (Ly) in the bronchial wall. (b) Section of human
jejunum showing lymphoid cells (Ly) stained green by a
fluorescent anti-leucocyte monoclonal antibody, in the
mucosal epithelium (ME) and in the lamina propria (LP). A
red fluorescent anti-IgA conjugate stains the cytoplasm of
plasma cells (PC) in the lamina propria and detects IgA in the

surface mucus, altogether a super picture! (c) Low power view
of human tonsil showing the MALT with numerous secondary
follicles (SF) containing germinal centres. (d) Peyer's patches
(PP) in mouse ileum. The T-cell areas are stained brown by a
peroxidase-labelled monoclonal antibody to Thy 1. ((a) was
kindly provided by Dr P. Lydyard, (b) by Prof. G. Janossy, (c)
by Mr C. Symes and (d) by courtesy of Dr E. Andrew.)

Facing page

Figure 6.4. *Spleen. (a) Diagrammatic representation. (b) Low*
power view showing lymphoid white pulp (WP) and red pulp
(RP). (c) High power view of secondary follicle (SF) with
germinal centre (GC) surrounded by periarteriolar (T-cell)
lymphoid tissue, showing arteriole (A), marginal zone (MZ)
and red pulp (RP). (d) Localization of the thymus-independent
antigen, ficoll, on the marginal zone macrophages. The ficoll is

visualized by labelling with the red fluorescent dye
tetramethyl-rhodamine. (e) Preferential localization of a
thymus-dependent antigen (conjugated to green fluorescein)
on the follicular dendritic cells (ignore orange fluorescence).
((b) photographed by Dr P.M. Lydyard, (c) by Dr K.A.
MacLennan, (d) and (e) kindly provided by Prof. J.H.
Humphrey.)

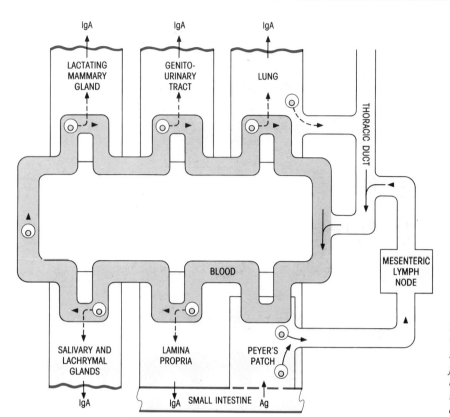

Figure 6.6. *Circulation of lymphocytes within the mucosal associated lymphoid system. Antigen-stimulated cells move from Peyer's patches (and probably lung and maybe all the mucosal member sites) to colonize the lamina propria and the other mucosal surfaces (～～～).*

as ficoll, which, as the name suggests, are capable of stimulating antibody production without intervention from T-cells (figure 6.4d).

In primed animals, antigens complex with circulating antibody and perhaps fix C3 so that they localize very effectively on the surface of the follicular dendritic cells within the germinal centres of secondary follicles (figure 6.4e). These cells have very elongated processes which can make contact with numerous lymphocytes and their surface receptors for Ig Fc, and C3b enable them to trap the complexed antigen very efficiently and hold the antigen on their surface for extended periods, in keeping with the memory function of secondary follicles. Evidence for this notion may be derived from animals effectively depleted of complement by injection of cobra venom factor which contains the reptilian equivalent of C3b. This fires the alternative pathway by forming a complex with factor B but because of its insensitivity to the mammalian C3b inactivator, it persists long enough to discharge the feedback loop to exhaustion and deplete C3 completely. Such mice can neither localize antigen—antibody complexes on their follicular dendritic cells, nor generate B-memory cells in response to T-dependent antigens (see p. 95).

T-cells seem to communicate with a different

species of dendritic antigen presenter, the interdigitating cell of the lymph node paracortical area; this is illustrated in figure 6.7 which shows the large area of close contact with the membranes of the surrounding T-lymphocytes rather well. Some of these, at least, derive from the dendritic Langerhans' cells of the skin which are thus able to transport antigen from the periphery for effective presentation to the lymph node T-cells.

Unlike the macrophages which in a sense are 'brutal microbe crunchers', the dendritic cells are not phagocytic although the interdigitating cells may have just whatever limited powers of degradation are required for the processing of antigen for T-cell recognition.

THE ACTIVATION OF T-CELLS

The surface markers of immunocompetent T- and B-lymphocytes

T- and B-cells differ in certain ways in their mode of activation and it is helpful for this discussion, and for general knowledge, to compare the *surface markers* of these cell types which naturally reflect the

Figure 6.7. *Interdigitating cell (IC) in the thymus-dependent area of the rat lymph node. This is thought to be an antigen-presenting cell derived from the Langerhans' cell in the skin which travels to the node in the afferent lymph as a 'veiled' cell bearing antigen on its profuse surface processes. Intimate contacts are made with the surface membranes (arrows) of the surrounding T-lymphocytes (TL). The cytoplasm of the IC contains relatively few organelles and does not show Birbeck granules (racket-shaped cytoplasmic organelles, characteristic of the Langerhans' cell), but these granules appear after antigenic stimulation (× 2000). (From Kamperdijk E.W.A., Hoefsmit E.Ch.H., Drexhage H.A. & Balfour B.H. (1980). In* Mononuclear Phagocytes, *3rd edn. Van Furth R. (ed.). Rijhoff Publishers, The Hague. Courtesy of authors and publishers.)*

93

different ways in which they communicate with extracellular moieties. The main characteristics of human T- and B-cells are set out in table 6.1. The most clear-cut difference is established by reagents which recognize the antigen receptors, anti-CD3 (T3) for T-cells and anti-immunoglobulin for B-cells, and in laboratory practice these are the markers used to enumerate the two lymphocyte populations. Quite often, the adventitious formation of rosettes with sheep erythrocytes (figure 2.5e) is used for the detection and separation of T-cells. Attention should also be drawn to the so-called 'non-specific mitogens' which activate populations of T- or B-cells in a way which is unrelated to the antigen specificity of the lymphocyte receptors because they react with constant, as distinct from highly variable, structures on the cell surface. For this reason, they are often termed polyclonal B- or T-cell activators.

Monoclonal antibodies also help to define specialized T-cell subsets of which the most prominent are shown in table 6.2 with their murine counterparts. CD4 (T4) and L3T4 are markers of helper T-cells and are probably involved in forming subsidiary links with class II MHC to strengthen the cellular

Table 6.1. *Comparison of human T- and B-cells.*

	T	B
% in peripheral blood	65–80	8–15
ANTIGEN RECEPTOR MARKERS: Surface Ig *CD3(T3)	 − ++	 ++ −
OTHER RECEPTORS: Sheep cell rosettes (CD2 T11) Fcγ receptors C3b receptors (CR1, CR2) EBV receptors Measles receptors	 ++ + (some) ± − ++	 − ++ ++ + (= CR2) −
MHC: Class I Class II	 ++ only activated cells	 ++ ++
POLYCLONAL ACTIVATION:	anti-T3 concanavalin A phytohaemagglutinin (PHA) pokeweed mitogen (PWM)	anti-Ig Staph. aureus str. Cowan 1 EBV pokeweed mitogen (PWM)

* The CD markers on the lymphocyte surface are defined by a cluster of monoclonal antibodies all reacting with the same molecule. Thus CD3 is best known by one of the monoclonals which first defined it, viz. T3.

CONSEQUENCES OF ANTIGEN RECOGNITION

Table 6.2. *T-cell subsets in man and mouse.*

	HUMAN	MOUSE
Pan T markers	CD3 (T3) CD2 (T11)	Thy1
T-helper/T-delayed hypersensitivity	CD4 (T4)	L3T4
	CD5 (T1)	Ly1
T-cytotoxic/suppressor	CD8 (T8)	Ly2

Homologous markers on human and mouse cells are linked.

interactions with the cell-presenting antigen. Similarly, the CD8 (T8) and Ly2 molecules on cytolytic T-cells connect with MHC class I (figure 7.12).

The activation of T-cells requires two signals

Antibodies to the T-cell receptor, either anti-idiotype or anti-T3, when insolubilized by coupling to Sepharose, will not activate resting T-cells on their own. Addition of interleukin-1 (IL-1) now readily induces RNA and protein synthesis, the cell enlarges to a blast-like appearance, interleukin-2 (IL-2) synthesis begins and the cell moves from G_0 into the G_1 phase of the mitotic cycle. Thus, two signals are required for the activation of a resting T-cell (figure 6.8). Antigen in association with MHC class II on the surface of antigen-presenting cells is clearly capable of fulfilling these requirements. Ternary complex formation between the T-cell receptor, antigen and MHC provides a signal through the receptor/T3 complex and presumably exposes the T-cell to high local concentrations of IL-1 from the antigen-presenting cell.

The biochemical repercussions of these activation signals are complicated, but figure 6.9 makes some attempt to set out a minimally accepted overall scheme leading to synthesis of RNA and protein, including IL-2. The very earliest detectable events involve increased turnover of phosphatidyl inositol compounds and a rapid increase in cytoplasmic calcium concentration either through the opening of a Ca^{2+} channel in the plasma membrane or more probably by mobilization of intracellular stores under the influence of inositol triphosphate, itself derived by the action of an activated phospholipase on phosphatidyl inositol diphosphate. The other cleavage product, diacylglycerol, activates a calcium-dependent protein kinase *c* linked to the formation

of IL-2. Further breakdown of diacyglycerol to arachidonic acid leads through mediators of the 5-lipoxygenase pathway to increased cyclic-GMP formation and this greatly enhances the activity of cGMP-dependent protein kinase(s) responsible for phosphorylation of a number of substrates, including non-histone acidic nuclear proteins critical for gene expression. cGMP has also been implicated in the activation of DNA-dependent RNA polymerases and the initiation of ribosomal and other RNA synthesis.

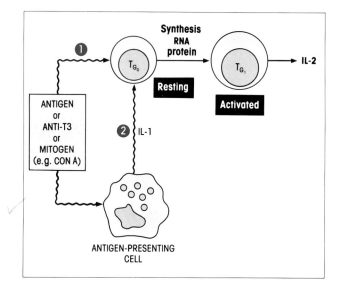

Figure 6.8. *Activation of resting T-cells requires two signals.*

THE ACTIVATION OF B-CELLS

B-cells respond to three different types of antigen

1. Type 1 thymus-independent antigens

Certain antigens such as bacterial lipopolysaccharides, at a high enough concentration, have the ability to activate a substantial proportion of the B-cell pool polyclonally, i.e. without reference to the antigen specificity of the surface receptor hypervariable regions. At low concentrations, which do not cause polyclonal activation, those B-cells with Ig receptors *specific* for these antigens will focus them passively on their surface and be stimulated by their inherent mitogenic power (figure 6.13a).

94

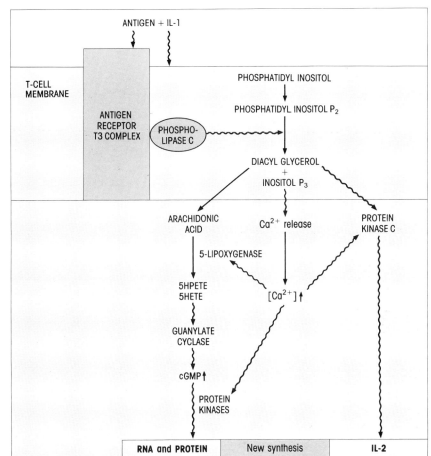

Figure 6.9. *Biochemical pathways of T-cell activation. The crucial event stimulated by antigen plus interleukin-1 would seem to be activation of the phospholipase which splits phosphatidyl inositol diphosphate to the reactive products diacylglycerol and inositol triphosphate. The increased intracellular Ca^{2+} concentration activates a number of different enzyme systems which lead finally to new synthesis of RNA, protein and interleukin-2 (5HPETE, 5, hydroperoxyeicosatetraenoic acid; 5HETE, 5, hydroxyeicosatetraenoic acid; cGMP, cyclic 3', 5'-guanosine monophosphate). (The arachidonic acid sequence is distilled from a review by Hadden J.W. & Coffey R.G. In* **Mechanisms of Lymphocyte Activation and Immune Regulation** *Gupta S., Paul W. and Fauci A (eds). Plenum Press, N.Y. In press.)*

2. Type 2 thymus-independent antigens

Certain linear antigens which are not readily degraded in the body and which have an appropriately spaced, highly repeating determinant—pneumococcus polysaccharide, D-amino acid polymers and polyvinylpyrrolidone, for example—are also thymus-independent in their ability to stimulate B-cells directly without the need for T-cell involvement. They persist for long periods on the surface of specialized macrophages located at the subcapsular sinus of the lymph nodes and the splenic marginal zone, and can bind to antigen-specific B-cells with great avidity through their multivalent attachment to the complementary Ig receptors which they cross-link (figure 6.13b).

In general, the thymus-independent antigens give rise to predominantly IgM responses and relatively poor, if any, memory.

3. Thymus-dependent antigens—the need for collaboration with T-helper cells

Many antigens are thymus-dependent in that they provoke little or no antibody response in animals which have been thymectomized at birth and have few T-cells. In general, antigens cannot fulfil the molecular requirements for direct stimulation, they may be univalent with respect to the specificity of each determinant, they may be readily degraded by phagocytic cells and they may lack mitogenicity. If they bind to B-cell receptors they will sit on the surface just like a hapten and not trigger the B-cell (figure 6.10). Cast your mind back to the definition of a hapten—a small molecule like dinitrophenyl (DNP) which binds to preformed antibody (e.g. the surface receptor of a specific B-cell) but fails to stimulate antibody production (i.e. stimulate the B-cell). Remember also that haptens become immunogenic when coupled to an appropriate carrier protein (p. 55). We now know that the carrier functions to stimulate T-helper cells which cooperate with B-cells to enable them to respond to the hapten by providing some accessory signals (figure 6.10). It should also be evident from figure 6.10 that while one determinant on an antigen is behaving as a hapten in binding to the B-cell, the other determinants subserve a carrier function in recruiting T-helper cells.

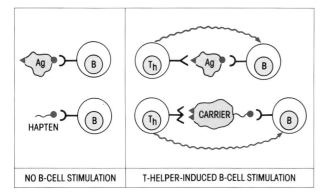

| | | NO B-CELL STIMULATION | T-HELPER-INDUCED B-CELL STIMULATION |

Figure 6.10. *T-helper cells cooperate through carrier determinants to help B-cells respond to hapten or equivalent determinants on antigens by providing accessory signals. (For simplicity we are ignoring the MHC component in T-cell recognition, but we won't forget it.)*

	Priming injection	Boosting injection	Secondary response to hapten (DNP)
1	BSA-DNP	BSA-DNP	+++
2	BSA-DNP	OVA-DNP	±
3	BSA-DNP + OVA	OVA-DNP	+++
4	BSA-DNP	BSA + OVA-DNP	±

Figure 6.11. *The role of carrier priming in the secondary response to hapten. The boosting injection only produces a secondary hapten response when the hapten is physically linked to a carrier to which the animal is already primed (after Rajewsky): BSA, bovine serum albumin; DNP, dinitrophenyl; Ova, chicken ovalbumin.*

It is worthwhile examining the evidence on which these assertions are based. The first experiment in figure 6.11 shows that boosting with a hapten-carrier conjugate produces a secondary antibody response (not altogether surprising). The second shows that boosting with the hapten on a second carrier is ineffective unless the animal had already been separately primed to the second carrier (experiment 3). The last experiment shows that if the hapten and carrier are not physically linked together, they are not able to induce a secondary response. The roles of cooperating carrier-primed T-cells in the secondary response to carrier-hapten conjugates are revealed by the adoptive transfer experiments in figure 6.12.

Antigen processing by B-cells

The need for physical linkage of hapten and carrier strongly suggests that T-helpers must recognize the carrier determinants on the responding B-cell in order to provide the relevant accessory stimulatory signals. However, since T-cells only recognize processed membrane-bound antigen in association with MHC molecules, the T-helpers cannot recognize native antigen bound simply to the Ig-receptors of the B-cell as naïvely depicted in figure 6.10. All is not lost, however, since primed B-cells can present antigen to T-helper cells—in fact, they work at much lower antigen concentrations than conventional presenting cells because they can focus antigen through their surface receptors. They must therefore be capable of 'processing' the antigen and the current view is that antigen bound to surface Ig is taken into endosomes together with class II MHC and then recycled to the surface in processed form associated with the class II molecules where it is available for recognition by specific T-helpers (figure 6.13c). The need for the physical union of hapten and carrier is now revealed; the hapten leads the carrier to be processed in the cell which is programmed to make anti-hapten antibody and, following stimulus by the T-helper recognizing processed carrier, it will carry out its programme and ultimately produce antibodies which react with the hapten (is there no end to the wiliness of nature?!).

The nature of B-cell activation

Cross-linking of B-cell surface receptors, for example by anti-IgM conjugated to insoluble Sepharose particles, induces the early activation events. The involvement of antigen-presenting cells in the activation process is still not clearly defined. The polymeric type-2 thymus-independent antigens with repeating determinants firmly cross-link Ig receptors to form a stable matrix, but they are normally presented on specialized macrophages which produce an assortment of possible accessory factors like IL-1 and C3. The latter is of interest since antibodies to the CR2 receptor for C3b are mitogenic for B-cells and, furthermore, the polyclonal activator Epstein Barr (EB) virus is known to bind to this receptor.

96

Figure 6.12. *The secondary response of B-cells primed to dinitrophenyl (DNP) depends upon help from T-cells sensitized to carrier determinants. Spleen cells from primed mice were fractionated into T-cells by nylon wool filtration or panning off B-cells with anti-Ig plates; B-cell fractions were obtained by killing T-cells with anti-Thy 1 plus complement. Appropriate mixtures of T- and B-cells were transferred to irradiated hosts of the same strain and then challenged with either of the two hapten-carrier conjugates. BSA, bovine serum albumin; Ova, ovalbumin.*

	Adoptive transfer of secondary response to hapten			
Sensitization	BSA	OVA-DNP	OVA	BSA-DNP
Adoptive transfer	T-CELLS	B-CELLS	T-CELLS	B-CELLS
Challenge	BSA-DNP	+++		±
	OVA-DNP	±		+++

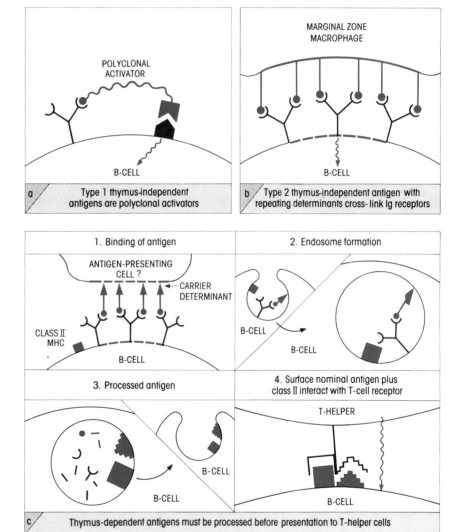

Figure 6.13. *B-cell recognition of three types of antigen.* ⟿ *, activation signal;* Ⲩ *, surface Ig receptor;* − − − − *, cross-linking of receptors.*

a / Type 1 thymus-independent antigens are polyclonal activators

b / Type 2 thymus-independent antigen with repeating determinants cross-link Ig receptors

1. Binding of antigen

2. Endosome formation

3. Processed antigen

4. Surface nominal antigen plus class II interact with T-cell receptor

c / Thymus-dependent antigens must be processed before presentation to T-helper cells

Be that as it may, Ig receptor cross-linking leads to a series of changes which probably closely parallel those seen in T-cell activation, active turnover of phosphatidyl inositol phosphates, formation of inositol triphosphate with mobilization of intracellular Ca^{2+}, and of diacylglycerol and activation of protein kinase c (cf. figure 6.9). The other event which is of importance for T-dependent antigens is an early increase in the surface expression of class II MHC molecules. Since T-dependent antigens are usually univalent with respect to B-cell receptors, it is not easy to see how Ig receptors can be cross-

CONSEQUENCES OF ANTIGEN RECOGNITION

linked unless this was to occur weakly through some type of linked array of native antigen on an initial antigen-presenting cell prior to B-cell processing (cf. figure 6.13c). Of course, it is also possible that Ig receptors undergo spontaneous endosome recycling and that no stimulus is received by the B-cell until a helper T-cell reacts with the processed antigen and class II MHC on its surface. The nature of the T-cell activating signal is not entirely clear but one of the T-cell products, B-cell stimulatory factor (BSF-1), must be a strong candidate since it is capable of bringing resting B-cells to the activated G_1 state described above.

Like the activated T-cell, the stimulated B-lymphocyte also acquires a number of surface receptors for growth factors derived from T-helpers and the stage is now set for the proliferation which characterizes the next phase in the immune response.

Clonal expansion is achieved by T-cell soluble factors

Thymus-independent polyclonal activators drive B-cells into division independently of Ig receptors through their innate mitogenic potential, while type-2 thymus-independent antigens presumably get the B-cells cycling through Ig receptor cross-linking together with macrophage accessory factors. Our discussion will focus on the T-dependent responses which actually have much greater flexibility in terms of antibody class, affinity, memory and probably clone size.

The first expansion occurs in the helper-T population which express surface receptors of high affinity for interleukin-2 (IL-2) and proliferate in response to IL-2 produced either by themselves or perhaps by another subpopulation (figure 6.14).

The T-cell blasts also produce an impressive array of other soluble factors (lymphokines) which can induce changes in the status of many other cell types, B-cells, cytotoxic T-cell precursors, macrophages, endothelial cells and so on. For this reason they are often referred to as *inducer* cells. However, in the present context we will restrict ourselves to the expansion of newly activated B-cells. They express surface receptors for BSF-1 which, in addition to activating G_0 B-cells, can also act as a growth factor (previously called BCGF-I (IL-4), i.e. B-cell growth factor) and the cells proliferate under the influence of the high local concentrations of BSF-1 produced by the closely adherent T-cells (figure 6.12c), and presumably to a lesser extent by other

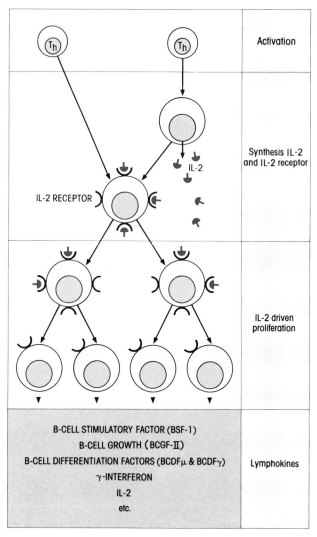

Figure 6.14. *Activated T-blasts expressing surface receptors for interleukin-2 proliferate in response to IL-2 produced by itself or by another T-cell subset. Expansion is controlled through down-regulation of the IL-2 receptor by IL-2 itself. The expanded population secretes a wide variety of biologically active lymphokines.*

T-cells in the vicinity. Further clonal expansion of B-cells is engineered by a second B-cell growth factor BCGF-II (figure 6.15). Under particular experimental conditions *in vitro*, IL-2, IFNγ and IL-1 have all been shown to have some capacity to synergize with these B-cell growth factors but the extent of their contribution under physiological conditions *in vivo* is still perhaps contentious.

Further T-cell factors bring about maturation of effector cells

After clonally expanding the activated B-blasts, differentiation factors bring about maturation to cells with effector function. The B-cell differentiation factor BCDFμ promotes the formation of plasma cells with a high rate of secretion of IgM. BCDFγ brings about class switch to IgG together with the changes required for a high rate of synthesis and secretion of antibody (figure 6.15). Obscurity still surrounds the signals which guide cells along the pathway to memory and encourage the abnormally high mutation rate in the Ig variable region genes which precedes this, but people think this ought to happen within the secondary follicle germinal centre.

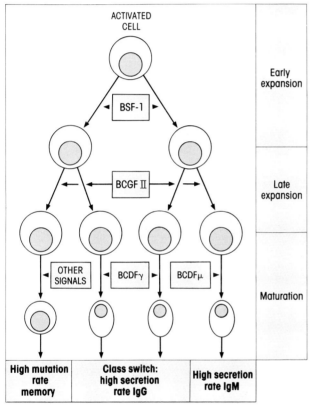

Figure 6.15. *Clonal expansion and maturation of activated B-cells under the influence of T-cell derived soluble factors. c-Myc expression, which is maximal 2 h after antigen or anti-μ stimulation, parallels sensitivity to BCGF II; transfection with c-myc substitutes for anti-μ. The origin of the signals for memory cell differentiation is unknown.*

SUMMARY

Lymphocytes mediate acquired immune responses which involve a first phase of induction or activation, a second phase of clonal proliferation and a final phase in which a proportion of the lymphocytes become effector cells and the remainder an expanded population of memory cells able to provide secondary responses.

The immune response occurs most effectively in structured secondary lymphoid tissue. The lymph nodes filter and screen lymph flowing from the body tissues while spleen filters the blood. B- and T-cell areas are separated. B-cell structures appear in the lymph node cortex as primary follicles or secondary follicles with germinal centres after antigen stimulation; T-cells occupy the paracortical area; plasma cells synthesizing antibody appear in medullary cords which penetrate the macrophage-lined medullary sinuses. Lymphoid tissue guarding the gastro-intestinal tract is unencapsulated and somewhat structured (tonsils, Peyer's patches, appendix) or present as diffuse cellular collections in the lamina propria. Together with the subepithelial accumulations of cells lining the mucosal surfaces of the respiratory and genito-urinary tracts, they form the 'secretory immune system' which bathes the surface with protective IgA antibodies. Bone marrow is a major site of antibody production. Lymphocyte recirculation between the blood and lymphoid tissues is guided by specialized homing receptors on the surface of the high-walled endothelium of the postcapillary venules.

Antigen is presented to lymphocytes by macrophages and by specialized antigen-presenting cells in T- and B-cell areas. Dendritic cells in secondary follicles bind immune complexes firmly and persistently and are linked with B-cell memory.

T- and B-cells are readily distinguished by surface markers, T3 (CD3) on T-cells and surface Ig on B-cells. T-cells also form spontaneous rosettes with sheep erythrocytes.

Activation of T-cells requires two signals, one through the T-cell T3 complex, the other interleukin-1 (IL-1) from antigen-presenting cells. Cleavage of phosphatidyl inositol diphosphate leads to mobilization of intracellular Ca^{2+}, activation of protein kinases and subsequent synthesis of RNA and protein including interleukin-2 (IL-2).

B-cells respond to three different types of antigen, thymus-independent type-1 (polyclonal activators), thymus-independent type-2 (polymeric non-degradable) and thymus-dependent which require T-helper recognition of one determinant on the antigen (carrier) to help a B-cell respond to another determinant (hapten) on the same molecule. B-cells process antigen which binds to their Ig receptors and re-express it on their surface with class II MHC. B-cells are activated either by non-specific polyclonal activation, or Ig receptor cross-linking associated with a macrophage signal, or by a signal from helper T-cells recognizing nominal antigen plus class II MHC. A strong candidate for this signal is B-cell stimulatory factor (BSF-1) known to be capable of activating resting G_0 B-cells. These events lead to phosphatidyl inositol diphosphate breakdown and comparable cascade reactions to those seen in activation of T-cells.

Activated T-cells secrete IL-2 which drives division in cells expressing IL-2 receptors. The T-cells produce a series of lymphokines: BSF-1 and then B-cell growth factor (BCGF-II) clonally expand the activated B-cells, B-cell differentiation factor μ (BCDFμ) matures the cells into high secretion rate IgM producers while BCDFγ causes class-switching and high rates of IgG secretion.

Further reading

Feldmann M., Lamb J.R. & Woody J.N. (eds) (1985) *Human T-Cell Clones.* Humana Press, Clifton, N.Jersey, USA.

Gupta S., Paul W. & Fauci A. (eds) (1987) *Mechanisms of Lymphocyte Activation and Immune Regulation.* Plenum Press, New York.

Hamaoka T. & Ono S. (1986) Regulation of B-cell differentiation. *Ann. Rev. Immunol.,* **4**, 167.

Henry K. & Farrer-Brown G. (1981) *Colour Atlas of Thymus and Lymph Node Histology with Ultrastructure.* Wolfe Medical Publications, London.

Melchers F. & Andersson J. (1986) Factors controlling the B-cell cycle. *Ann. Rev. Immunol.,* **4**, 13.

THE ACQUIRED IMMUNE RESPONSE

II – Production of Effectors

THE SYNTHESIS OF HUMORAL ANTIBODY

Detection and enumeration of antibody-forming cells

Immunofluorescence

Cells containing antibody within their cytoplasm can be identified by the 'sandwich' technique (see figure 5.20c). For example, a cell making antibodies to tetanus toxoid if treated first with the antigen will subsequently bind a fluorescein-labelled anti-tetanus antibody and can then be visualized in the fluorescence microscope.

Plaque techniques

Antibody-secreting cells can be counted by diluting them in an environment in which the antibody formed by each individual cell produces a readily observable effect. In one of the most widely used techniques, developed from the original method of Jerne and Nordin, the cells from an animal immunized with sheep erythrocytes are suspended together with an excess of sheep red cells and complement within a shallow chamber formed between two microscope sides. On incubation the antibody-forming cells release their immunoglobulin which coats the surrounding erythrocytes. The complement will then cause lysis of the coated cells and a plaque clear of red cells will be seen around each antibody-forming cell (figure 7.1). Direct plaques obtained in this way largely reveal IgM producers since this antibody has a high haemolytic efficiency. To demonstrate IgG synthesizing cells it is necessary to increase the complement binding of the erythrocyte–IgG antibody complex by adding a rabbit anti-IgG serum; this develops the 'indirect plaques' and can be used to enumerate cells making antibodies in different immunoglobulin subclasses, provided the appropriate rabbit antisera are available. The method can be extended by coating an antigen such as pneumococcus polysaccharide on to the red cell, or by coupling hapten groups to the erythrocyte surface.

In the 'Elispot' modification, the antibody-forming cell suspension is incubated on a dish of immobilized antigen. The secreted antibody is captured locally and is visualized after removal of the cells, by treatment with peroxidase-labelled anti-Ig, and development of the colour reaction by incorporating the substrate in a gel which is poured over the floor of the dish. Limited diffusion of the coloured reaction product in the gel provides a series of macroscopic spots which can be readily enumerated (figure 7.2).

Protein synthesis

In the normal antibody-forming cell there is a rapid turnover of light chains which are present in slight excess. Defective control occurs in many myeloma cells and one may see excessive production of light

	COMPLEMENT
Secreted antibody coats surrounding red cells	Coated erythrocytes are lysed by complement to form plaque with antibody-forming cell at centre

Figure 7.1. *Jerne plaque technique for enumerating antibody-forming cells (Cunningham modification). (a) The* **direct** *technique for cells synthesizing IgM haemolysin is shown. The* **indirect** *technique for visualizing cells producing IgG haemolysins requires the addition of anti-IgG to the system. The difference between the plaques obtained by direct and indirect methods gives the number of 'IgG' plaques. The* **reverse plaque** *assay enumerates total Ig producing cells by capturing secreted Ig on red cells coated with anti-Ig. Multiple plaque assays can be carried out by a modification using microtitre plates. (b) Photograph of plaques which show as circular dark areas (some of which are arrowed) under dark-ground illumination. They vary in size depending upon the antibody affinity and the rate of secretion by the antibody-forming cell. (Courtesy of Mr C. Shapland, Ms P. Hutchings & Dr D. Male.)*

chains or complete suppression of heavy chain synthesis. Interchain disulphide bridges may form while the heavy chains are still attached to the ribosomes (figure 7.3) but the sequence in which the intermediates arise varies with the nature of the immunoglobulin. Using 'pulse and chase' techniques with radioactive amino acids it was found that the build-up of both light and heavy chains proceeds continuously starting from the N-terminal end. Furthermore, isolation of the mRNA for each type of chain has shown them to be of appropriate size to allow synthesis of the complete peptides. The evidence therefore confirms the present view that the messenger regions for variable and constant regions are spliced together before leaving the nucleus.

Differential splicing mechanisms also provide a rational explanation for the co-expression of surface IgM and IgD with identical V regions on a single cell (figure 7.4), and for the switch from production of membrane-bound IgM receptor to secretory IgM in the antibody-forming cell (figure 7.5).

Class switching occurs in individual B-cells

The synthesis of antibodies belonging to the various immunoglobulin classes proceeds at different rates. Usually there is an early IgM response which tends to fall off rapidly. IgG antibody synthesis builds up to its maximum over a longer time period. On secondary challenge with antigen, the time course of the IgM response resembles that seen in the primary. By contrast, the synthesis of IgG antibodies rapidly accelerates to a much higher titre and there is a relatively slow fall-off in serum antibody levels (figure 7.6). The same probably holds for IgA and in a sense both these immunoglobulin classes provide the main *immediate* defence against future penetration by foreign antigens.

There is evidence that individual cells can switch over from IgM to IgG production. Several days after immunization with salmonella flagella, isolated cells taken into micro-drop cultures were shown to produce both IgM and IgG immobilizing antibodies. In another study it was shown that antigen challenge of irradiated recipients receiving relatively small numbers of lymphoid cells, produced splenic foci of cells, each synthesizing antibodies of different heavy chain class bearing a single idiotype; the common idiotype suggests that each focus is derived from a single precursor cell whose progeny can form antibodies of different class.

Antibody synthesis in most classes shows considerable dependence upon T-cooperation in that the responses in T-deprived animals are strikingly deficient; such is true of mouse IgG1, IgA, IgE and part of the IgM antibody responses. Immunopotentiation by complete Freund's adjuvant, a water-in-oil emulsion containing antigen in the aqueous phase and a suspension of killed tubercle bacilli in the oily phase (p. 181), seems to occur, at least in part, through the activation of helper T-cells which stimulate antibody production in T-dependent classes. The prediction from this that the response to T-independent antigens (e.g. pneumococcus polysaccharide, p. 95) should not be potentiated by Freund's adjuvant is borne out in practice; furthermore, as mentioned previously, these antigens evoke primarily IgM antibodies and poorly defined immunological memory as do T-dependent antigens injected into T-cell deficient neonatally thymectomized hosts.

Thus, in rodents at least, the switch from IgM to IgG and other classes appears to be largely under T-cell control presumably mediated by soluble factors such as B-cell differentiation factor γ (p. 99). These bring about the transfer of a given *VDJ* gene segment from $\mu\delta$ to an alternative constant region gene by utilizing specialized switch region sequences (figure 7.7), so yielding antibodies of the same specificity but of different class.

Figure 7.2. *'Elispot' (from ELISA technique) system for enumerating antibody-forming cells. The picture shows spots formed by hybridoma cells making autoantibodies to thyroglobulin revealed by alkaline phosphatase-linked anti-Ig (courtesy of P. Hutchings). Increasing numbers of hybridoma cells were added to the top two and bottom left-hand wells which show corresponding increases in the number of 'Elispots'. The bottom right-hand well is a control using a hybridoma of irrelevant specificity.*

Is the specificity of antibody secreted by the progeny the same as that of the surface immunoglobulin of the clonal parent?

The answer is, often yes, often partially and sometimes no. You may think that a trifle cryptic so let's

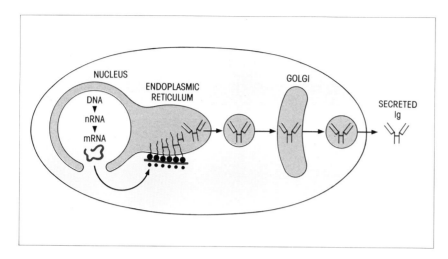

Figure 7.3. *Synthesis of mouse IgG2a immunoglobulin. As the H-chains near completion, adjacent peptide chains can spontaneously cross-link through their constant regions. It is thought that the light chains may aid release of the terminal chains from the ribosome by forming the L−H−H molecule. Combination with a further light chain would yield the full immunoglobulin L−H−H−L (based on Askonas B.A. & Williamson A.R. (1986) Biochem. J. 109, 637). The order in which the interchain disulphide bridges are formed varies in different immunoglobulins depending on the relative strengths of the bonds as assessed by susceptibility to reduction. Surface receptor Ig would be inserted by its hydrophobic sequences into the membrane of the endoplasmic reticulum as it was synthesized.*

104

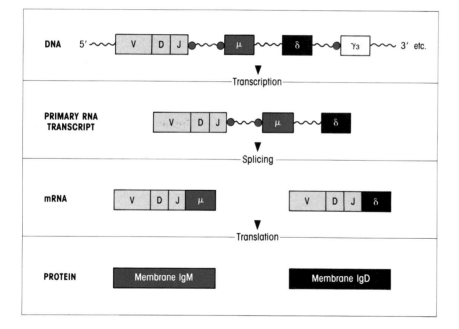

Figure 7.4. *Surface membrane IgM and IgD receptors of identical specificity appear on the same cell through differential splicing of the composite primary RNA transcript. For simplicity the leader sequence has been omitted.* ∿∿∿ = *introns.*

recapitulate. The clonal selection hypothesis predicts an affirmative answer to our question because it postulates that each lymphocyte is programmed to make only one antibody, that it puts the antibody as a receptor on its surface so that antigen will bind to it, and that as a result the cell is selectively triggered for antibody formation; as it only knows how to make one antibody, the specificity should be identical with the original surface receptor.

The one-cell one-antibody idea does seem O.K.

With immunofluorescent techniques, individual immunoglobulin cells can be stained for either κ or λ chains but not both, and in the heterozygous rabbit, for the maternal allotypic marker or the paternal but never both together (*allelic exclusion*). Furthermore, plasma cell tumours only produce one, and not more than one, myeloma protein. Similar restrictions apply to the staining of surface Ig on B-lymphocytes.

That these surface immunoglobulins can behave as antibodies is suggested by the ability of a small percentage of lymphocytes to bind specific antigens such as sheep cells (forming 'rosettes') or radioactive salmonella flagellin. This binding can be blocked by anti-immunoglobulin sera. Humphrey has further shown that the percentage of cells binding

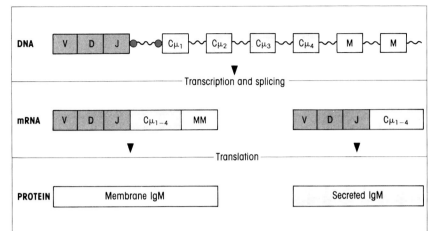

Figure 7.5. *Splicing mechanism for the switch from the membrane to the secreted form of IgM. The hydrophobic sequence encoded by the exons M−M which anchors the receptor IgM to the membrane is spliced out in the secreted form (leader sequences again omitted for simplicity).*

Figure 7.6. *Synthesis of IgM and IgG antibody classes in the primary and secondary responses to antigen.*

antigen is increased in primed and decreased in tolerant animals.

When a soluble antigen like polymerized flagellin binds to a specific cell it causes patching and capping of the surface Ig in just the same way as an anti-Ig serum (cf. p. 19). If the antigen-capped cells are now stained with fluorescent anti-Ig, all the Ig is found in the cap, there being none on the remainder of the lymphocyte surface, i.e. when antigen reacts with a cell, all the Ig molecules on the cell surface combine with the antigen showing that they have similar specificity. Exactly the same result is seen if an anti-idiotype is used for capping, i.e. all the surface Ig molecules on a given cell have the same idiotype. So far so good.

Figure 7.7. *Class-switching to produce antibodies of identical specificity but different immunoglobulin isotype (in this example from IgM to IgG₁) is achieved by a 'looping out' process which utilizes the specialized switch sequences (●) and leads to a loss of the intervening DNA (μ, δ and γ3). Rare examples of mutant clones expressing an isotypic gene 5' of the parent heavy chain gene suggest that switching to constant region genes on the sister chromatid may sometimes occur.*

PRODUCTION OF EFFECTORS

The surface antibody does appear to be related to the specificity of the secreted immunoglobulin

If the production of a given antibody depends upon its representation as a surface Ig in the pool of antigen-sensitive B-cells, then positive or negative selection for cells of that specificity prior to antigen challenge should have profound effects on subsequent reactivity. Indeed that is just what happens. Depletion of antigen-specific cells by reaction with their surface receptors abrogates the further ability of that population to respond to antigen (figure 7.8). Likewise, a high percentage of cells isolated by virtue of their specific binding to a hapten like DNP, secrete anti-DNP when stimulated under kindly conditions *in vitro*. If more is wanted, then it can be shown rather cleverly that surface and cytoplasmic Ig in secreting cells share a common idiotype. First stain the surface Ig of the living cells at 4°C with fluorescein-labelled anti-idiotype and then fix with glutaraldehyde and stain the cytoplasm of

the cytocentrifuged cells with anti-idiotype conjugated with rhodamine. Double staining proves the point. Well now, why could the initial question not be answered unequivocally in the affirmative? The answer lies in somatic mutation.

Class-switched B-cells are subject to high mutation rates after the initial response

The reader will no doubt recollect that this point was made in Chapter 3 when discussing the generation of diversity, but in the present context it is important to note that such mutations occurring in the hypervariable regions before or during the generation of memory cells can give rise to antibodies with a different combining affinity to that of the parent cell. Randomly, some mutated daughter cells will have higher affinity for antigen, some the same or lower and others perhaps none at all. Similarly, mutations in the framework regions may be 'silent' or, if they perturb the ability of the molecule to fold properly, give rise to non-functional molecules.

Antibody affinity

The effect of antigen dose

Other things being equal, the binding strength of an antigen for the surface antibody receptor of a B-cell will be determined by the usual affinity constant of the reaction:

$$Ag + (surface)Ab \rightleftharpoons AgAb$$

and the reactants will behave according to the Law of Mass Action (cf. p. 61).

It may be supposed that when an appropriate number of antigen molecules are bound to the antibody receptors on the cell surface, the lymphocyte will be stimulated to develop into an antibody-producing clone. When only small amounts of antigen are present, only those lymphocytes with high-affinity antibody receptors will be able to bind sufficient antigen for stimulation to occur and their daughter cells will, of course, also produce high-affinity antibody. Consideration of the antigen–antibody equilibrium equation will show that, as the concentration of antigen is increased, even antibodies with relatively low affinity will bind more antigen; therefore at high doses of antigen the lymphocytes with lower-affinity antibody receptors will also be stimulated and, as may be seen from

Figure 7.8. *Depletion of cells with surface receptors for antigen removes subsequent ability to respond to that antigen. (a) Primed cells (blue) depleted by reaction between surface Ig on the lymphocytes and insolubilized antigen packing the column. Further control, ovalbumin-coated beads. (b) Primed cells (blue) destroyed by radiation 'suicide' through binding highly radioactive antigen to surface Ig. Further control, unlabelled antigen (TGAL). BSA = bovine serum albumin; Ova = ovalbumin; TGAL = poly-lysine with poly-alanine side chains randomly tipped with tyrosine and glutamine.*

figure 7.9, these are more abundant than those with receptors of high affinity. Furthermore, there is a strong possibility that cells with the highest affinity will bind so much antigen, as to become tolerized (cf. p. 131). Thus, in summary, low amounts of antigen produce high-affinity antibodies, whereas high antigen concentrations give rise to an antiserum with low to moderate affinity.

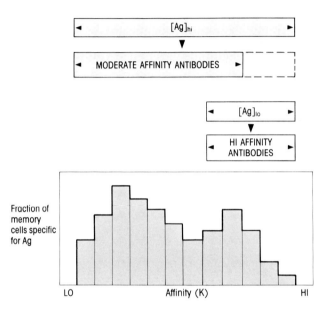

Figure 7.9. *Relationship of antigen concentration to affinity of antibodies produced. Low concentrations of antigen ($[Ag]_{lo}$) bind to and stimulate a range of high affinity memory cells and the resulting antibodies are of high affinity. High doses of antigen ($[Ag]_{hi}$) are able to bind sufficiently to the low affinity cells and to stimulate them, whilst the highest affinity cells may bind an excess of antigen and be tolerized; the resulting antiserum will have a population of low to moderate affinity antibodies.*

Maturation of affinity

In addition to being brisker and fatter, secondary responses tend to be of higher affinity, which from our point of view is a particularly felicitous state of affairs. There are probably two main reasons for this maturation of affinity after primary stimulation. First, once the primary response gets under way and the antigen concentration declines to low levels, only successively higher affinity cells will bind sufficient antigen to maintain proliferation. Second, at this stage the cells are mutating madly and any mutants with an adventitiously higher affinity will bind antigen well and be positively selected for by its persistent clonal expansion.

It is worth noting that responses to thymus-independent antigens which have poorly developed memory with very rare mutations do not show this phenomenon of affinity maturation. Overall, the ability of T-cell helpers to facilitate responses to non-polymeric, non-polyclonally activating antigens, to induce expansive clonal proliferation, to effect class switching and, lastly, to fine-tune responses to higher affinity has provided us with bigger, better and more flexible immune responses.

The monoclonal antibody revolution

A fantastic technological breakthrough has been achieved by Milstein and Köhler who devised a technique for the production of 'immortal' clones of cells making single antibody specificities by fusing normal antibody-forming cells with an appropriate B-cell tumour line. These so-called 'hybridomas' are selected out in a tissue culture medium which fails to support growth of the parental cell types, and by successive dilutions or by plating out, single clones can be established (figure 7.10). These clones can be propagated in spinner culture or grown up in the ascitic form in mice when quite prodigious titres of monoclonal antibody can be attained. Remember that even in a good antiserum, over 90% of the Ig molecules have little or no avidity for the antigen, and the 'specific antibodies' themselves represent a whole spectrum of molecules with different avidities directed against different determinants on the antigen. What a contrast is provided by the monoclonal antibodies where all the molecules produced by a given hybridoma are identical (figure 4.9): they have the same Ig class and allotype, the same variable region, structure, idiotype, affinity and specificity for a given epitope.

Whereas the large amount of non-specific, relative to antigen-specific, Ig in an antiserum means that background binding to antigen in any given immunological test may be uncomfortably high, the problem is greatly reduced with a monoclonal antibody preparation since all the Ig is antibody, thus giving a much superior 'signal : noise' ratio. By being directed towards single epitopes on the antigen, monoclonal antibodies frequently show high specificity in terms of their low cross-reactivity with other antigens. Occasionally, however, one sees quite unexpected binding to molecules which react poorly, if at all, with a specific antiserum directed to the original antigen. The reason for this has already been discussed (p. 63). Suffice it to say here that the problem can be circumvented by using a group

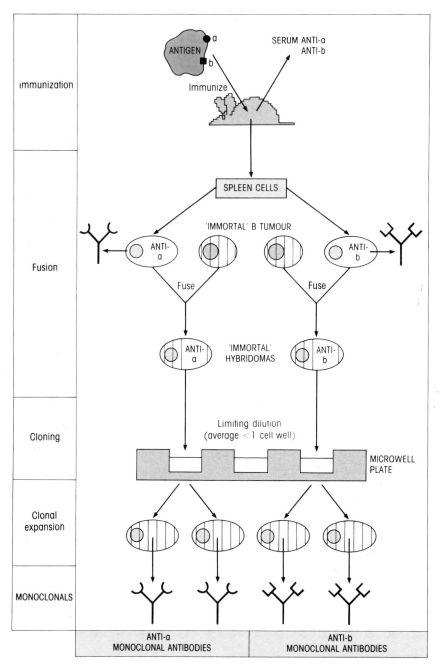

Figure 7.10. *Production of monoclonal antibodies. Mice immunized with an antigen bearing (shall we say) two epitopes, **a** and **b**, develop spleen cells making anti-**a** and anti-**b** which appear as antibodies in the serum. The spleen is removed and the individual cells fused in polyethylene glycol with constantly dividing (i.e. 'immortal') B-tumour cells selected for a purine enzyme deficiency and often for their inability to secrete Ig. The resulting cells are distributed into micro-well plates in HAT (hypoxanthine, aminopterin, thymidine) medium which kills off the perfusion partners, at such a high dilution that **on average** each well will contain less than one hybridoma cell. Each hybridoma being the fusion product of a single antibody-forming cell and a tumour cell will have the ability of the former to secrete a single species of antibody and the immortality of the latter enabling it to proliferate continuously, clonal progeny providing an unending supply of antibody with a single specificity—the monoclonal antibody. In this example, we considered the production of hybridomas with specificity for just two epitopes, but the same technique enables monoclonal antibodies to be raised against complex mixtures of multiepitopic antigens. Fusions using rat cells instead of mouse may have certain advantages in giving a higher proportion of stable hybridomas, and monoclonals which are better at fixing human complement, a useful attribute in the context of therapeutic application to humans involving cell depletion.*

of overlapping monoclonals reacting with the same determinant or a combination of monoclonals to more than one determinant on the same antigen.

A tremendous advantage of the monoclonal antibody as a reagent is that it provides a single standard material for all laboratories throughout the world to use in an unending supply if the immortality and purity of the cell line is nurtured; antisera raised in different animals, on the other hand, may be as different from each other as chalk and cheese. The monoclonal approach again shows a clean pair of heels relative to conventional strategies in the production of antibodies specific for individual components in a complex mixture of antigens, which, for example, one may wish to do in trying to identify which of a set of antigens on a given parasite can generate antibodies which are protective for the host. Whereas in the prehybridoma era we would have tried to purify individual antigens from the complex mixture and then raised antibodies to each component, now we would make a large number of hybridomas from the spleen of an animal immunized with the complete antigen mixture and separate the individual hybridomas by simple cloning. It must be clear that we now have in our hands a really powerful technique whose applications are truly legion. Some of these are touched upon in table 7.1 to give the reader an inkling of what is possible but the potential defies the imagination; the separation of individual cell types with specific surface markers (lymphocyte subpopulations, neural cells, etc.), diagnosis of lymphoid and myeloid malignancies, tissue typing, radioimmunoassay, serotyping of micro-organisms, elucidation of the fine structure of the antibody combining site and the basis for variability, immunological intervention with passive antibody, anti-idiotype inhibition or 'magic bullet' therapy with cytotoxic agents coupled to antitumour-specific antibody—these and many other areas will all be transformed by hybridoma technology.

Hybridomas producing human antibodies would be particularly valuable for therapeutic purposes. It is possible to fuse human antibody-forming cells with mouse tumour lines but the mixed hybrids tend to be unstable and shed chromosomes. Progress in finding an effective human tumour line as a partner is still not altogether satisfactory. One of the commonly used cell lines tends to fuse only with a highly selected population of B-cells which make IgMκ immunoglobulin. An alternative is to transform antigen-enriched lymphocytes to cell lines by polyclonal stimulation with EB virus and then to

Table 7.1. *Some applications of monoclonal antibodies.*

ENUMERATION OF HUMAN LYMPHOCYTE SUBPOPULATIONS	Anti-T3 identifies all mature T-cells Anti-T4 identifies subset containing T-helpers Anti-T8 identifies cytotoxic/suppressor T-cells
CELL DEPLETION	Cocktail of anti-T3 monoclonals + complement kills T-cells in human bone marrow to prevent graft vs host reaction (p. 228)
CELL ISOLATION	Separation of murine Lyt1 + ve T-cells by monclonal anti-Lyt1 in the FACS (p. 81)
PROBING FUNCTION OF CELL SURFACE MOLECULES	Anti-T8 inhibits killing by cytotoxic T-cells Anti-Ia monoclonal inhibits T-cell response to macrophage-processed Ag
BLOOD GROUPING	Anti-A monoclonal provides more reliable standard reagent than conventional antisera
DIAGNOSIS IN CANCER	Monoclonal anti-T-ALL allows differentation from non-T-ALL (cf. p.144) Follicle centre cell lymphoma identified by peroxidase-labelled anti-common ALL in tissue sections
IMAGING	Radioactive anti-carcinoembryonic antigen (p. 232) used to localize colonic tumours or secondaries by scanning
IMMUNORADIOMETRIC ASSAY	Good discrimination for assay of antigen by monoclonals to more than one site
ANALYSIS OF COMPLEX ANTIGEN MIXTURES	Identification of the 'protective' antigen in parasite suitable for vaccine production Identification of antigenic 'patch' on acetyl choline receptor involved in experimental myasthenia gravis (p. 268)
ANALYSIS OF EMBRYOLOGICAL RELATIONSHIPS	Separate monoclonals to neurons of neural tube and neural crest origin help to define embryological derivation of cells in nervous system Monoclonals to Ag on chick prosencephalon reveal a concentration gradient on the dorso-ventral axis of the retina, ? positional information for forming specific synapses
MONOCLONAL MUTANTS	Mutants lacking Fc structures used for *in vivo* neutralization of toxic drugs e.g. digoxin overdose, or for defining biological roles of Fc domains
FUSED HYBRIDOMAS	Producing antibodies with dual specificity
ANALYSIS OF IMMUNE RESPONSE	Gives data on repertoire and on mutation events (the original reason for developing the hybridoma technology)
ARTIFICIAL ENZYMES	Monoclonal antibodies which recognize the transitional state of the reactants in a reversible reaction can theoretically simulate an enzyme — early days but big potential

clone or fuse with a plasmacytoma line, but again the responding population tends to be a restricted subset. Perhaps there are wider possibilities for immortalization of B-cells by transfection with SV40 DNA containing the T-antigen oncogene which has

PRODUCTION OF EFFECTORS

so far been used successively with rabbit B-cells. Also, we must not forget that mouse monoclonals can be made more human by recombinant DNA manipulations.

CELL-MEDIATED IMMUNITY HAS TWO ARMS

In combating intracellular infections by acquired immune responses, two different types of effector T-cells are generated: T-helpers and cytolytic T-cells. Their functions are summarized in figure 7.11.

T-helper cells produce soluble mediators (lymphokines)

Activation

Primed T-helpers are stimulated through recognition of surface-bound nominal antigen plus MHC class II by the T-cell receptor T3 complex and, as we have discussed fairly extensively, this leads to proliferation and the secretion of a battery of lymphokines.

This process is often monitored by measuring the proliferative response of the cells to antigen *in vitro* and in the case of human peripheral blood lymphocytes, this will be almost entirely attributable to T-cells. The alternative is to assay lymphokine release and the favourite used to be migration inhibition factor (MIF). The system, which the more historically minded can read about in greater detail in earlier editions, involved packing a mixture of lymphocytes and macrophages into capillary tubes which were then incubated overnight with antigen in dishes; the cells would migrate out of the capillaries to form a fan of cells on the floor of the dish and any reduction in the area of migration was attributable to MIF. A simpler and more reliable assay is to follow IL-2 production using the IL-2-dependent proliferation of selected T-cell lines, but inevitably these biological tests will be overtaken by the radioimmunoassays for IFNγ, and presumably for IL-2

110

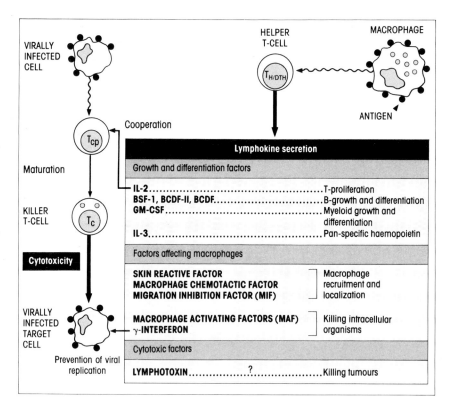

Figure 7.11. *The cell-mediated immune response. This operates through the generation of cytotoxic T-cells and the release of lymphokines through the stimulation of two distinct T-subpopulations, the cytotoxic cell precursor (T_{cp}) and the T-helper/inducer/delayed type hypersensitivity cells ($T_{h/dth}$). Different lymphokines may be produced by different lymphocyte subsets, and at this time it is not possible to say whether cells mediating delayed-type hypersensitivity (the skin manifestation of a cell-mediated immune response) represent a distinct subpopulation from the helpers. The intense proliferation induced by antigenic stimulation has not been shown but is essential for amplification of the response. Other lymphokines which activate osteoclasts and fibroblasts have been described.*

CHAPTER 7

now that recombinant products and monoclonal antibodies are available.

The helper T-cells belong to the subset bearing the T4 (CD4) marker in the human, and L3T4 in the mouse, and since anti-T4 blocks activation, T4 must play some part in the process. Although not formally demonstrated, it seems likely that T4 interacts in some way with class II molecules on the stimulator cell. In support is the observation that the cytotoxic cells used to type DP specificities (one of the human class II D-region molecules) are T4 positive. The T4 could act in a 'docking' or accessory binding capacity to augment low-affinity interactions, but the ability of anti-T4 to inhibit the activation of T-helpers by Sepharose-linked anti-T3 rather implies that the T4 molecule is involved in some regulatory signalling process. LFA-1 (leucocyte function accessory-1 molecule) also figures in the equation somewhere since anti-LFA-1 is inhibitory and it may assist the cellular interactions by some subsidiary binding or orienting mechanism which is at present obscure (figure 7.12).

Do different T-cell subsets make different lymphokines?

There is not a broad concensus on the answer but a report at the 1986 International Immunology Congress (the latest information available at the time of writing) maintained that, given sound bioassay techniques, T-helper clones could be divided into two types: T_{H1} make IL-2 and IFNγ but not BSF-1,

while T_{H2} secreted BSF-1 but not IL-2 or IFNγ. Both made IL-3 and GM-CSF (cf. figure 7.11). T_{H1}, but not T_{H2}, are alleged to mediate delayed-type hypersensitivity, the term given to the skin reaction obtained on antigen challenge of individuals with specific T-cell-mediated immunity (cf. Chapter 12). In passing, it should also be noted that not all T4-positive cells are T-helpers, but more of that in the following chapter. We should now discuss the most prominent lymphokines in more detail.

Growth and differentiation factors

B-cell promoting factors were considered previously. *Interleukin-2* is utterly pivotal for the amplification of activated T-cell subsets. It is a single peptide of molecular weight 15.5 kD which acts only on cells which express high-affinity IL-2 receptors. These receptors are not present on resting cells, but 9 hours after polyclonal activation the genes for IL-2 receptor begin to be transcribed, and only after a further 15 hours are the IL-2 genes themselves expressed (figure 7.13). With the availability of pure IL-2 it was possible to show that activated T-cells expressed $2-4 \times 10^3$ IL-2 receptors of exceedingly high affinity per cell but, in addition, a further $30-60 \times 10^3$ low-affinity IL-2 receptors, although both types reacted with the *Tac* monoclonal antibody. Separation of an activated T-cell population into those with high- and low-affinity receptors showed clearly that an adequate number of high-affinity receptors were mandatory for the mitogenic

111

Figure 7.12. *Scandalously crude representation of the molecules involved in the interactions between T-helpers and T-killers with their antigen-specific target cell. T_R = T-cell antigen-specific receptor; I and II refer to MHC class; 'LFA-1' and 'LFA-2' are given apostrophes to indicate that we are not sure of the identity of the human equivalents of the murine molecules bearing those labels. Murine equivalents of T4 and T8 are L3T4 and Ly2 respectively.*

Figure 7.13. *Sequential transcription of genes for the c-myc proto-oncogene, IL-2 receptor (IL-2ᵣ), γ-interferon (IFNγ) and IL-2 following polyclonal activation of resting human T-cells. The transcriptions are unaffected by the presence of cycloheximide showing that they are independent of protein synthesis and therefore that the c-myc protein itself, for example, is not involved.*

action of IL-2. It is the skewed cellular distribution of these high-affinity receptors which is responsible for the asynchronous division of activated T-cells on addition of IL-2. The numbers of these receptors on the cell increase under the action of antigen and of IL-2, and as antigen is cleared, so the receptor numbers decline and, with that, the responsiveness to IL-2. It should be appreciated that although IL-2 is an immunologically non-specific T-cell growth factor, it only functions appropriately in specific responses because unstimulated T-cells do not express IL-2 receptors.

Two of the lymphokines influence haemopoietic cells. Whereas *GM-CSF* is restricted in its action to promoting the growth of mixed neutrophil and macrophage colonies from bone marrow stem cells in agar cultures, *IL-3* acts as a panspecific haemopoietin which promotes the formation of colonies of erythroid cells, megakaryocytes and mast cells in addition. Furthermore, IL-3 can persuade even mature cells like macrophages and mast cells to divide. *In vivo* it acts locally and in the gut, for example, T-cell responses induce a proliferation of IL-3-dependent mast cells in the vicinity. The physiological role of IL-3 may well be to recruit many of the bone-marrow-derived accessory cells required for an effective immune response at a given site.

Although identified originally through its antiviral effects, γ-interferon has proved to be a pleiotrophic lymphokine with multiple effects on the growth and differentiation of a wide variety of cell types. For example, it can induce the differentiation of myeloid cells from bone marrow and from chronic myelogenous leukaemia which then express the surface Fcγ receptors, enzymes and functional abilities of more mature monocytes. A distinctive property of great significance is the induction of class II

MHC expression on endothelial cells and a wide variety of epithelial cells and tumour cell lines; it also enhances expression of class I genes. These are changes aimed at facilitating interaction between immune T-lymphocytes and non-lymphoid cells as in viral infections for example. The further roles of this versatile lymphokine in activating macrophages and inhibiting tumour growth will be discussed below.

Macrophage-related lymphokines

Since T-cells and macrophages have an important working partnership in the fight against intracellular infections, it is not surprising to learn that major T-cell soluble factors are dedicated to establishing a link with the mononuclear phagocytes. The *skin reactive factor* which induces an erythematous reaction when injected intradermally could play a role in the production of local changes which facilitate recruitment of monocytes from the circulation. Circulating and tissue mononuclear phagocytes are attracted to the site of T-cell activation by a *macrophage chemotactic factor* and held there by the *migration inhibition factor* (*MIF*) (see above) which binds to fucose-containing glycolipids on the macrophage surface. The accumulated macrophages are now subjected to *macrophage activating factor* (*MAF*) which switches on their formidable microbicidal armamentarium and makes them inhospitably lethal for any organisms which are ingested. Although there may be more than one MAF, it has been established unequivocally that IFNγ itself is a potent activator and the recombinant molecule can mimic MAF preparations faithfully. It is interesting to note also that IFNγ can affect the growth of intracellular parasites in cells other than macrophages; for example, it inhibits the growth of *Rickettsia prowazekii* in mouse fibroblast cultures.

The cytotoxic lymphokine

Lymphotoxin, a product of both T4 and T8 families, kills or is cytostatic for fibroblasts and a number of cell lines *in vitro*, but transformed cells are even more sensitive. Recent work with cloned products reveals a synergism between IFNγ and lymphotoxin (figure 7.14) in which IFNγ sets up the cell for destruction by inducing the formation of lymphotoxin receptors. The ability of lymphotoxin-producing cells to kill both themselves and other T-cells hints at a possible role in immunoregulation.

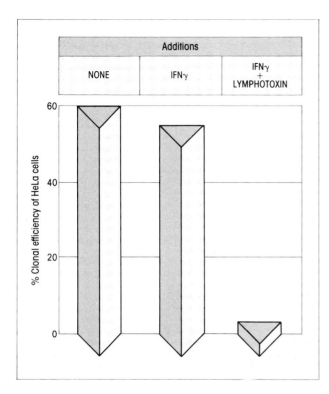

	Additions	
NONE	IFN-γ	IFN-γ + LYMPHOTOXIN

Figure 7.14. *Synergism of γ-interferon (IFNγ) and lymphotoxin in the growth inhibition of the HeLa tumour cell line (data from Stone-Wolff D.S. et al. (1984)* **J. Exp. Med.** *159, 828).*

Killer T-cells

Cytolytic T-cells represent the other major arm of the cell-mediated immune response and are generally thought to be of strategic importance in the killing of virally infected cells and possibly in contributing to the postulated surveillance mechanisms against cancer cells.

The cytotoxic cell precursor cells recognize antigen on the surface of cells in association with class I MHC, and like B-cells they require help from T-cells which somehow must see the antigen in association with class II MHC. The helper cells provide IL-2 for clonal expansion of the precursor cells and some as yet ill-defined differentiation factors which bring about maturation to a cytolytic effector. The frequency of the precursor cells can be measured by *limiting dilution techniques* and one such study is shown in detail in figure 7.15 because this approach is widely used to determine precursor frequency in different systems. In essence, the method depends upon the fact that if one takes several replicate aliquots of a given cell suspension which would be expected to contain *on average* one precursor per

aliquot, then Poisson distribution analysis shows that 37% of the aliquots will contain *no* precursor cells (through the randomness of the sampling). Thus, if aliquots are made from a series of dilutions of a cell suspension and incubated under conditions which allow the precursors to mature and be recognized through some amplification scheme, the dilution at which 37% of the aliquots give negative responses will be known to contain an average of one precursor cell per aliquot and one can therefore calculate the precursor frequency in the original cell suspension.

The lethal process

Cytolytic T-cells which are generally of the T8 or Ly2 subset bind to the target cell intimately through T-receptor recognition of antigen plus class I MHC, the interaction being assisted by some association between T8 and class I and by less well-defined accessory molecules such as LFA-1 and LFA-2 (figure 7.12). MHC recognition is important for this binding but it does not seem to be involved in the signals leading to cell death, since B-cell hybridomas making anti-T3 or antibodies to the T-receptor idiotype are killed by cytolytic T-cells independently of their MHC haplotype; what does appear to be vital is an intimate signalling to the T-receptor or the T3 transducer.

Following activation of the killer cell, most of the cytoplasmic granules rapidly become localized between the nucleus and the target cell. As we have argued earlier (cf. p. 13), there is evidence for exocytosis of the granule contents which are thought to cause lesions in the target cell membrane and death by colloid osmotic lysis, although not all would agree that this is the whole story.

SUMMARY

Antibody-forming cells can be detected by immunofluorescent and plaque techniques. Ig peptide chains are synthesized as a single unit starting at the N-terminal end. The switch from membrane-bound to secreted IgM involves loss by RNA-splicing of the hydrophobic membrane 'anchor'.

IgM antibody responses reach an early peak and decline; IgG levels are quantitatively much higher and more persistent and dominate the secondary response. Generally speaking, T-dependent antigens through the action of T-helper cells and their

113

Figure 7.15. *Limiting dilution analysis of cytotoxic T-cell precursor frequency in spleen cells from a BALB/c mouse stimulated with irradiated C57BL/6 spleen cells as antigen. BALB/c splenic responder cells were set up in 24 replicates at each concentration tested together with antigen and excess of T-helper factors. The generation of cytotoxicity in each well is looked for by adding ⁵¹Cr-labelled tumour cells (EL-4) of the C57BL/6 haplotype; cytotoxicity is then revealed by measuring the release of soluble ⁵¹Cr-labelled intracellular material into the medium. (From Simpson E. & Chandler P. In* **Handbook of Experimental Immunology,** *Weir D.M. (ed.) (1986), figure 68.2. Blackwell Scientific Publications, Oxford, with permission.)*

(a) The points show the percentage of specific lysis of individual wells. The dotted line indicates 3 standard deviations above the medium release control, and each point above that line is counted as positive for cytotoxicity.

(b) The data replotted in terms of the percentage of negative wells at each concentration of responder cells over the range in which the data titrated (5 × 10³/well to 0.625 × 10³/well). The dotted line is drawn at 37% negative wells and this intersects the regression line to give a precursor (Tₖₚ) frequency of 1 in 2327 responder cells. The regression line has an r² value of 1.00 in this experiment.

114

soluble factors, give bigger antibody responses than T-independent antigens, and furthermore, involve isotype class-switching and the generation of memory.

The evidence that one cell is programmed to make one antibody and that this provides the receptor for selection by antigen, is sound. However, the final specificity of the progeny may differ somewhat from that of the parent due to the fact that class-switched B-cells undergo surprisingly high mutation rates as they mature into memory cells. Selection of high-affinity cells arising by mutation leads to higher affinity antibody responses. Low doses of antigen provoke higher affinity antibody responses than high doses.

Immortal hybridoma cell lines making monoclonal antibodies provide powerful new immunological reagents and insights into the immune response.

The T-cell-mediated immune response has two arms, T-helpers which make a range of soluble effector molecules (lymphokines) and cytotoxic T-cells which are themselves responsible for direct killing, usually of virally-infected cells.

T-helpers belong to the T4 subset in the human, L3T4 in the mouse, and their activation may be followed by proliferation or selected lymphokine release. Several lymphokines affect growth and differentiation of other cells. BSF-1, BCGF-II and BCDF guide the B-cell response. Interleukin-2 (IL-2) is pivotal for T-cell expansion and acts on high-affinity surface receptors. Although IL-2 is a non-specific T-cell growth factor, it promotes specific immune responses because resting T-cells lack the IL-2 receptor. GM-CSF promotes growth of myeloid colonies from bone marrow stem cells in agar, but IL-3 is a panspecific haemopoietin which acts on all haemopoietic precursors and even on mature cells. γ-Interferon has a multiplicity of effects; it induces the differentiation of myeloid cells and promotes expression of class II MHC molecules on endothelial cells, a variety of epithelial cells and many tumour cell lines so facilitating interactions between T-lymphocytes and non-lymphoid cells.

γ-Interferon also plays a role as a major macrophage activating factor stimulating a full range of microbicidal mechanisms which enable the phagocytes to kill intracellular organisms. Other lymphokines, skin-reactive factor, macrophage chemotactic factor and migration inhibition factor all act to localize mononuclear phagocytes at the antigen site for activation.

γ-Interferon also acts synergistically with the cellular poison, lymphotoxin by inducing the expression of lymphotoxin receptors in the target cell.

Cytotoxic lymphocytes develop from precursors which are activated by antigen plus MHC class I and are expanded and mature by the action of IL-2 and ill-defined maturation factors produced by helper T-cells. The precursor frequency can be estimated by the method of limiting dilution analysis.

Cytolytic T-cells which belong to the T8 (or Ly2) subsets, bind to their targets through recognition of antigen + class I by the T-cell receptor; interaction with class I is facilitated by T8. A rapid rearrangement of cytoplasmic granules with cytotoxic potential occurs and exocytosis releases the contents onto the membrane of the target cell. Lesions are produced and the twilight and demise of the cell ensues.

Further reading

Goding J.W. (1986) *Monoclonal Antibodies: Principles and Practice*. Academic Press, London.
Lennox E.S. (ed.) (1984) Clinical applications of monoclonal antibodies. *Brit. Med. Bull.* Churchill Livingstone, UK.
Pick E. (ed.) Series *Lymphokines*. Academic Press, New York.

115

THE ACQUIRED IMMUNE RESPONSE

III – Control

Antigen is a major factor in control

The acquired immune response evolved so that it would come into play when contact with an infectious agent was first made. The appropriate antigen-specific cells expand, the effectors eliminate the antigen and then the response quietens down and leaves room for reaction to other infections. Feedback mechanisms must operate to limit antibody production; otherwise, after antigenic stimulation, we would become overwhelmed by the responding clones of antibody-forming cells and their products, a clearly unwelcome state of affairs as may be clearly seen in multiple myeloma where control over lymphocyte proliferation is lost. It makes sense for antigen to be a major regulatory factor and for antibody production to be driven by the presence of antigen, falling off in intensity as the antigen concentration drops. There is abundant evidence to support this view. Antigens can stimulate lymphocytes through their surface receptors directly as witnessed by proliferation of T-cell clones presented with antigen *in vitro* and formation of a clone of antibody-forming cells from a single B-cell precursor cultured with antigen and T-cell soluble factors under limiting-dilution conditions. Furthermore, clearance of antigen by injection of excess antibody during the course of an immune response leads to a dramatic drop in antibody synthesis and the number of antibody-secreting cells.

Antibody exerts feedback control

A useful control mechanism is to arrange for the product of a reaction to be an inhibitor and this type of negative feedback is seen with antibody. Thus we see examples of antibody diverting antigen to immunogenically inoffensive sites in the body to prevent primary sensitization in the protection against rhesus immunization afforded by administration of anti-D to mothers at risk (p. 202) and the inhibitory effect of maternal antibody on the peak titres obtained on vaccinating infants. Removal of circulating antibody by plasmapheresis during an on-going response leads to an increase in synthesis, whereas injection of preformed IgG antibody markedly hastens the fall in the number of antibody-forming cells (figure 8.1) consistent with feedback control on overall synthesis. It is unlikely that this is achieved by simple neutralization of antigen since whole IgG is so much more effective than its $F(ab')_2$ fragment in switching off the reaction; there is some evidence that cross-linking the antigen and Fc receptors on the B-cell through surface-bound antigen enables the IgG to block the productive phase of the T-dependent B-cell response.

By contrast, injection of IgM antibodies enhances the response (figure 8.1), but since antibodies of this isotype appear at an early stage after antigen challenge, they would be useful in boosting the initial response.

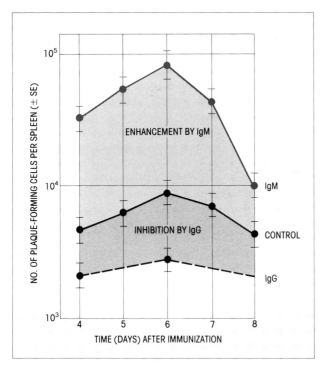

Figure 8.1. *Time course of enhancement of antibody response to sheep red cells (SRBC) due to injection of preformed IgM, and of suppression by preformed IgG antibodies. Mice received medium containing monoclonal IgM anti-SRBC, IgG anti-SRBC or medium alone i.v. 2 hours prior to immunization with 10^5 SRBC. (Data provided by J. Reiter, P. Hutchings, P. Lydyard and A. Cooke.)*

T-cell regulation

T-helper cells

We have deliberated at length on the role of T-helper cells in the facilitation of cytotoxic T-cell and B-cell responses, and in the production of class-switching and memory responses. We should perhaps note that the T-helpers do not expand B-cell

and Tc-cell clone sizes indefinitely since the maturation factors inhibit the action of the proliferative lymphokines.

Different T-cells have surface receptors for the Fc regions of the various Ig classes and a role for these in isotype-specific help has been sought. Thus T-cell lines from Peyer's patches produced many more IgA-producing B-cells from Peyer's patch precursors than did splenic T-cell lines. However, the bias was for help to IgA-precommitted B-cells rather than inducing a class-switch to IgA since Peyer's patch T-cells did not markedly enhance IgA production by splenic B-cells. Evidence for the production of IgE-binding factors from Fcε-receptor bearing T-cells which enhance B-cell secretion of IgE has been obtained; intriguingly, lipomodulin produced by another T-cell is said to block glycosylation of the IgE-binding factor so that it now becomes a *suppressor* of IgE synthesis.

T-suppressor cells

We have now raised the question of suppression as distinct from help and perhaps it is inevitable that Nature, having evolved a functional set of T-cells which promote immune responses, should also develop an opposite set whose job would be to prevent the helpers from getting out of hand. Suppressor T-cells were first brought to the serious attention of the immunological fraternity by a phenomenon colourfully named by its discoverer, 'infectious tolerance'. Quite surprisingly it was shown that if mice are made unresponsive by injection of a high dose of sheep red cells, their T-cells will suppress specific antibody formation in normal recipients to which they have been transferred (figure 8.2). It may not be apparent to the reader why this result was at all surprising, but at that time antigen-induced tolerance was regarded essentially

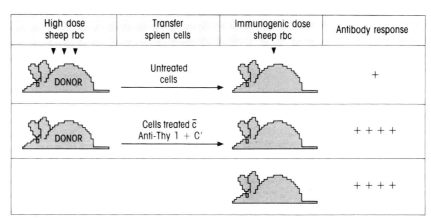

Figure 8.2. *Demonstration of T-suppressor cells. Spleen cells from a donor injected with a high dose of antigen, depress the antibody response of a syngeneic animal to which they have been transferred. The effect is lost if the spleen cells are first treated with anti-Thy 1 serum plus complement showing that the suppressors are T-cells (after Gershon R.K. & Kondo K. (1971) Immunology 21, 903: in these studies mice were thymectomized, irradiated and reconstituted with bone marrow and thymocytes).*

High dose sheep rbc	Transfer spleen cells	Immunogenic dose sheep rbc	Antibody response
DONOR	Untreated cells		+
DONOR	Cells treated c̄ Anti-Thy 1 + C'		+ + + +
			+ + + +

ACQUIRED RESPONSE – CONTROL

117

as a negative phenomenon involving the depletion or silencing of clones rather than a state of *active* suppression. Over the years, T-suppressors have been shown to modulate a variety of humoral and cellular responses, the latter including delayed-type hypersensitivity, cytolytic T-cells and antigen-specific T-cell proliferation. However, suppressor systems are not exactly straightforward.

Initiation is by suppressor-inducer cells

There is a general agreement that the suppressor circuits are initiated by cells of helper phenotype, i.e. CD4 or Ly1, called suppressor-inducer cells. Taking a broad view, the helper cells may be looked upon as general inducers of all the effector cells for cell-mediated and humoral immunity and it would be consistent with such a scheme that the T-suppressors should be generated by and react against cells occupying this pivotal position (figure 8.3). The CD4$^+$ population displays heterogeneity when analysed for cell surface markers by monoclonal antibodies; proliferative responses to recall antigens and help for B-cell stimulation by the polyclonal activator pokeweed mitogen (PWM) resides in the UCHL1 positive set while the ability to induce suppression in PWM responses is a property of the UCHL1$^-$, Leu8$^+$ T-cells (the labels refer to the monoclonal antibodies used).

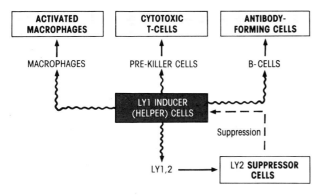

Figure 8.3. *Immunoregulatory feedback circuit showing the central position of Ly1 cells in the induction (〜〜▶) of T-dependent responses and in the generation of T-suppressors which in turn inhibit the Ly1 cells. The inducer population is heterogeneous.*

Class II MHC restriction of induction

The suppressor-inducers are activated by contact with antigen presented by cells which in the spleen are characterized by adherence for plastic or glass surfaces and the possession of the notorious class II-related I-J determinants. Now the I-J story is somewhat confused but we have to make some sense out of it because the polymorphism it defines is linked in a clear way with the function of the suppressor circuits. Originally I-J was identified by antisera obtained by reciprocal hyperimmunization of the BI0.A(3R) and (5R) strains with unfractionated spleen cells. After appropriate absorptions, the antisera so obtained recognized a proportion of the total T-cell populations which proved to be associated with suppressor activity. Since the 3R and 5R strains only differed as a result of a recombination event mapping close to I-E, I-J was thought to be encoded by genes in this region. Unfortunately, DNA sequencing showed that this region was already fully occupied with genes for I-E and C4 and there was no room for a further gene product. Some considerable light was shed on this conundrum by experiments which showed that bone marrow cells of $H-2^b$ haplotype developing in the thymus of $H-2^{b \times k}$ hosts developed I-J molecules of *host* (i.e. H-2^b *and* H-2^k) phenotype and vice versa. Thus the I-J specificity is imposed by the I-E region haplotype rather than being encoded by it. Since the thymus selects for T-cells with receptors which recognize host MHC, it is possible that the I-J antisera are directed to the determinants (idiotype) on the T-cell receptors restricted to I-E molecules, and maybe also to the T-cell receptors which are anti-idiotypic to them. On this view, anti-I-J is an anti-idiotypic serum reacting with the series of idiotypically related receptors associated with I-E recognition (figure 8.4 may help!).

These considerations, together with the fact that most, but by no means all, T-helper clones are I-A rather than I-E restricted, has led to Mitchison's suggestion that in the majority of cases (but not necessarily in all), T-helpers use I-A and suppressors I-E. Strands of evidence which accord with this hypothesis derive from the enhancement of antigen-specific proliferative responses of putatively suppressed T-cells resulting from addition of anti-I-E, and in human cases by addition of anti-DQ (although note, DQ is structurally equivalent to I-A).

Detailed analysis of murine responses to antigens such as hen egg-white lysozyme tells us that certain determinants can evoke very strong suppressor rather than helper responses depending on the mouse strain, and also, that T-suppressors directed to one determinant can switch off helper and antibody responses to other determinants on the same molecule. Thus mice of H-2^b haplotype respond poorly to lysozyme because they develop dominant

118

Figure 8.4. *The nature of I-J on suppressor T-cells. Stem cells acquire the I-J haplotype of the environment within which they mature (note they also acquire the I-J specificity of their own haplotype). One explanation is that I-J collectively describes idiotypes on the suppressor cells (and the complementary anti-idiotypic cells) selected by the host class II molecules during ontogeny.*

suppression; however, if the three N-terminal amino acids are removed from the antigen, H-2^b mice now make a splendid response showing that the T-suppression directed against the determinant associated with the N-terminal region had switched off the response to the remaining determinants on the antigen. This must imply that the antigen itself must act as a form of bridge to allow communication between T-suppressor and cells reacting to the other determinants.

The effectors of suppression

Cells which mediate suppression are far more vulnerable than helpers to adult thymectomy, X-irradiation and cyclophosphamide. For example, adult thymectomy in the mouse has little effect on the T-helper population but does lead to a fall in the T-suppressors, thereby increasing the response to T-independent antigens and preventing the fall-off in IgE antibody to haptens coupled with Ascaris extracts which occurs in intact animals. They are of the Ly2$^+$, I-J$^+$ phenotype in the mouse and belong to the CD8$^+$(T8) subset in the human.

The mechanisms by which suppression is brought about are not exactly clear. It has not proved easy to

clone T-suppressors. Evidence for T-cell V gene rearrangements is still fragmentary. The soluble factors which allow communication between cells in the suppressor circuit have not yet been cloned and their physiological status *in vivo* is still uncertain. Antigen-specific effectors acting during induction of responses and others acting at later stages have been described, all requiring antigen plus I-J for their actions. Interaction can also occur through recognition of an idiotype on the T-helper receptors by an anti-idiotype on the suppressors. These could be linked to the major regulatory immunoglobulin idiotypes to be discussed shortly since neonatal suppression of the B-cell idiotype by treatment with anti-μ serum or anti-idiotype prevents the development of the anti-idiotype suppressors. There is also general agreement that a non-specific T-acceptor cell is finally recruited and is triggered by antigen to release non-specific suppressor factors which can turn off responses to unrelated antigens in the close vicinity. Adherent cells (? macrophages plus dendritic antigen-presenting cells) are also able to function as acceptor cells for soluble suppressor factors produced by the final effectors and binding of these factors could lead to loss of ability to present antigen if, for example, they blocked synthesis of IL-1. It seems to me that interaction of suppressors with antigen on the surface of antigen-presenting cells would account for the regulation of helper cells binding to other antigen determinants (figure 8.5) and also explain how suppressors recognizing antigen plus I-E could influence helpers binding to antigen plus I-A (assuming it needs explaining). Such a reaction could also be responsible for *antigenic competition*, the situation in which one T-dependent antigen can block the response to another.

It is important not to lose track of the so-called 'natural suppressor cells' such as those provoked by total lymph node irradiation (cf. p. 224) and I would like to draw attention to a report that NK cells lacking the Thy 1 (mouse T-cell marker) can inhibit the one-way mixed lymphocyte reaction (p. 222) or the primary IgM response to sheep cells *in vitro*, by suppressing dendritic cells which have already reacted with the antigen; this offers a further opportunity for feedback control since IFNγ and IL-2 produced by T-helpers can activate NK cells.

Further complexity is introduced by the concept of the 'contrasuppressor' cell which competes with and antagonizes the action of suppressors for T-helpers. The mouse effector is an Ly1$^+$ I-J$^+$ T-cell with binding sites for the lectin *Vicia villosa* and there is evidence for a CD8$^+$(T8$^+$) cell with the same

119

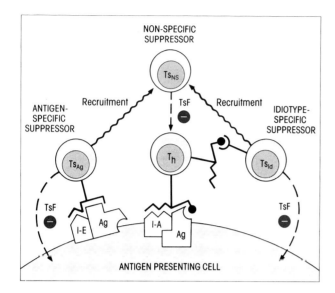

NON-SPECIFIC
SUPPRESSOR

Ts_NS

ANTIGEN-
SPECIFIC
SUPPRESSOR

Recruitment   TsF   Recruitment   IDIOTYPE-
SPECIFIC
SUPPRESSOR

Ts_Ag   T_h   Ts_Id

TsF   TsF

I-E   Ag   I-A   Ag

ANTIGEN PRESENTING CELL

Figure 8.5. *Possible mechanism for interaction of antigen and idiotype-specific suppressors operating through an antigen-presenting cell (tongue in cheek). For those likely to read the literature on this topic, one suppressor loop is thought to involve a cascade starting with the inducer (Ts_1; antigen-specific) which through a soluble factor TsF_1, triggers the transducer (Ts_2; idiotype-specific) which itself produces TsF_2 leading to recruitment of the effector (Ts_3). Time will tell how many different suppressor systems operate* in vivo *and how complex they will prove to be.*

120

lectin-binding ability subserving a similar function in the human.

Effector T-cells are guided to the appropriate target by MHC surface molecules

One may well ask why the complicated process of MHC recognition by T-cells evolved; why can't the T-cell just see the antigen alone without all this MHC fuss? The reason is that a T-cell works by recognizing antigen on the surface of a cell with which it is going to communicate and it is pointless for it to perceive either free antigen or antigen idly sitting on some basement membrane. The role of the MHC molecules is to make sure that the T-cell makes contact with antigen on the surface of the *appropriate* target cell.

Let us explore this point by looking at the role of cytotoxic T-cells in viral infection. When a cell is first infected with virus, there is an eclipse phase during which the machinery of the cell is being switched for viral replication and the only marker of the complete microbe is the viral antigen on the cell surface. At this stage, killing of the cell by a cytotoxic T-cell will prevent viral replication.

How does the killer T-cell know when it has reached its target? It has to recognize two features before striking: one is the presence of viral antigen and the other is its location on the surface of a body cell; it does not want to dissipate its efforts on extracellular free virus. This dual recognition function is carried out by the T-cell receptor which identifies both the surface viral antigen and the class I MHC molecules which are present on nearly every cell in the body and can therefore be used as markers for cells as such. Thus the killer cell operates on the basis that:

surface **viral** antigen + class I MHC ≡ **virally** infected cell

In other words, viral antigen is the code for 'viral infection' and class I molecules are the code for 'cell', and that is why T-cell receptors have to see both antigens.

The situation is quite different with intracellular bacteria and protozoa which do not go through an eclipse phase after phagocytosis by macrophages but are held as infectious entities; lysis by cytotoxic T-cells will merely release the organisms, not kill them. A separate strategy utilizing the delayed-type hypersensitivity T-cell population is required and, in this case, the effector T-lymphocyte recognizes the infected macrophage by the presence of microbial antigen on the surface in association with a class II molecule which is now a code for 'macrophage'. This interaction triggers the release of lymphokines which enable the macrophage to kill the intracellular parasites (p. 160). Similarly, in T−B cooperation, the B-cell is recognized through its class II molecule associated with the foreign antigen while T-cells mediating suppression utilize I-J and possibly I-E in the mouse and equivalent molecules in the human. In summary, each antigen-specific T-lymphocyte subset has to communicate with a particular cell type in order to make the *appropriate* immune response and it does so by recognizing not only foreign antigen but also the particular MHC molecule used as a marker of that cell (table 8.1).

Table 8.1. *Guidance of T subpopulations to appropriate target cell by MHC molecules.*

Function	Cell interaction	MHC marker on target cell
T-help	T-B	II
T-proliferation	T-macrophage	II
T-delayed sensitivity	T-macrophage	II
T-suppression	T-T	I-J(II?)
T-cytotoxic	T-infected cell	I

CHAPTER 8

Idiotype networks

Jerne's network hypothesis

The hypervariable loops on the immunoglobulin molecule which go to form the antigen combining site have individual characteristic shapes which can be recognized by the appropriate antibodies as idiotypic determinants (cf. p. 35). There are hundreds of thousands, if not more, of different idiotypes in one individual.

Jerne reasoned brilliantly that the great diversity of idiotypes would to a considerable extent mirror the diversity of antigenic shapes in the external world. Thus, he said, if lymphocytes can recognize a whole range of foreign antigenic determinants, they should be able to recognize the idiotypes on other lymphocytes. They would therefore form a large network or series of networks depending upon idiotype–anti-idiotype recognition between lymphocytes of the various T- and B-subsets (figure 8.6) and the response to an external antigen perturbing this network would be conditioned by the state of the idiotypic interactions.

Evidence for idiotypic networks

There is no doubt that the elements to form an idiotypic network are present in the body. Individuals can be immunized against idiotypes on their own antibodies, and such autoanti-idiotypes have been identified during the course of responses induced by antigens. For example, when certain strains of mice are injected with pneumococcal vaccines, they make an antibody response to the phosphoryl choline groups in which the germ-line-encoded idiotype T15 dominates. If the individual antibody-forming cells are examined by plaque assays at different times after immunization, waves of T15$^+$ and of anti-T15 (i.e. autoanti-idiotype) cells are demonstrable. Similarly, immunization with

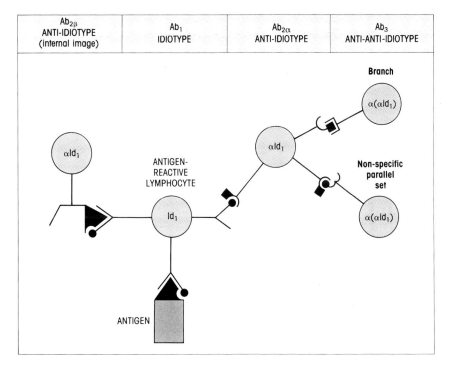

Figure 8.6. *Elements in an idiotypic network in which the antigen receptors on one lymphocyte reciprocally recognize an idiotype on the receptors of another. T-helper, T-suppressor and B-lymphocytes interact through idiotype–anti-idiotype reactions; either stimulation or suppression may result. One of the anti-idiotype sets, Ab$_{2\beta}$, may bear an idiotype of similar shape to (i.e. provides an **internal image** of) the antigen. The same idiotype (●) may be shared by two receptors of different specificity (since the several hypervariable regions provide a number of potential idiotypic determinants and a given idiotype does not always form part of the epitope binding site, i.e. the paratope), so that the anti-(anti-Id$_1$) does not necessarily bind the original antigen. (The following abbreviations are often employed: α as a prefix = anti; Id = idiotype; Ab$_1$ = Id; Ab$_{2\alpha}$ = αId not involving the paratope; Ab$_{2\beta}$ = in internal image αId involving the paratope; Ab$_3$ = α(αId).)*

the acetylcholine agonist BISQ followed by fusion of the spleen cells to produce hybridomas, yielded a series of anti-BISQ monoclonals (idiotypes) and a smaller number of anti-idiotypic monoclonals of which a surprising proportion behaved as internal images of BISQ in their ability to stimulate acetylcholine receptors (figure 8.7).

Anti-idiotypic specificities can be demonstrated on both T-helpers and T-suppressors. For example, during the induction of suppression to the p-azophenylarsonate group by intravenous injection of hapten-conjugated lymphocytes, antigen-specific Ts_1 suppressors bearing the major cross-reactive idiotype CRI_A (p. 35) appear first, but these give rise to second-order Ts_2 anti-idiotype suppressor cells. Antigen and idiotype specific T-helpers have been demonstrated in the response to various antigens, the former MHC-restricted and the latter not, and both are required for optimal antibody synthesis.

Furthermore, idiotypic interactions can modulate the immune response. Quite low doses of anti-idiotype, of the order of nanograms, can greatly enhance the expression of that idiotype in the response to a given antigen, whereas doses in the microgram range lead to suppression (figure 8.8).

Regulation by idiotype interactions

There has been a series of investigations based on the following protocol. Antigen is injected into $animal_1$ and the antibody produced, Ab_1 (idiotype), is purified and injected into $animal_2$. Ab_2 (anti-idiotype) so formed is purified and used to immunize $animal_3$ and so on (figure 8.9). Consistently, it is found that Ab_2 (anti-Id_1) recognizes an idiotype (Id_1) on Ab_1 which is also strongly present in Ab_3. Ab_4 behaves like Ab_2 in seeing the common idiotype on Ab_1 and Ab_3. None the less, although Ab_1 and Ab_3 share idiotypes, only a small fraction of Ab_3 reacts with the original antigen. This is the result one would expect if the idiotype was a cross-reacting Id (public Id) present on a variety of antibodies (and by implication B-cell receptors) of different specificities. As may be seen in figure 8.9, the anti-Id_1 (Ab_2), when injected into $animal_3$, would react with all B-cells bearing Id_1 and presumably trigger them to produce Id_1 antibodies, only a fraction of which have specificity for the original antiserum.

Such frequently occurring and usually germ-line-encoded idiotypes seem to be provoked fairly readily with anti-Id and are therefore candidates for

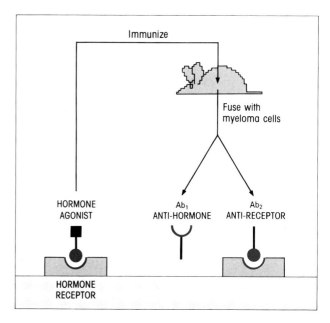

Figure 8.7. *The spontaneous production of autoanti-idiotype during immunization with a hormone agonist. Hybridomas obtained from the immunized mouse secrete anti-hormone and anti-idiotype which reacts with the hormone receptor; this indicates a close relationship between hormone, receptor, anti-hormone and anti-idiotype implying some connection between autoantibodies within the idiotype network and hormone systems.*

regulatory Id which can be under some degree of control by a limited idiotypic network. Germane to this idea are the observations that, late in immunization, antibodies with utterly distinct specificities, directed against totally different epitopes on the same antigen, often bear a common or cross-reacting idiotype. Presumably, the first clone of antibodies to be formed which bears a dominant cross-reacting Id generates a population of regulatory T-helper cells which recognize this Id; from the complex mixture of B-lymphocytes activated by the other epitopes on the antigen, these T-helpers in turn selectively recruit those with Id positive receptors (figure 8.10). We can now see how the antigen and idiotype specific T-helpers synergize in the antibody response, the latter expanding Id positive clones induced by the former.

While there would be a large measure of agreement with the view that relatively closed Id—anti-Id circuits involving major germ-line idiotypes contribute to a regulatory system, there is probably much less support for a full 'Jernerian' network extending functionally to the myriad private idiotypes. Given that regulation can occur through interaction with public or cross-reactive idiotypes, what is its importance relative to antigen-mediated

Figure 8.8. *Modulation of a major idiotype in the antibody response to antigen by anti-idiotype. In the example chosen, the idiotype is present in a substantial proportion of the antibodies produced in controls injected with irrelevant Id plus antigen (i.e. this is a public or cross-reacting Id; p. 35). Pretreatment with 10 ng of a monoclonal anti-Id greatly expands the Id^+ antibody population whereas prior injection of 10 μg of anti-Id completely (or almost completely) suppresses expression of the idiotype without having any substantial effect on total antibody production due to a compensatory increase in Id^- antibody clones.*

123

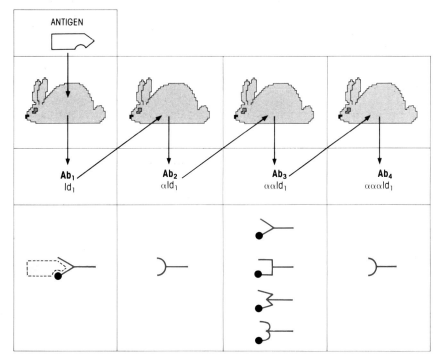

Figure 8.9. *Ab_1 produced by the antigen is injected into a second animal to produce Ab_2; this in turn is purified and injected into animal$_3$ and so on. Ab_2 and Ab_4 both react with an idiotype (●) on Ab_1 and Ab_3 but only a fraction of Ab_3 reacts with the original antigen. Bona & Paul (**Immunol. Today** 1982, 3, 230) interpret the results in terms of a common regulatory idiotype Id_1 shared by many antibodies other than those reacting with the original antigen but recruited by the injection of anti-Id_1 (Ab_2) which stimulates the range of lymphocytes whose receptors bear this common or cross-reacting idiotype. On this basis, one can understand the paradoxical finding of Oudin & Cazenave that not all the Ig molecules bearing a given Id in response to an antigen can function as specific antibody. The presence of large amounts of Id_1 in Ab_3 also suggests that the linear relationship through the cross-reacting Id_1 is dominant, with relatively insignificant branching through the variety of 'private' idiotypes on Ab_2 molecules (cf. figure 8.6) because of the low frequency of such idiotypes and their anti-idiotypes.*

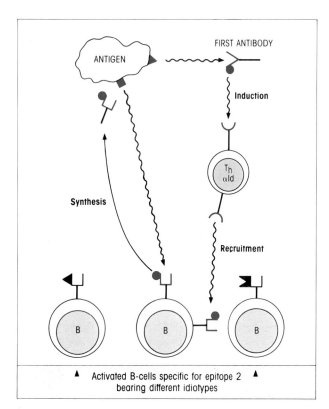

Figure 8.10. *Role of anti-idiotypic T-helper in recruiting antibodies with specificities for the different epitopes on an antigen but bearing the same public or cross-reacting idiotype. The first antibody bearing a cross-reacting Id induces αId T-helpers which are assumed to recruit Id⁺ B-cells already activated by antigen; if resting Id⁺ cells were recruited the amount of non-specific Ig synthesized might be wastefully high. It is also possible that recruitment might operate via anti-idiotypic antibodies which could act on Id⁺ B-cells to increase their surface class II and improve their 'cooperability' with T-helpers. It is worth considering whether memory αId T-helpers could be responsible for the phenomenon of 'original antigenic sin' in which a second infection with influenza virus involving an antigenically related but not identical strain generates antibodies with a higher titre for the strain which produced the first infection.*

control? Although the answer will vary with different antigens, it may turn out that in general the antigen-directed systems will dominate, with idiotypic networks providing accessory amplification and suppressive loops since (i) it seems most likely that antigen recognition and elimination were the driving forces behind selection for an adaptive immune response and therefore one wants the system to be sensitive to the presence and concentration of antigen, and (ii) there would seem to be little point in Id and anti-Id squabbling about control of the response after antigen had been eliminated. The Id network could allow the response to 'tick over' for

extended periods and maintain the memory-cell population, while the presence of primed T-helpers directed against a common Id on the various memory B-cells specific for a given antigen would increase their rate of mobilization during a secondary response.

The germ-line idiotypic network may have a fundamental role to play in the maintenance of the *V* gene repertoire and in determining the initial state of the immune system before the encounter with antigen as we shall discuss in the next chapter.

Manipulation of the immune response through idiotypes

The idiotypic network provides interesting opportunities to manipulate the immune response, particularly in hypersensitivity states such as autoimmune disease, allergy and graft rejection. However, normally the B-cell response is so diverse that suppression by anti-Id is likely to prove difficult; even when the response is dominated by a public Id and that Id is suppressed, compensatory expansion of Id negative clones ensures that the fall in the total antibody titre is relatively undramatic (cf. figure 8.8). Perhaps ways can be developed to restrict this Id negative compensation, particularly if the total number of idiotypes is small as might perhaps be the case with IgE antibody synthesis in patients with atopic allergy. Conceivably, T-helper cells may express a narrow spectrum of idiotypes thereby being more susceptible to suppression by Id auto-immunization which in any case may produce far more widespread effects within the internal network than treatment with anti-Ids from other species which may see only a small part of the system. In this respect, reports that 'vaccination' with irradiated lines of helper T-cells specific for brain or thyroid antigens prevents the induction of experimental autoimmunity against the relevant organ, are encouraging. Sporadic success has been obtained with the strategy of autoimmunizing rats of strain A with antibodies (AαB) raised in A against the transplantation antigens of strain B so that the T-cell-mediated rejection of a subsequent strain B graft is suppressed, presumably because the anti-idiotypic response (anti-[AαB]) inactivates lymphocytes capable of recognizing the graft by virtue of the AαB receptors on their surface. A totally different approach would be to use monoclonal anti-Id of the 'antigen internal image' set (figure 8.6) to stimulate antigen-specific T-suppressors capable of turning off B-cells directed to other epitopes on the antigen through bridging by the antigen itself (cf. figure 8.5).

Since we know that under suitable conditions anti-Id can also stimulate antibody production, it might be possible to use 'internal image' monoclonal anti-Ids as 'surrogate' antigens for immunization in cases where the antigen is difficult to obtain in bulk—for example, antigens from parasites such as filaria or the weak embryonic antigens associated with some cancers. Another example is where protein antigens obtained by chemical synthesis or gene cloning fail to fold into the configuration of the native molecule; this is not a problem with the anti-Id which by definition has been selected to have the shape of the antigenic epitope.

At this stage, if the reader is feeling a little groggy, try a glance at figure 8.11 which attempts a summary of the main factors currently thought to modulate the immune response.

The influence of genetic factors

Some genes affect general responsiveness

Mice can be selectively bred for high or low antibody responses through several generations to yield two lines, one of which consistently produces high-titre antibodies to a variety of antigens and the other, antibodies of relatively low titre (figure 8.12; Biozzi & colleagues). Out of the ten or so different genetic loci involved, one or more affect macrophage behaviour. The two lines are comparable in their ability to clear carbon particles or sheep erythrocytes from the blood by phagocytosis, but macrophages from the high responders retain a far higher proportion of added antigen in a relatively undegraded (and presumably) immunogenic form on their surface (cf. p. 64). On the other hand, the low responders survive infection by *Salmonella typhimurium* better and their macrophages support much slower replication of listeria (cf. p. 159) showing a dichotomy in the ability of macrophages to subserve humoral as compared with cell-mediated immunity.

Immune response linked to immunoglobulin genes

A large proportion of the antibodies made by the A/J strain of mice in response to the hapten p-azophenylarsonate, bear a major cross-reacting idiotype (CRI$_A$) somewhat coarsely referred to by the immunological cognoscenti as the ARS idiotype. Breeding experiments have shown that the capacity to produce this idiotype is inherited and is linked to the genetic markers for the immunoglobulin constant region, i.e. as might be expected, the gene encoding the idiotype occurs on the chromosome carrying the genes for the constant region. Thus, since we inherit genes which enable us to make particular antibodies one might suppose that the capacity to produce an antibody response would be limited by the repertoire of specificities encoded by the genes on this chromosome. However, since the mechanisms for generating antibody diversity from the available genes are so powerful, immunodeficiency is unlikely to occur as a consequence of a poor Ig variable region gene repertoire.

125

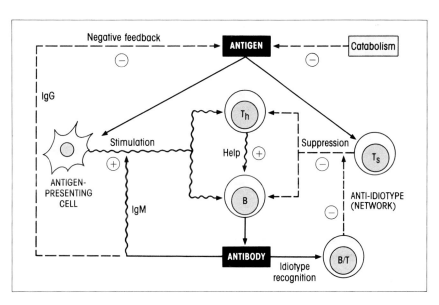

Figure 8.11. *Regulation of the immune response. T_h = T-helper cell; T_s = T-suppressor cell. T-help for cell-mediated immunity will be subject to similar regulation. Some of these mechanisms may be interdependent; for example, one could envisage anti-idiotypic antibody acting in concert with a suppressor T-cell by binding to its Fc receptor, or suppressor T-cells with specificity for the idiotype on T_h or B-cells. To avoid too many confusing arrows, I have omitted the recruitment of B-cells by anti-idiotypic T-helpers and direct activation of anti-idiotype T-suppressors by idiotype-positive T-helpers.*

Figure 8.12. *Breeding of high and low antibody responders (after Biozzi and colleagues). A group of wild mice (with crazy mixed-up genes) are immunized with sheep red blood cells (RBC) a multideterminant antigen. The antibody titre of each individual mouse is shown by a circle. The male and female giving the highest titre antibodies (●) were bred and their litter challenged with antigen. Again, the best responders were bred together and so on for 20 generations when all mice were high responders to sheep RBC and a variety of other antigens. The same was done for the poorest responders (●) yielding a strain of low responder animals.*

The immune response can be influenced by the major histocompatibility complex

There was much excitement when it was first discovered that the antibody responses to a number of thymus-dependent antigenically simple substances are determined by genes mapping to the MHC. For example, mice of the H-2^b haplotype respond well to the synthetic branched polypeptide (T,G)-A--L (cf. p. 106), whereas H-2^k mice respond poorly.

We say that mice of the H-2^b haplotype (i.e. a particular set of H-2 genes) are high responders to (T,G)-A--L because they possess the appropriate Ir gene. With another synthetic antigen, (H,G)-A--L, having histidine in place of tyrosine, the position is reversed, the 'poor (T,G)-A--L responders' now giving a good antibody response and the 'good (T,G)-A--L responders' a weak one, showing that the capacity of a particular strain to give a high or low response varies with the individual antigen (table 8.2). These relationships are only apparent when antigens of highly restricted structure are studied because the response to each single determinant is controlled by an Ir gene and it is highly unlikely that the different determinants on a complex antigen will all be associated with consistently high or consistently low responder Ir genes; rather one would expect an average of randomly high and low responder genes since the various determinants on most thymus-dependent complex antigens are structurally unrelated. Thus H-2 linked immune responses have been observed not only with relatively simple polypeptides, but also with transplantation antigens from another strain and autoantigens

where merely one or two determinants are recognized as foreign by the host. With complex antigens, H-2 linkage is usually only seen when the dose administered is so low that just one immunodominant determinant is recognized by the immune system. In this way, reactions controlled by Ir genes are distinct from the overall responsiveness to a variety of complex antigens which is a feature of the Biozzi mice (above).

Table 8.2. *H-2 haplotype linked immune responses to synthetic peptides.*

ANTIGEN	H-2 HAPLOTYPE				
	b	*k*	*d*	*a*	*s*
(TG)-A--L	Hi	Lo	Int	Lo	Lo
(HG)-A--L	Lo	Hi	Int	Hi	Lo

The Ir genes map to the I region and control T—B cooperation

Table 8.3 gives some idea of the type of analysis used to map the Ir genes. The three high responder strains have individual *H-2* genes derived from prototypic pure strains which have been interbred to produce recombinations within the H-2 region. The only genes they have in common are I-A^k and H-$2D^b$; since the B.10 strain bearing the H-$2D^b$ gene is a low responder, high response must be linked in this case to possession of I-A^k. The I-region molecules must almost certainly represent the Ir gene product since a point mutation in the I-A subregion in one strain led to a change in the class II molecule

Table 8.3. *Mapping of the Ir gene for (H,G)−A−−L responses by analysis of different recombinant strains.*

Strain	H-2 region					(H,G)-A--L Response
	K	I-A	I-E	S	D	
A	k	k	k	b	b	Hi
A.TL	s	k	k	k	b	Hi
B.IO.A(4R)	k	k	b	b	b	Hi
B.IO	b	b	b	b	b	Lo
A.SW	s	s	s	s	s	Lo

at a site affecting its polymorphic specificity and changed the mice from high to low responder status with respect to their thymus-dependent antibody response to antigen *in vivo*. The mutation also greatly reduced the proliferation of T-cells from immunized animals when challenged *in vitro* with antigen plus appropriate presenting cells, and there is a good correlation between antigen-specific T-cell proliferation and the responder status of the host. The implication that responder status may be linked to the generation of T-helpers is amply borne out by adaptive transfer studies showing that irradiated $(H\text{-}2^b \times H\text{-}2^k)$ F1 mice make good antibody responses to (T,G)-A--L when reconstituted with antigen-primed B-cells from another F1 plus T-cells from a primed $H\text{-}2^b$ (high responder); T-cells from the low responder $H\text{-}2^k$ mice only supported poor antibody responses. This also explains why these H-2 gene effects are seen with thymus-dependent but not T-independent antigens.

The mechanism by which class II molecules influence responder status is still not completely clear. Two major hypotheses have been espoused.

(a) Defective presentation. On this view the class II on the macrophage of the poor responder phenotype is unable to form the correct association with the nominal antigen to present a given determinant effectively to the specific T-cell (so-called 'determinant selection'). However, isolation of T-cell clones from high responders immunized with the antigen on low responder macrophages, which can be stimulated by antigen presented on poor responder macrophages, suggests that these macrophages can present antigen if the right T-cells are there to see it.

(b) Defective T-cell recognition. This holds that poor response is due to a class II-induced 'hole' in the T-cell repertoire so that the antigen-class II duo cannot be perceived. Jerne postulated that T-cells start out with a set of receptors which recognize major histocompatibility polymorphic determinants and that diversity is generated in the thymus, through T-cells with self-reacting receptors being forced to mutate until they no longer recognize self. On this basis, poor responder phenotypes would produce mutant receptors which were unable to recognize structures for the particular

antigen. The 'cross-tolerance' hypothesis of Ebringer provides an alternative mechanism by which MHC products could drive holes in the T-cell repertoire; originally, it was postulated that low response resulted from similarity in shape between the antigen and the individual's own MHC to which tolerance had, of course, already been established. This would predict that the F1 cross between high and low responder strains would be a low responder whereas the opposite is usually the case. A modification of this hypothesis states that tolerance occurs to self-molecules in association with an MHC component and that in the low responder, the antigen resembles some self-component in the context of the low responder MHC which tolerizes the relevant T-cells, whereas this is not true for the high responder MHC. Taking the (T,G)-A--L case as an example, this would imply that in the low responder $H\text{-}2^k$:

$$\text{self-X} \leftrightarrow \text{I-A}^k \equiv (T,G)\text{-A--L} \leftrightarrow \text{I-A}^k$$

and in the high responder $H\text{-}2^b$:

$$\text{self-X} \leftrightarrow \text{I-A}^b \not\equiv (T,G)\text{-A--L} \leftrightarrow \text{I-A}^b$$

(where the arrows indicate an association between the self-molecule X, and the class II MHC).

On this basis, the T-cells clonally restricted to the high responder phenotype $H\text{-}2^b$, and which recognize antigen in the context of this haplotype, will not be tolerized in the $(H\text{-}2^b \times H\text{-}2^k)$ F1, which will therefore be a responder (got it?—if not, don't worry—too much!).

In some instances, I-region low response may be due to the generation of a dominant T-suppressor population which overwhelms the helpers (cf. figure 8.5). This phenomenon may prove to be relatively common.

Factors influencing the genetic control of the immune response are summarized in figure 8.13.

Are there regulatory immuno-neuroendocrine networks?

There is a danger, as one focuses more and more on the antics of the immune system, of looking at the body as a collection of myeloid and lymphoid cells roaming around in a big sack and of having no regard to the integrated physiology of the organism (Are there really people who are so myopic? I can hear you say). Within the wider physiological context, attention has been drawn increasingly to interactions between immunological and neuro-endocrine systems.

Immune processes can be influenced by neuroendocrine factors

Immunological cells have the receptors which enable them to receive signals from a whole range of hormones: corticosteroids, insulin, growth hor-

127

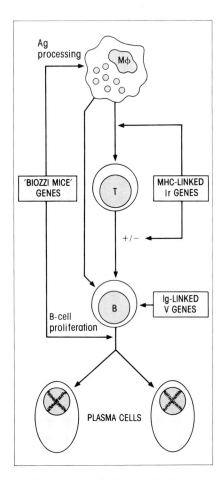

Figure 8.13. *Genetic control of the antibody response.*

coids, androgens, oestrogens and progesterone depress immune responses whereas growth hormone, thyroxine and insulin do the opposite. To give one example, 10–15-fold variations in blood glucocorticoid levels induced by adrenalectomy and stress were mirrored reciprocally by changes in the number of antibody-secreting cells. Sex differences are especially notable in autoimmune diseases.

Immunological organs are innervated by autonomic and primary sensorial neurons, and neonatal (but not adult) sympathectomy with 6-hydroxydopamine and surgical denervation of the spleen enhance immune responses. At a more physiological level, stress and circadian rhythms modify the functioning of the immune system and there is a very popular observation concerning modulation of the delayed-type hypersensitivity Mantoux reaction in the skin by hypnosis. Elegant demonstration of nervous system control is provided by studies showing suppression of conventional immune responses and enhancement of NK cell activity by classical Pavlovian conditioning. There is every possibility that the numerous investigations alleging an adverse effect of psychological factors such as bereavement upon immune function are leading us with tiny faltering steps to a new age of 'psychoimmunology'.

Immunological influences on neuroendocrine mechanisms

Glucocorticoid levels in the blood are reported to increase to immunosuppressive levels at the time of the peak response to antigen challenge. Interleukin-1 (figure 8.14) and a not fully characterized lympho-

mone, oestradiol, testosterone, β-adrenergic agents, acetylcholine, endorphins and enkephalins. There is an extensive literature concerning their influence on immune function, but by and large, glucocorti-

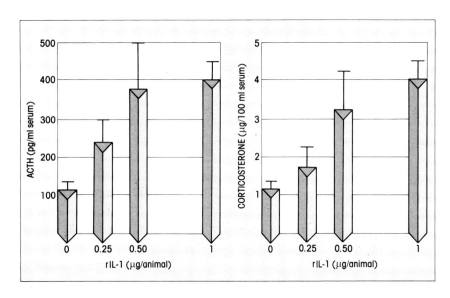

Figure 8.14. *Enhancement of ACTH and corticosterone blood levels in C3H/HeJ mice 2 hours after injection of recombinant IL-1 (values are means ± S.E.M. for groups of 7–8 mice). The significance of the mouse strain used is that they lack receptors for bacterial lipopolysaccharide (LPS) so the effects cannot be attributed to LPS contamination of the IL-1 preparation. (Reprinted from Besedovsky H., del Rey A., Sorkin E. & Dinarello C.A. (1986)* **Science, 233,** *652, with permission. Copyright 1986 by the AAAS.)*

kine are capable of stimulating glucocorticoid synthesis and do so through the pituitary–adrenal axis.

IL-1 increases slow-wave sleep when introduced into the lateral ventricle of the brain and both IL-1 and interferon produce pyrogenic effects through their action on the temperature-controlling centre. The significance of IgFc binding to pituitary ACTH-producing cells has still not been revealed.

Circuits

Two network interactions between the immune and neuroendocrine systems have been reasonably well established. The first would involve the increased synthesis of glucocorticoids under the influence of IL-1, a lymphokine and possibly a thymus hormone, generated during the immunological response. In turn, the glucocorticoids would exert feedback suppression by influencing several processes including production of IL-1 and IL-2 (figure 8.15a).

A second circuit involves the seemingly intimate relationships between hormone receptor, hormone, anti-hormone and anti-idiotype (figure 8.15b). This point has come to our attention already in discussing the production of anti-receptor antibodies during immunization with an acetylcholine agonist (figure 8.7) and is of relevance to the pathogenesis of autoimmune disorders directed against hormone receptors (see p. 258).

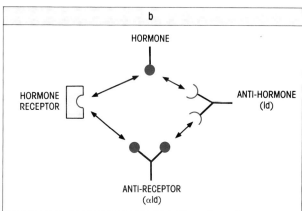

Figure 8.15. *Two immunological circuits involving neurological and endocrinological systems. (a) Glucocorticoid feedback through IL-1 and lymphokine production (after Besedovsky and colleagues). (b) Autoantibodies to hormones and their receptors (cf. figure 8.7).*

129

Immunological tolerance avoids self-reactivity

Events in the neonatal period

Over 40 years ago Owen made the intriguing observation that non-identical (dizygotic) twin cattle, which shared the same placental circulation and whose circulations were thereby linked, grew up with appreciable numbers of red cells from the other twin in their blood; if they had not shared the same circulation at birth, red cells from the twin injected in adult life would be rapidly eliminated by an immunological response. From this finding Burnet & Fenner conceived the notion that potential antigens which reach the lymphoid cells during their developing immunologically immature phase in the perinatal period can in some way specifically suppress any future response to that antigen when the animal reaches immunological maturity. This,

they considered, would provide a means whereby unresponsiveness to the body's own constituents ('self') could be established and thereby enable the lymphoid cells to make the important distinction between 'self' and 'non-self'. On this basis, any foreign cells introduced into the body around the perinatal period should trick the animal into treating them as 'self' components in later life and the studies of Medawar and his colleagues have shown that *immunological tolerance* or unresponsiveness can be artificially induced in this way. Thus neonatal injection of CBA mouse cells into newborn A strain animals suppresses their ability to immunologically reject a CBA graft in adult life (figures 8.16

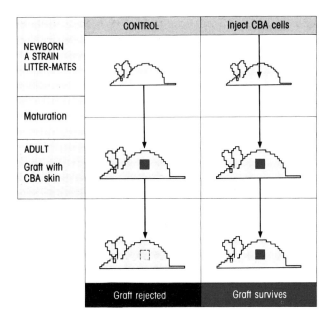

	CONTROL	Inject CBA cells
NEWBORN A STRAIN LITTER-MATES		
Maturation		
ADULT Graft with CBA skin		
	Graft rejected	Graft survives

Figure 8.16. *Induction of tolerance to foreign CBA skin graft in A strain mice by neonatal injection of antigen (after Billingham R., Brent L. & Medawar P.B. (1953)* Nature *172, 603). The effect is antigen specific since the tolerant mice can reject third-party grafts normally.*

and 8.17). Tolerance can also be induced with soluble antigens; for example, rabbits injected with bovine serum albumin at birth fail to make antibodies on later challenge with this protein.

Events in the adult

It is now recognized that tolerance can be induced in the adult as well as the neonate, although in general much higher doses of antigen are required (figure 8.18). Surprisingly, repeated injection of *low* doses of certain antigens such as bovine serum albumin (BSA) which are weakly immunogenic, established a state of tolerance as revealed by a poor antibody response on challenge with BSA in a strongly antigenic form (in complete Freund's adjuvant—see p. 181). It was shown subsequently that this 'low zone tolerance' could also be achieved with more powerful antigens provided an immunosuppressive drug such as cyclophosphamide was given to inhibit antibody synthesis during the low dose treatment.

Thus, there is a 'low zone' and a 'high zone' in terms of antigen predosage for tolerance induction. Elegant studies by Weigle and co-workers have pin-pointed the T-cell as the target for tolerance at low antigen levels while both B- and T-lymphocytes are made unresponsive at high antigen dose (table 8.4). Thus, for 'thymus-dependent' antigens at dose levels where the T-cells play a major cooperative role in antibody formation, the overall immunological performance of the animal will reflect the degree of reactivity of the T-cell population. In other words, the T-cells guide the reaction and when they are tolerant the B-cells will not respond. The implications for self-tolerance are that the concentrations at which autologous molecules circulate, will determine the cellular compartment which is tolerized (figure 8.19).

Protein antigens are more tolerogenic (able to induce tolerance) when in a soluble rather than an aggregated or particulate form which can be readily taken up by macrophages, and it seems that molecules are more likely to be tolerogenic if they escape processing by macrophages before presentation to

Figure 8.17. *CBA skin graft on fully tolerant A strain mouse showing healthy hair growth eight weeks after grafting (courtesy of Prof. L. Brent).*

CHAPTER 8

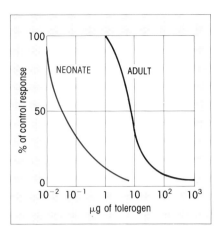

Figure 8.18. *Relative susceptibility of neonatal versus adult B-cells to tolerization by different doses of T-dependent antigen fluorescein-conjugated human IgG. The degree of tolerance was assessed by the antibody response relative to controls after challenge with antigen. Neonatal B-cells are tolerized at concentrations 100-fold lower than those effective against adult cells.*

the lymphocyte. Persistence of antigen is required to maintain tolerance. In Medawar's experiments the tolerant state was long lived because the injected CBA cells survived and the animals continued to be chimaeric (i.e. they possessed both A and CBA cells). With non-living antigens such as BSA, tolerance is gradually lost, the most likely explanation being that, in the absence of antigen, newly recruited immunocompetent cells which are being generated throughout life are not being rendered tolerant. Since recruitment of newly competent T-lymphocytes is drastically curtailed by removal of the thy-

Table 8.4. *Effect of antigen dose on tolerance induction in T- and B-cells.*

Tolerogen administered (mg)	% Tolerance induced		
	T-CELLS	B-CELLS	DONOR SPLEEN
0.1	96	9	62
0.5	99	56	97
2.5	99	70	99

After induction of tolerance to aggregate-free human IgG in mice, the reactivity of thymocytes and bone marrow cells (containing B-cells) was assessed by transfer to irradiated recipients of either bone marrow or thymus respectively from normal donors followed by IgG in an immunogenic form. The degree of tolerance induced in the donor is shown in the final column. Low antigen doses tolerize the T-cells. B-cells become unresponsive at higher doses. The T-cell activity largely dictates the response of the spleen as a whole (from Chiller J.M., Habicht G.S. & Weigle W.O. (1971) Science 171, *183).*

mus, it is of interest to note that the tolerant state persists for much longer in thymectomized animals.

Mechanism of tolerance induction

Immunological 'silence'

It is self-evident that the immune system will be tolerant of its own body components if it cannot communicate with them—we might then speak of a state of immunological 'silence'. Since virtually all body components are likely to be T-dependent because they lack the molecular qualities of T-independence (p. 94), they will not become immunogenic unless they associate with class II MHC. Soluble circulating materials can become associated with class II with some efficiency through capture and processing by B-cells; however, if there is a relatively low concentration of the component *and* the B-cells have a relatively low affinity, the signal to the T-helpers will probably not be adequate for triggering. Turning to surface molecules on cells which normally lack class II, e.g. TSH receptors on the thyroid, it is clear that 'silence' will dominate since they would be incapable of activating self-reactive T-cells (unless they were shed from the surface in large amounts and then presented by class II positive macrophages).

Immunological silence would also result if an individual has no genes coding for lymphocyte receptors directed against particular self-determinants; analysis of the experimentally induced autoantibody response to cytochrome *c* suggests that only those parts of the molecule which show species variation are autoantigenic whereas the highly conserved regions where the genes have not altered for a much longer time appear to be silent, supposedly because the autoreactive specificities have had time to disappear.

Clonal deletion

The restriction of each lymphocyte to a single specificity makes the job of establishing self-tolerance that much easier simply because it just requires a mechanism which functionally deletes self-reacting cells and leaves the remainder of the repertoire unscathed. The mechanism requires self-antigens to select the relevant clones since there is no other way to recognize them. The exceptional vulnerability of the neonate to tolerance induction has led to the suggestion that, during lymphyocyte development, the cell goes through a phase in which contact

131

with antigen leads to death or permanent inactivation. In support of this view, the surface Ig of very early B-cells can be capped at much lower concentrations of anti-IgM than are required by adult cells and remarkably, after endocytosis of the caps, the surface receptors are resynthesized by the adult cells but not by the early B-lymphocytes which are now effectively aborted through their inability to 'see' antigen. Even if they do ultimately resynthesize their receptors, they can still have been functionally inactivated; mice tolerized at birth with DNP linked to human IgG grow up with B-cells which can be isolated on DNP-immunoadsorbents through their surface receptors, yet cannot be activated to make anti-DNP as can similarly isolated cells from normal animals. Like the aged roué wistfully drinking in the visual attractions of some young belle, these tolerized lymphocytes can 'see' the antigen but lack the ability to do anything about it.

132

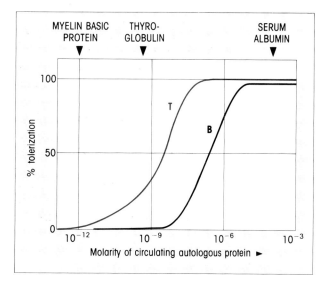

Figure 8.19. *Relative susceptibility of T- and B-cells to tolerance by circulating autologous molecules. Those circulating at low concentration induce no tolerance; at intermediate concentration, e.g. thyroglobulin, T-cells are moderately tolerized; molecules such as albumin which circulate at high concentrations tolerize both B- and T-cells.*

An ingenious mechanism based upon the idea of a 'veto' cell has been introduced to eliminate autoreactive cytotoxic T-cells, it being envisaged that such cells have the power to make cytolytic T-cells which recognize them commit suicide but leave the 'veto' cell unharmed.

Tolerance can be maintained by T-suppressor cells

Tolerance to protein antigens, induced at low concentrations, has been shown in at least one case to be mediated by T-suppressors directed against T-helpers and a suppressor mechanism will probably prove to be the most common basis for this phenomenon. The inferior immunogenicity of soluble, as distinct from aggregated or particulate, antigen has been ascribed to weak stimulation of T-helpers in contrast to effective activation of suppressor cells.

Helplessness of B-cells

We have already seen (cf. figure 8.19), that T-cells are more readily tolerized than B-cells and, as a result, a number of self-reacting B-cells are present in the body which cannot be triggered by T-dependent self-components since the T-cells required to provide the necessary T−B help are already tolerant —you might describe the B-cells as helpless. If we think of the determinant on a self-component which combines with the receptors on a self-reacting B-cell as a hapten and another determinant which has to be recognized by a T-cell as a carrier (cf. figure 6.10), then tolerance in the T-cell to the carrier will prevent the provision of T-cell help and the B-cell will be unresponsive.

If Bretscher and Cohn are correct in their hypothesis that two signals are needed for B-cell triggering but that a single signal through the Ig receptor alone leads to tolerance, there may be further consequences of helplessness, because if the self-reactive determinants cross-link B-cell receptors in the absence of T-cell signals, the B-cell should become tolerized; in fact, B-cell tolerance to haptenic determinants is readily produced when the hapten is presented to the B-cell on a thymus-independent carrier or on a carrier such as autologous IgG, to which the individual is already tolerant.

The concept of a single signal leading to tolerance may be extended to T-cells since there is evidence that if they are stimulated in the absence of IL-2 or in the presence of antibodies to MHC class II, prolonged unresponsiveness will be the outcome.

It is likely that self-tolerance involves all these mechanisms to varying degrees and that while clonal deletion is of prime importance early in life, T-suppression becomes a dominant factor later (figure 8.20). It should be stressed that these terms, early and late, apply to the life of the lymphocyte, not of the host. If an adult is irradiated and reconstituted with immature lymphocytes in the form of

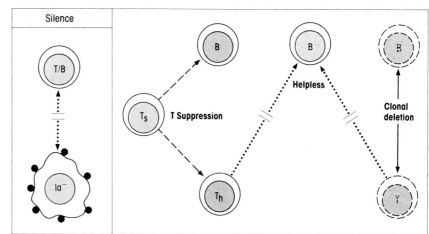

Figure 8.20. *Mechanisms of self-tolerance. Unresponsiveness will result if self-components and lymphocytes will not speak to each other (self-determinant (●) on Ia negative cell or lymphocyte lacks receptors), if T- or B-cells are T-suppressed or clonally deleted, or if T-dependent B-cells are deprived of T-help.*

bone marrow cells, the animal behaves as a neonate with respect to the ease of tolerance induction with low doses of antigen.

SUMMARY

Regulation of the antibody response is strongly influenced by antigen concentration; since the response is largely antigen driven, as effective antigen levels fall through catabolism and antibody feedback, the synthesis of antibody wanes.

T-cells regulate B-lymphocyte responses not only through cooperative help but also by T-cell suppressor networks which are initiated by inducer cells of T-helper phenotype. There is class II restriction governing these interactions but the precise molecular mechanisms are uncertain. Antigen-specific, idiotype-specific and non-specific suppressors all contribute. Effector T-cells are guided to their targets by MHC surface molecules, cytotoxic T-cells by class I, T-helpers by class II and T-suppressors by 'I-J'.

Lymphocytes can interact with the idiotypes on the receptors of other lymphocytes to form a network (Jerne). Idiotypes which occur frequently and are shared by a multiplicity of antibodies (public or cross-reacting Id) are targets for regulation by anti-idiotypes in the network thus providing a further mechanism for control of the immune response. The network offers the potential for therapeutic intervention to manipulate immunity.

A number of varied genetic factors influence the immune response. Approximately ten genes control the overall antibody response to complex antigens: some affect macrophage antigen handling and some the rate of proliferation of differentiating B-cells. Genes coding for antibodies of given specificities may be inherited together with (i.e. linked to) genetic markers for the heavy chain. Immune response genes linked to the major histocompatibility locus define the class II products on the T- and B-cells and antigen-presenting cells which control the interactions required for T—B collaboration.

Immunological, neurological and endocrinological systems can all interact and regulatory interdependent circuits are being described.

Immunological tolerance can be induced by exposure to antigens in neonatal and (less readily) in adult life. T-cells are more readily tolerized than B-cells leaving T-dependent B-cells 'helpless'. Elimination of specific cells or generation of T-suppressors may occur, while unresponsiveness to some self-components results from immunological 'silence'.

133

Further reading

Dorff M. & Benacerraf B. (1984) Suppressor cells and immunoregulation. *Ann. Rev. Immunol.,* **2,** 127.
Male D.K., Champion B. & Cooke A. (1987) *Advanced Immunology.* Gower Medical Publishing, London.
Moller G. (ed.) (1984) Idiotype networks. *Immunol. Rev.,* **79.**
Schwartz R. (1986) Immune response genes of the murine MHC. *Adv. Immunol.,* **38,** 31.

THE ACQUIRED IMMUNE RESPONSE
IV – Development

DEVELOPMENT OF THE IMMUNE SYSTEM IN EARLY LIFE

The multipotential haemopoietic stem cell

Haemopoiesis originates in the early yolk sac but as embryogenesis proceeds, this function is taken over by the fetal liver and finally by the bone marrow where it continues throughout life. The haemopoietic stem cell which gives rise to the formed elements of the blood (figure 9.1) can be shown to be multipotent, to seed other organs and to renew itself through the creation of further stem cells. Thus an animal can be completely protected against the lethal effects of high doses of irradiation by injection of bone marrow cells which will re-populate its lymphoid and myeloid systems. The stem cells differentiate within the micro-environment of sessile cells under the influence of various so-called colony-stimulating factors. These are now being cloned and we can expect very important advances in this area in the near future.

The thymus provides the environment for T-cell differentiation

The gland is organized into a series of lobules based upon meshworks of epithelial cells derived em-bryologically from an outpushing of the gut endo-derm of the third pharyngeal pouch and which form well-defined cortical and medullary zones (figure 9.2). The epithelial cells are known to syn-thesize a series of peptidic thymus hormones of which four have been well characterized and sequenced: thymulin, α_1 and β_4-thymosin, and thy-mopoietin (and its active pentapeptide TP-5). They mostly seem capable of promoting the appearance of T-cell differentiation markers and a variety of T-cell functions on culture with bone marrow cells *in vitro*, but while it seems clear that they will be concerned with the many differentiation steps within the thymus, the details are still lacking.

The specialized large epithelial cells in the outer cortex are known as 'nurse' cells because they can each be associated with large numbers of lympho-cytes which do appear to be lying within their cytoplasm. The epithelial cells of the deep cortex have branched dendritic processes rich in class II MHC. They connect through desmosomes to form a network through which cortical lymphocytes must pass on their way to the medulla (figure 9.2). The cortical lymphocytes are densely packed compared with those in the medulla, many are in division and a surprising number are in the throes of dying as evidenced by their pyknotic nuclei. On their way to the medulla, the lymphocytes pass a cordon of 'sentinel' macrophages at the cortico-medullary junction. A number of bone-marrow-derived inter-digitating dendritic cells are present in the medulla and the epithelial cells have broader processes than

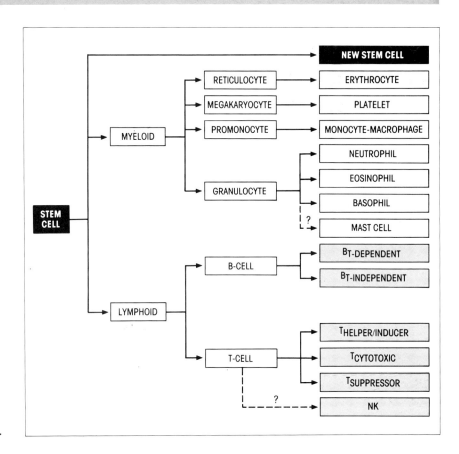

Figure 9.1. *The multipotential haemopoietic stem cell and its progeny.*

135

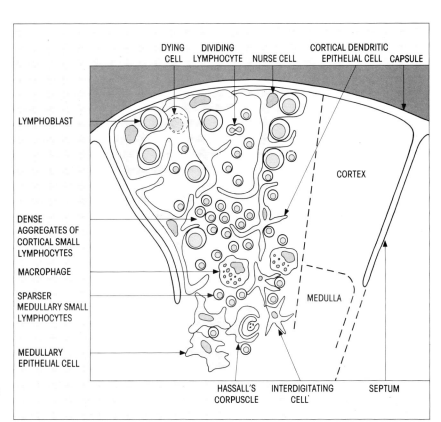

Figure 9.2. *Cellular features of a thymus lobule. See text for description. (Adapted from Hood L.E., Weissman I.L., Wood W.B. & Wilson J.H. (1984)* Immunology, *2nd edn. p.261. Benjamin/Cummings Publishing Co., California.)*

their cortical counterparts and express high levels of both class I and class II MHC. Whorled, possibly degenerate aggregates of epithelial cells form the highly characteristic Hassall's corpuscles beloved of histopathology examiners. The medullary lymphocytes possess a 20-α-hydroxyl steroid dehydrogenase and are therefore far less vulnerable to the cytolytic effects of cortisone than the cortical lymphocytes.

The differentiation of T-cells within the thymus

The evidence that bone marrow stem cells differentiate in the thymus to become immunocompetent T-cells comes from experiments on the reconstitution of irradiated hosts. An irradiated animal is restored by bone marrow grafts through the immediate restitution of granulocyte precursors; in the longer term also through reconstitution of the T- and B-cells destroyed by irradiation. However, if the animal is thymectomized before irradiation, bone marrow cells will not reconstitute the T-lymphocyte population (figure 9.3).

By day 11−12 in the mouse embryo, lymphoblastoid stem cells from the bone marrow begin to colonize the periphery of the epithelial thymus rudiment. If the thymus is removed at this stage and incubated in organ culture, a whole variety of mature T-lymphocytes will be generated. This is not seen if 10-day thymuses are cultured and shows that the lymphoblastoid colonizers give rise to the immunocompetent small lymphocyte progeny.

Differentiation is accompanied by changes in surface markers

The incoming prothymocyte attracted to the thymus by chemotactic factors stains positively for the enzyme Tdt (figure 9.4) which is thought to be involved in the insertion of nucleotide sequences at the N-terminal region of D and J variable region segments to increase diversity (cf. p. 50). The cortical thymocytes soon express a cortex specific marker (T6 in the human; TL in the mouse), the permanent T-cell markers (T1 and T11; Thy 1) and the *combined* markers for helper/inducer and cytotoxic/suppressor populations (T4, T8; L3T4, Ly2). Gradually, nearly all the cells express the T-cell receptor with α and β chains linked to T3. The cells move across the cortico-medullary junction presumably to the medulla where the T4 and T8 markers segregate in

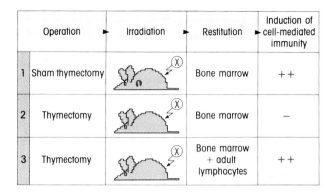

	Operation ►	Irradiation ►	Restitution ►	Induction of cell-mediated immunity
1	Sham thymectomy	(X)	Bone marrow	+ +
2	Thymectomy	(X)	Bone marrow	−
3	Thymectomy	(X)	Bone marrow + adult lymphocytes	+ +

Figure 9.3. *Maturation of bone marrow stem cells under the influence of the thymus to become immunocompetent lymphocytes capable of cell-mediated immune reactions. X-irradiation (X) destroys the ability of host lymphocytes to mount a cellular immune response but the stem cells in injected bone marrow can become immunocompetent and restore the response (1) unless the thymus is removed (2), in which case only already immunocompetent lymphocytes are effective (3). Incidentally, the bone marrow stem cells also restore the levels of other formed elements of the blood (red cells, platelets, neutrophils, monocytes) which otherwise fall dramatically after X-irradiation and such therapy is crucial in cases where accidental or therapeutic exposure to X-rays or other anti-mitotic agents seriously damages the haemopoietic cells.*

parallel with differentiation into separate immunocompetent populations of T-helpers and T-cytotoxic/suppressors. We have discussed the heterogeneity of these T-cell subsets and further subdivision into functional cytotoxic precursors and suppressors has been possible with selected monoclonal antibodies.

The precise lineage of NK cells is still in doubt. They express the markers T3, T8 and T11 which are normally restricted to T-cells, they have IL-2 receptors and are driven to proliferate by IL-2 and they can produce IFNγ. Data on T-receptor V gene rearrangement is rather mixed. They must be related to T-cells in some way.

Receptor rearrangement

The rearrangement of V, D, J and C region genes required to generate the T-cell receptor (p. 49) has not yet taken place at the prothymocyte stage. If one follows the stages of differentiation in organ cultures of mouse thymus, 35% of T-cells show D-J rearrangements in β- or γ-genes at day 15; subsequently, there is simultaneous appearance of V_β and V_γ mRNA and finally there is expression of V_β and V_α but little V_γ. The gene product is seen first in the cytoplasm and then appears at the cell surface (figure 9.5). Sections of 17-day-old thymus stained

136

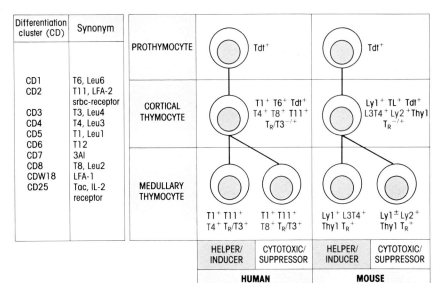

Differentiation cluster (CD)	Synonym
CD1	T6, Leu6
CD2	T11, LFA-2 srbc-receptor
CD3	T3, Leu4
CD4	T4, Leu3
CD5	T1, Leu1
CD6	T12
CD7	3Al
CD8	T8, Leu2
CDW18	LFA-1
CD25	Tac, IL-2 receptor

Figure 9.4. *Cell surface differentiation markers of thymic T-lymphocytes in the human and mouse. For reference purposes, a table showing the clusters of overlapping monoclonal antibodies defining given surface molecules is given. Tdt = terminal deoxynucleotidyl transferase; T_R = T-cell α, β receptor linked to T3; srbc = sheep red blood cell. Equivalent human and mouse markers are: T1/Ly1; T4/L3T4; T8/Ly2; T6/TL?*

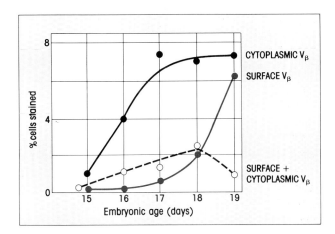

Figure 9.5. *Expression of V_β in the cytoplasm and on the surface of differentiating intrathymic T-cells assessed by immunofluorescent staining. β-chains detected with monoclonal Ab F23.1 which recognizes V_β on only 1 out of 3−4 adult T-cells, i.e. the total number of cells expressing V_β is likely to be much higher than indicated. (Data from Owen J.J.T., Kingston R. & Jenkinson E.J. (1986)* **Immunology 59**, *23, adapted with permission.)*

with anti-V_β show clustering of positive cells which could be indicative of clonal expansion events.

The imprinting of MHC restriction

T-cells acquire their ability to utilize self-MHC molecules for antigen recognition in the thymus. If an (H-2^k × H-2^b) F1 animal is sensitized to an antigen, the primed T-cells can recognize that antigen on presenting cells of either H-2^k or H-2^b haplotype, i.e. they can use either parental haplotype as a recognition restriction element. However, if bone

marrow cells from the (H-$2^{k×b}$) F1 are used to reconstitute an irradiated F1 which had earlier been thymectomized and given an H-2^k thymus, the subsequently primed T-cells can only recognize antigens in the context of H-2^k, not of H-2^b (figure 9.6). Thus the phenotype of the thymus imprints H-2 restriction on the differentiating T-cells.

It will also be seen in figure 9.6 that incubation of the thymus graft with deoxyguanosine, which destroys the cells of macrophage and dendritic cell lineage, has no effect on imprinting suggesting that this function is carried out by epithelial cells.

Induction of self-tolerance

If stem cells in bone marrow of H-2^k haplotype are cultured with fetal thymus of H-2^d origin, the maturing cells become tolerant to II-2^d as shown by their inability to give a mixed lymphocyte proliferative response when cultured with stimulators of H-2^d phenotype; third-party responsiveness was not affected. Studies with deoxyguanosine-treated thymus showed that the cells responsible for tolerance induction were probably of the macrophage or dendritic cell type (table 9.1).

It seems likely that T-cells which react strongly with self, i.e. bind with high affinity to H-2 plus other autologous molecules of the surface of these intrathymic macrophage/dendritic cells, will be eliminated, whereas those capable of reacting with H-2 plus foreign antigens will only bind with poor affinity to H-2 alone and will therefore survive. In this respect, one can appreciate that the blood-thymus barrier established by the impermeability

Thymectomize b × k mice	Graft with thymus of haplotype	Irradiate and reconstitute with b × k bone marrow	Prime with KLH	Proliferative response of primed T-cells to KLH on antigen-presenting cells of haplotype	
				H-2^b	H-2^k
	b × k	⟶		+ +	+ +
	b	⟶		+ +	−
	dGuo-treated b	⟶		+ +	−
	k	⟶		−	+ +
	dGuo-treated k	⟶		−	+ +

Figure 9.6. *Imprinting of H-2 T-helper restriction by the thymus. Host mice were F1 crosses between strains of haplotype H-2^b and H-2^k. They were thymectomized and grafted with 14 day fetal thymuses, irradiated and reconstituted with F1 bone marrow. After priming with the antigen, keyhole limpet haemocyanin (KLH), the proliferative response of lymph node T-cells to KLH on antigen-presenting cells of each parental haplotype was assessed. In some experiments the thymus lobes were cultured in deoxyguanosine (dGuo) which destroys intrathymic cells of macrophage/dendritic cell lineage. (From Lo D. & Sprent J. (1986)* Nature 319, 672.)

of cortical capillaries to high molecular weight substances, enables thymocytes to differentiate in a micro-environment free of foreign antigens.

In summary, it looks as though the thymic epithelial cells are concerned (as one of their jobs) with establishing the specificity of H-2 restriction, whereas the macrophage/dendritic cells may be concerned with tolerance induction to self.

Table 9.1. *Induction of tolerance in bone marrow stem cells by incubation with deoxyguanosine-sensitive cells in the thymus. These cells can be replaced by progenitors in the bone marrow inoculum (Jenkinson E.J., Jhittay P., Kingston R. & Owen J.J. (1985)* Transplantation 39, 331).

Bone marrow stem cells	Deoxyguanosine-treated thymus	Tolerance induction to H-2 haplotype		
		k	d	b
k	d	+	−	−
k + d	d	+	+	−

B-cells differentiate in the fetal liver and then in bone marrow

The B-lymphocyte precursors are present among the islands of haemopoietic cells in fetal liver by 8–9 weeks of gestation in man and 14 days in the mouse. Production of B-cells wanes and is taken over by the bone marrow for the remainder of life. Using the modified culture conditions recently introduced by Whitlock and Witte, it is now possible to grow bone marrow cells *in vitro* and achieve the growth of pre-B and B-cells. Although pre-B cells comprise only a minor subpopulation of the cells in those cultures, it is possible to analyse the different stages in their development by rescue with the Abelson murine leukaemia virus (A-MuLV), a replication-defective retrovirus capable of transforming pre-B cells at various points in their development into clones.

Phenotypic changes in differentiating B-cells

The early rapidly dividing pre-B cells display cytoplasmic μ chains but no light chains (figure 9.7). Subsequently, the light chains are expressed and, in the immature B-cell, the receptor for which the cell is finally programmed is inserted into the plasma membrane as a specific IgM molecule.

At the next stage of differentiation, the cell develops a commitment to producing a particular antibody class and either bears surface IgM alone or in combination with IgA or IgG. The further addition of surface IgD now marks the readiness of the virgin B-cell for priming by antigen. Some cells, therefore, bear surface Ig of three different classes; M, G and D or M, A and D, but all Ig molecules on a single cell have the same idiotype and therefore are derived from the same V_H and V_L genes. IgD is lost on antigenic stimulation so that memory cells lack this Ig. At the terminal stages in the life of a fully mature plasma cell, virtually all surface Ig is shed. Injection of anti-μ (anti-IgM heavy chain) into chick embryos prevents the subsequent maturation of IgM and IgG antibody-producing cells, whereas

138

CHAPTER 9

| HAEMOPOIETIC STEM CELL | B-CELL PRECURSOR | PRE-B-CELLS | IMMATURE B-CELL | MATURE B-CELL |

Figure 9.7. *Differentiation markers of developing B-cells. Monoclonal antibodies define the surface molecules B220, BP-1 and BP-3. FcR = Fcγ receptor; C3R = C3b receptor. (After Cooper M.D. In* **Progress in Immunology VI.** *Cinader B. and Miller R.G. (eds) (1986) p. 18, Academic Press.)*

anti-γ inhibits only IgG development. Although we have seen earlier that T-helpers can induce class-switching, it is also the case that some isotype switching probably occurs independently of antigen as a result of micro-environmental factors. In the embryonic chicken bursa, a regular switch from IgM to IgG is observed and it seems possible that local influences in the gut will prove to be responsible for the predominant development of IgA bearing cells. These cells are generated in Peyer's patches, pass into the blood via the thoracic duct and return to populate the diffuse lymphoid tissue in the lamina propria of the gut.

Other differentiation markers are recorded in figure 9.7 and it is not surprising to see class II MHC molecules appear on the immunocompetent B-cell bearing in mind their importance for T-cell collaboration.

There is a minor population of B-cells which, in addition to surface Ig, express the T-cell markers CD5 (T1) or Ly1 depending upon the species. The progenitors of this subset move from the bone marrow to the peritoneal cavity fairly early in life and their possible relationship to idiotype networks and autoantibody production will be discussed at a later point.

The sequence of immunoglobulin gene rearrangements

By analysis of Abelson-MuLV-transformed clones of pre-B cells, it has proved possible to unravel the orderly cascade of Ig gene rearrangements which occur during differentiation.

1 Initially, the *D-J* segments on *both* heavy chain coding regions (one from each parent) rearrange (figure 9.8).

2 A *V-DJ* recombinational event now occurs on one chain. If this proves to be a *non-productive* rearrangement (i.e. adjacent segments are joined in an incorrect reading frame or in such a way as to generate a termination codon downstream from the splice point), then a second *V-DJ* rearrangement will occur on the sister heavy chain region. If a productive rearrangement is achieved, the pre-B cell expresses cytoplasmic μ chains.

3 The next set of Ig gene rearrangements occur on the κ light chain gene loci and these involve *V-J* recombinations on first one and then the other κ allele until a productive $V_κ$-*J* rearrangement is accomplished. Were that to fail, an attempt would be made to achieve productive rearrangement of the λ alleles.

4 The IgM molecule now prohibits any further gene shuffling.

Allelic exclusion

Since each cell has chromosome complements derived from each parent, the differentiating B-cell has four light and two heavy chain gene clusters to choose from. Once the *V.D.J.* DNA rearrangement has occurred within one light and one heavy chain cluster, the V genes on the other four chromosomes are held by some mechanism in the embryonic state so that the cell is able to express *only one light and one heavy chain*. This so-called *allelic exclusion* is essential for clonal selection to work since the cell is then only programmed to make the one antibody it uses as a

GERM LINE	V — D — J — C_H (MATERNAL) V — D — J — C_H (PATERNAL)	
STAGE 1	V — DJ — C_H V — DJ — C_H	
STAGE 2	VDJ — C_H ⊖ V — DJ — C_H	OR	V~DJ — C_H VDJ — C_H	▶ μ
STAGE 3	μ ⊕ VJ — $C_κ$ V — J — $C_κ$	OR	V~J — $C_κ$ VJ — $C_κ$	▶ IgM
STAGE 4	VJ — $C_κ$ ⊖ ---- IgM ---- ⊖ V — J — $C_κ$	V — J — $C_λ$ V — J — $C_λ$

UNREARRANGED ☐   PRODUCTIVE ☐   NON-PRODUCTIVE ⬚

Figure 9.8. *Postulated sequence of B-cell gene rearrangements and mechanism of allelic exclusion (see text).*

140

cell surface receptor to recognize antigen. Furthermore, this gene exclusion mechanism prevents the formation of molecules containing two different light or two different heavy chains which would have non-identical combining sites and therefore be functionally monovalent with respect to the majority of antigens; such antibodies would be non-agglutinating and would tend to have low avidity because the bonus effect of multivalency could not operate.

Two mechanisms have been postulated to account for allelic exclusion. The stochastic (random) model proposed that because of a high probability of unproductive rearrangement, only one functional allele was likely to be created. The feedback model proposed that the creation of a functional Ig somehow inhibited subsequent rearrangement at allelic loci. Studies with transgenic mice in which a pre-rearranged μ-gene was successfully injected into fertilized mouse embryos, have provided support for the feedback model. Thus the presence of a functional μ-gene represses heavy chain gene rearrangements in pre-B cells (figure 9.8). Furthermore, the formation of associated heavy and light chains inhibits any subsequent light chain gene rearrangement.

Different specific responses can appear sequentially

The responses to given antigens in the neonatal period appear sequentially as though each species were programmed to rearrange its V genes in a definite order (figure 9.9).

B-cells change in responsiveness to negative signals with age

One has to distinguish between the age of a B-cell and the age of the host. At the earliest stages all the

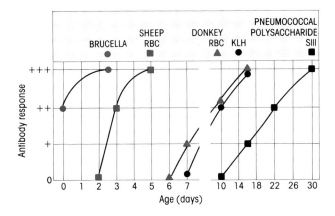

Figure 9.9. *Sequential appearance of responsiveness to different antigens in the neonatal rat. (RBC = red blood cell; KLH = keyhole limpet haemocyanin.)*

Figure 9.10. *Negative signalling to B-cells by receptor cross-linking. (a) After treatment with anti-IgM and washing, mature but not immature B-cells regenerate their receptors. (b) The immature B-cell is 'tolerized' by very low concentrations of receptor cross-linking agents such as multivalent antigens. The unresponsiveness induced in mature cells by high concentrations probably represents a different mechanism such as receptor blockade. PFC = antibody synthesizing plaque-forming cell. (Reproduced from Nossall G.J.V. (1986) Proc. Roy. Soc. 228B, 225, with permission.)*

B-cells are young, but as the animal ages and these B-cells mature, stem cells continually differentiate to form new B-cells.

Early and mature B-cells differ strikingly in their responsiveness to anti-IgM or multivalent antigens. These reagents cross-link the surface receptors causing patching, capping and eventually internalization (cf. figure 2.5f). Whereas mature B-cells re-synthesize their surface receptors within 24 hours, the immature lymphocytes fail to regenerate surface IgM as though they had received some negative 'tolerogenic' signal (figure 9.10a). This phenomenon occurs at very low antigen concentrations, and it is tempting to relate the change in sensitivity for this negative signalling with age of the cell (figure 9.10b) to its susceptibility for tolerance induction to self-components (c.f. p. 131, figure 8.18).

The idiotype network in early life

If the spleens of fetal mice which are just beginning to secrete immunoglobulin are fused with myeloma cells to produce hybridomas, an unusually high proportion are inter-related as idiotype–anti-idiotype pairs. This high level of idiotype connectivity is not seen in later life and suggests that these early cells, mostly Ly1 B, are programmed to synthesize germ-line gene specificities which have network relationships and that the network may be concerned with the stability of the Ig gene pool and possibly the amplification of the antibody repertoire by anti-idiotype-driven mutation in the non-Ly1 B-cell population. The specificities of these 'early' hybridomas are very similar to those of the 'natural' antibodies which appear spontaneously in germ-free animals not exposed to exogenous antigens, and it is noteworthy that several are IgM with low affinity for self-components such as DNA, IgG and cytoskeletal proteins, hinting perhaps at the use of these body components as points of reference to maintain the V genes encoding individual members of the idiotype network. Of course, by no means are all the Ly1 B specificities anti-self; many are directed to polysaccharide antigens of common pathogens, e.g. phosphoryl choline.

The overall response in the neonate

Lymph node and spleen remain relatively under-developed in the human even at birth except where there has been intra-uterine exposure to antigens as in congenital infections with rubella or other organisms. The ability to reject grafts and to mount an antibody response is reasonably well developed by birth but the immunoglobulin levels with one exception are low particularly in the absence of intra-uterine infection. The exception is IgG which is acquired by placental transfer from the mother, a process dependent upon Fc structures specific to this Ig class. This material is catabolized with a half-life of approximately 30 days and there is a fall in IgG concentration over the first three months accentuated by the increase in blood volume of the growing infant. Thereafter the rate of synthesis overtakes the rate of breakdown of maternal IgG and the overall concentration increases steadily. The other immunoglobulins do not cross the placenta and the low but significant levels of IgM in cord blood are synthesized by the baby (figure 9.11). IgM reaches adult levels by nine months of age. Only trace levels of IgA, IgD and IgE are present in the circulation of the newborn.

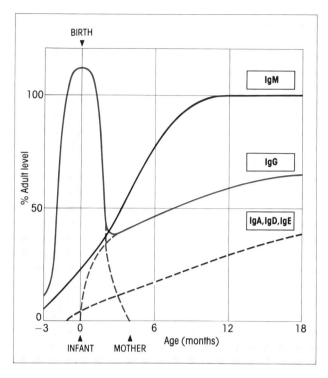

Figure 9.11. *Development of serum immunoglobulin levels in the human (after Hobbs J.R. (1969) In* **Immunology and Development,** *Adinolfi M. (ed.), p. 118. Heinemann, London).*

UNREGULATED DEVELOPMENT GIVES RISE TO LYMPHOPROLIFERATIVE DISORDERS

The cells involved in immune responses may undergo malignant transformation, giving rise to leukaemia, lymphoma or myeloma characterized by uncontrolled proliferation.

Deregulation of the *c-myc* proto-oncogene is a characteristic feature of many B-cell tumours

The realization that viral oncogenes are almost certainly derived from normal host genes concerned in the regulation of cellular proliferation, has led to the identification of many of these so-called proto-oncogenes. One of them, *c-myc* appears to be of crucial importance for entry of the lymphocyte, and probably many other cells, from the resting G_0 stage to the cell cycle. As we have earlier noted, increased

expression of *c-myc* is an early event associated with lymphocyte activation and it has been established that there is a strong relationship between the level of *c-myc* mRNA and the proliferative capacity of a cell population. It is also generally believed that shutdown of *c-myc* expression is linked to exit from the cycle and return to G_0.

Thus deregulation of *c-myc* expression will prevent cells from leaving the cycle and consign them to a fate of continuous proliferation. This is just what is seen in the neoplastic B-lymphoproliferative disorders where the malignant cells express high levels of *c-myc* protein usually associated with a reciprocal chromosomal translocation involving the *c-myc* locus. For example, Burkitt's lymphoma is a B-cell neoplasia with a relatively high incidence among African children in whom there is an association with the Epstein-Barr virus (EBV); in most cases studied, the *c-myc* gene located on chromosome 8 band q24 is joined by a reciprocal translocation event to the μ-heavy chain gene on chromosome 14 band q32 (figure 9.12). The two genes are connected in a transcriptionally opposing fashion so that *c-myc* is transcribed from the normal *c-myc* promoters, not those belonging to the μ chain. It is suggested that the normal mechanisms which down-regulate *c-myc* can no longer work on the

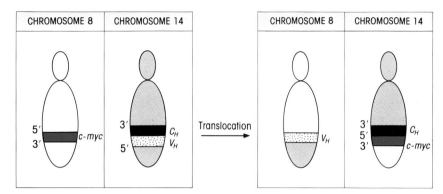

Figure 9.12. *Translocation of the* c-myc *gene to the μ-chain locus in Burkitt's lymphoma.*

translocated gene and so the cell is held in the cycling mode. Less frequently, *c-myc* translocates to the site of the kappa (chromosome 2) or lambda (chromosome 22) loci.

Chromosome translocations are common in lymphoproliferative disorders

Most lymphomas and leukaemias have visible chromosome abnormalities bound up with translocations to B-cell immunoglobulin or T-cell receptor gene loci but not necessarily involving *c-myc*. A reciprocal translocation between the μ-chain gene on chromosome 14 and an unknown oncogene on chromosome 18 has been identified in a follicular B-cell lymphoma, and another between the T-cell α-gene on chromsome 14 (q11) and another presumed oncogene on chromosome 11 in a T-acute lymphoblastic leukaemia (T-ALL). In a further case of T-cell leukaemia, an inversion on chromosome 14 brought the μ-chain locus at band q32 to the T-receptor α-gene at q11 with the possibility of producing a chimaeric receptor consisting of V_H-$C_α$/$V_β$$C_β$ chains.

The lack of proliferative control engendered by deregulation of *c-myc* and other similar events induced by chromosomal translocations is permissive for the progression towards neoplasia but is not in itself sufficient to bring about malignant transformation. Thus, transgenic mice harbouring a *c-myc* gene driven by the μ-heavy chain enhancer ($E_μ$-*myc* mice) have hyperplastic expansions of the pre-B cell population in the bone marrow and spleen during the pre-neoplastic period and yet do not develop tumours until 6−8 weeks of age and then they are monoclonal not polyclonal, suggesting that a random second event is required before autonomy is achieved.

Different lymphoid malignancies show maturation arrest at characteristic stages in differentiation

Lymphoid cells at almost any stage in their differentiation or maturation may become malignant and proliferate to form a clone of cells which are virtually 'frozen' at a particular developmental stage because of defects in maturation. The malignant cells bear the markers one would expect of normal lymphocytes reaching the stage at which maturation had been arrested. Thus, chronic lymphocytic leukaemia cells resemble mature B-cells in expressing surface class II and Ig, albeit of a single idiotype in a given patient. Using monoclonal antibodies directed against the terminal deoxynucleotidyl transferase (figure 9.14a), class II MHC, Ig and specific antigens on cortical thymocytes, mature T-cells and non-T, non-B acute lymphoblastic leukaemia cells, it has been possible to classify the lymphoid malignancies in terms of the phenotype of the equivalent normal cell (figure 9.13).

At one time it was thought that maturation arrest occurred at the stage when the cell first became malignant, but we now know that the tumour cells can be forced into differentiation by agents such as phorbol myristate acetate and the current view is that cells may undergo a few differentiation steps after malignant transformation before coming to a halt. The demonstration of a myeloma protein idiotype on the cytoplasmic μ chains of pre-B cells in the same patient certainly favours the idea that the malignant event had occurred in a pre-B cell whose progeny formed the plasma cell tumour. However, an alternative explanation could be transfection of normal pre-B cells by an oncogene complex from the myeloma cells possibly through a viral vector. With the exciting discovery of a C-type retrovirus

143

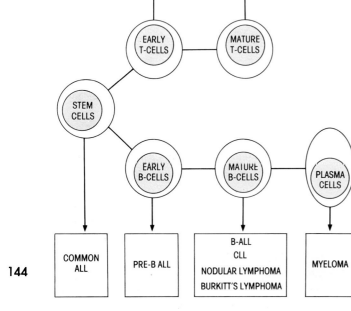

T-ALL	CUTANEOUS LYMPHOMA	MYCOSIS FUNGOIDES
T-LYMPHOBLASTIC LYMPHOMA	T-CLL	SÉZARY SYNDROME
	T-LYMPHOMA	

Figure 9.13. *Cellular phenotype of human lymphoid malignancies. ALL, acute lymphoblastic leukaemia; CLL, chronic lymphocytic leukaemia. (After Greaves M.F. & Janossy G.)*

144

associated with certain human T-cell leukaemias (HTLV), this is an interesting possibility. The virus is likely to have the same relationship to the T-cell as EB virus does to the B-cell, although what that is exactly is still unknown.

Immunohistological diagnosis of lymphoid neoplasias

With the availability of a range of monoclonal antibodies and improvements in immuno-enzymatic technology, great strides have been made in exploiting, for diagnostic purposes, the fact that malignant lymphoid cells display the markers of the normal lymphocytes which are their counterpart.

Leukaemias

This point can be made rather well if one looks at the markers used to distinguish between the various types of leukaemia (table 9.2). Whereas T-ALL and B-ALL cases have a poor prognosis, the patients

positive for the common acute lymphoblastic leukaemia antigen (CALLA; figure 9.14b) who include most childhood leukaemias, belong to a prognostically favourable group, many of whom are curable with standard therapeutic combinations of vincristine, prednisone and L-asparaginase. Bone marrow transplantation may help in the management of patients with recurrent ALL provided a remission can first be achieved.

Chronic lymphocytic leukaemia is uncommon in people under 50 and is usually relatively benign, although the 10–20% of patients with a circulating monoclonal Ig have a bad prognosis. Excessive numbers of CLL small lymphocytes are found in the blood (figure 9.14c, d and e) and, being derived from a single clone, they can be stained only with anti-κ *or* anti-λ. Their weak expression of CD5 suggests that they may be derived from the equivalent of the Ly1 B-cell population in the mouse.

Table 9.2. *Classification of lymphocytic leukaemia by immuno-enzymatic staining.*

Lymphocyte marker	Common ALL	Pre-B ALL	B-cell ALL	T-cell ALL	Chronic lymphocytic leukaemia
*CALLA	+	+	−	−	−
Cytoplasmic μ	−	+	−	−	−
Surface μ	−	−	+	−	+
Surface κ + λ	−	−	−	−	−
Pan-B	−	+	+	−	+
TdT	+	+	−	+	−
CD5 (T1)		−	−	+	+
CD2 (T11)	−	−	−	+	+
HLA-DR	+	+	+	−	+

* *Antigen-specific for lymphoid precursor cells and pre-B cells.*

Lymphomas

The extensive use of markers has greatly helped in the diagnosis of non-Hodgkin lymphomas. In the first place, the sometimes difficult distinction between a lymphoproliferative condition and carcinoma can be made with ease by using monoclonal antibodies to the leucocyte common antigen which will react with all lymphoid cells whether in paraffin or cryostat sections, and antibodies to cytokeratin which recognize most carcinomas (figure 9.14f). Second, the cell of origin of the lymphoma can be ascertained by panels of monoclonals which differentiate the cellular elements which form normal lymphoid tissue (table 9.3).

The majority of non-Hodgkin lymphomas are of B-cell origin and the feature which gives the game away to the diagnostic immunohistologist is the synthesis of monotypic Ig, i.e. of one light chain only (figure 9.14g); in contrast, the population of cells at a site of reactive B-cell hyperplasia will stain for both κ and λ chains (figure 9.14h).

Follicle centre cell lymphomas (figure 9.14g) imitating the reactive germinal centre account for over 50% of the B-lymphomas. They exhibit monotypic surface Ig and the larger centrocytes and centroblasts which make up two-thirds of the cases contain cytoplasmic Ig. They stain for MHC class II and weakly for CALLA (cf. table 9.2). Morphologically similar cells make up tumours variously labelled 'mantle zone lymphoma' or 'small cleaved cell lymphoma' but differ from follicle centre cells in positive surface staining for IgM *and* IgD, and CD5 and negativity for CALLA. Burkitt lymphoma lymphoblastoid cells (figure 9.14i) exhibit the common ALL antigen and surface IgM.

The overall prognosis for patients with non-Hodgkin lymphoma is poor even though improved by combined chemotherapy. Transplanted patients are 35 times more likely to develop lymphoma than normals, and there are indications that this cannot necessarily be attributed to the long-term immunosuppression.

Hodgkin's disease attacks the gross architecture of lymphoid tissue and is characterized by the bi-nucleate giant cells known as Reed—Sternberg cells (figure 9.14j) whose lineage is still disputed. Therapy depends upon the stage of the disease: patients with disease localized to lymphoid tissue above the diaphragm respond well to radiotherapy, while those with more widespread disease are treated more aggressively.

Plasma cell dyscrasias

Multiple myeloma

This is defined as a malignant proliferation of a clone of plasma cells in the bone marrow secreting a monoclonal Ig. The myeloma or 'M' component in serum is recognized as a tight band on paper electrophoresis (all molecules in the clone are of course identical and have the same mobility) and as an abnormal arc on immunoelectrophoresis with a 'bump' caused by the monoclonal protein (figure 9.15a and b). Since Ig-secreting cells produce an excess of light chains, it is to be expected that free light chains are present in the plasma of multiple myeloma patients, and indeed they can be recognized in the urine and give rise to amyloid deposits (see below). The characteristic 'punched out' osteolytic lesions in bones are thought to be due to release of osteoclastic factors by the abnormal plasma cells in the marrow. If untreated, the disease is rapidly progressive. With chemotherapy, the mean survival time from diagnosis is now about 5 years.

Marker	Follicle centre cells	Mantle zone cells	Plasma cells	T-cells	Macrophages	Interdigit-ating cells (T-cell area)	Follicular dendritic cells
Cytoplasmic Ig	±	−	+	−	−	−	−
J chain	±	−	±	−	−	−	−
Leucocyte common Ag (LCA)	+	+	+	+	+	+	?
HLA-DR	+	+	−	−	±	+	?
CALLA	+	−	−	−	−	−	−
Lysozyme	−	−	−	−	+	−	−
α1-Antitrypsin	−	−	−	−	+	−	−
S-100	−	−	−	−	−	+	−
Surface Ig	+	+	−	−	−	−	−
T-cell	−	−	−	+	−	±	−
Pan B-cell	+	+	±	−	−	−	−
C3b receptor	−	±	−	−	−	−	+

Table 9.3. *Immunohistochemical markers of normal lymphoid tissue (from Isaacson P.G. & Wright D.H. (1986). In* Immunochemistry: Modern Methods and Applications, *2nd edn. Polak J.M. & Noorden S. van (eds). Wright, Bristol, UK, with permission).*

(a)

(b)

(c)

(d)

(e)

(f)

LG

Ke

(g)

κ   λ

(h)

κ   λ

CHAPTER 9

(i)   (j)

(k)   (l)

Figure 9.14 facing page and above. *Immunodiagnosis of lymphoproliferative disorders. (a) Cytocentrifuged blast cells from a case of acute lymphoblastic leukaemia stained by anti-terminal deoxynucleotidyl transferase (TdT) using an immuno-alkaline phosphatase method (cells treated first with mouse monoclonal anti-TdT, then anti-mouse Ig and finally with an immune complex of anti-alkaline phosphatase + alkaline phosphatase before developing the enzymic reddish-purple colour reaction). Many strongly stained blast cells are seen together with unlabelled normal marrow cells. (b) Immuno-alkaline phosphatase staining of bone marrow cells from a case of acute lymphoblastic leukaemia, using monoclonal antibody specific for the common-acute lymphoblastic leukaemia antigen (anti-CALLA; antibody J5). The majority of cells are strongly labelled. Two non reactive cells are indicated by arrows. (c,d,e) Immuno-alkaline phosphatase labelling of blood smears from a case of chronic lymphocytic leukaemia with three monoclonal antibodies (anti-HLA-DR, anti-T3 antigen, and anti-T1 antigen): (c) HLA-DR antigen is present on all the leukaemic cells seen, but absent from a polymorph (arrowed); (d) three normal T-cells are labelled for the T3 antigen, but the leukaemic cells are negative; (e) T1 antigen is strongly expressed on two normal lymphocytes (arrowed), but also weakly expressed on the CLL cells. This pattern is typical of chronic lymphocytic leukaemia. (f) A case of gastric carcinoma (stained at the bottom using anti-cytokeratin, Ke) with a heavy lymphocytic infiltrate (top, stained with anti-leucocyte common antigen, LC). (g) Diffuse follicle centre type B-cell lymphoma showing λ light chain restriction; compare with (h) a reactive lymph node staining for both κ and λ light chains. (i) Burkitt's lymphoma showing 'starry sky' appearance. (j) Hodgkin's disease showing mixed cellularity and characteristic binucleate Reed–Sternberg cell with massive prominent nucleoli in the centre of the figure. (k) Amyloid deposits in kidney glomeruli visualized by Congo Red staining under polarized light. (l) A case of malignant lymphoma associated with macroglobulinaemia, showing lymphoplasmacytoid cells stained by the brown immunoperoxidase reaction for cytoplasmic IgM.*

((a)–(e) very kindly provided by Dr D. Mason, and (f)–(l) by Prof. P. Isaacson.)

'M' bands have been found in the sera of a number of individuals who have no clinical signs of myeloma; the comparative rarity with which invasive multiple myeloma develops in these people and the constant level of the monoclonal protein over a period of years suggests the presence of benign tumours of the lymphocyte-plasma cell series.

Figure 9.15. *Myeloma serum with an 'M' component.
(a) Agar gel electrophoresis showing strong band in γ-globulin region. (b) Immunoelectrophoresis against anti-IgG serum revealing the 'bump' or 'bow' in the precipitin arc. (Courtesy of Dr F.C. Hay.)*

Amyloid

148 Between 10 and 20% of patients with myeloma develop widespread amyloid deposits which contain the variable region of the myeloma light chain. Being identical, the variable region fragments polymerize and form the characteristic amyloid fibrils which are recognizable by their birefringence on staining with Congo Red (figure 9.14k). Other components in amyloid have not yet been characterized. The fibrils are relatively resistant to digestion and accumulate in the ground substance of connective tissue where they can lead to pathological changes in the kidneys, heart and brain. Amyloid can also be formed secondarily to chronic inflammatory conditions such as rheumatoid arthritis and familial Mediterranean fever but in this case involves the polymerization of a unique substance, Amyloid A (AA) protein derived from the N-terminal part of a serum precursor (SAA) of molecular weight 90 000. SAA behaves as an acute phase protein in that its concentration increases rapidly in response to tissue injury or inflammation. Levels rise with age and the minority of individuals with high values are those most likely to develop amyloid.

Waldenström's macroglobulinaemia

This disorder is produced by the unregulated proliferation of cells of an intermediate appearance called lymphoplasmacytoid cells which secrete a monoclonal IgM, the Waldenström macroglobulin (figure 9.14l). Remarkably, many of the monoclonal proteins have autoantibody activity, anti-DNA, anti-IgG (rheumatoid factor) and so on. It has been suggested that they are of the same lineage as CLL cells. Since the IgM is secreted in large amounts and is confined to the intravascular compartment, there is a marked rise in serum viscosity, the consequences of which can be temporarily mitigated by vigorous plasmapheresis. The disease runs a fairly benign course and the prognosis is quite good, although the appearance of lymphoplasmacytoid tumour cells in the blood is an ominous sign.

Heavy chain disease

Heavy chain disease is a rare condition in which quantities of abnormal heavy chains are excreted in the urine—γ chains in association with malignant lymphoma and α chains in cases of abdominal lymphoma with diffuse lymphoplasmacytic infiltration of the small intestine. The amino acid sequences of the N-terminal regions of these heavy chains are normal but they have a deletion extending from part of the variable domain through most of the C_H1 region so that they lack the structure required to form cross-links to the light chains. One idea is that the defect arises through faulty coupling of V and C region genes (cf. p. 139).

Immunodeficiency secondary to lymphoproliferative disorders

Immunodeficiency is a common feature in patients with lymphoid malignancies. The reasons for this are still obscure but it seems as though the malignant cells interfere with the development of the corresponding normal cells, almost as though they were producing some cell-specific chalone or transfecting suppressor factor.

Thus in multiple myeloma the levels of normal B-cells and of non-myeloma Ig may be grossly depressed and the patients susceptible to infection with pyogenic bacteria. Although the lineage of the Reed–Sternberg cell is still contentious, the main candidates are either T-cell or macrophage, and feedback suppressive influences on the normal counterpart would accord with the defects in cell-mediated immunity which are so striking even in early stage I or stage II patients. In fact, half the deaths in this malignant lymphoma are accounted for by infections with intracellular organisms such as *Pneumocystis* or cytomegalovirus.

THE EVOLUTION OF THE IMMUNE RESPONSE

Recognition of self is fundamental for multicellular organisms

For the selective processes of evolution to work effectively, it is essential that each multicellular organism maintains its individuality. It is not surprising, therefore, that mechanisms for the recognition and subsequent rejection of non-self can be identified as far down the evolutionary scale as the sponges (figure 9.16a) while there is unequivocal evidence for the ability of the lowly earthworm to reject tissues of other individuals of the same or different species (figure 9.16b).

Primitive discriminatory mechanisms must also come into play when amoebocytes, which are so widespread throughout invertebrate phylogeny, eliminate foreign material by phagocytosis.

Invertebrates have humoral defence mechanisms

In many phyla, phagocytosis is augmented by coating with agglutinins and bactericidins in the body fluids of non-immunized animals. Furthermore, it now appears that antisomes (as they are called) with some specificity can be *induced* by antigen administration; figure 9.17 provides an example of the response to a synthetic aromatic hapten on a carrier in the earthworm.

B- and T-cell responses are well defined in the vertebrates

Both B- and T-cell responses can be elicited even in the lowliest vertebrate studied, the California hagfish. This unpleasant cyclostome (which preys upon moribund fish by entering their mouths and eating the flesh from the inside) was originally considered 'the negative hero of the phylogeny of immunity' since, unlike the lamprey, a more advanced cyclostome, it appeared incapable of reacting immunologically. It now transpires that hagfish can make antibodies to haemocyanin and reject allografts, provided they are maintained at temperatures approaching 20°C (in general, poikilotherms make antibodies better at higher temperatures). The antibodies were present in a 28S macroglobulin fraction, but further up the evolutionary scale in the cartilaginous fishes, well-defined 18S and 7S immunoglobulins with heavy and light chains have now been defined.

Mechanisms for the generation of antibody diversity receive quite different emphasis as one goes from one species to another. We are already familiar with the mammalian system where multiple V genes are greatly amplified by a variety of recombinational events involving multiple D and J segments. The horned shark also has many V genes but the opportunities for combinatorial joining are tightly constrained by close linkage between individual V, D, J and C segments and this may be a factor in the restricted antibody response of this species. In sharp contrast, there seems to be only one operational V gene at the λ light chain locus in the chicken but this undergoes extensive somatic

149

Figure 9.16. *Recognition and rejection of non-self. (a) Parabiosed fingers of sponge from the same colony are permanently united but members of different colonies reject each other by 7–9 days. (b) A xenograft of body wall tissue from the earthworm* Eisenia *onto the earthworm* Lumbricus *is completely destroyed by 50 days.*

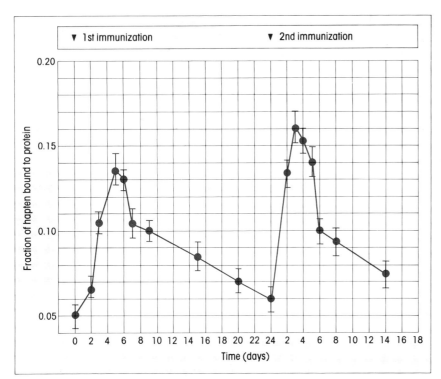

Figure 9.17. *Induction of protein specifically binding the hapten intensain after injection of earthworms with a hapten-KLH conjugate (10.5 μg for the first immunization and 6 μg for the second immunization). Each point represents the mean ± SD based upon results from at least six immunized earthworms. (Reprinted from Châteaureynaud-Duprat P. et al. (1985)* **Immunology** *56, 751, with permission.)*

diversification possibly utilizing non-functional adjoining V pseudogenes in a somatic gene-conversion-like process.

The evolution of distinct B- and T-cell lineages was accompanied by the development of separate sites for differentiation

The differential effects of neonatal thymectomy and bursectomy in the chicken on subsequent humoral and cellular responses paved the way for the eventual recognition of the separate lymphocyte lineages which subserve these functions. Like the thymus, the bursa of Fabricius develops as an embryonic outpushing of the gut endoderm, this time from hind- as distinct from fore- gut, and provides the micro-environment to cradle incoming stem cells

and direct their differentiation to immunocompetent B-lymphocytes. As may be seen from table 9.4, bursectomy had a profound effect on humoral antibody synthesis, but did not unduly influence the cell-mediated reactions responsible for tuberculin skin reactivity and graft rejection. On the other hand, thymectomy grossly impaired cell-mediated reactions and had some effect on antibody production.

The distinctive anatomical location of the B-cell differentiation site in a separate lymphoid organ in the chicken was immensely valuable to progress in this field because it allowed such experiments to be carried out. However, many years went by in a fruitless search for an equivalent bursa in mammals before it was realized that the primary site for B-cell generation was in fact the bone marrow itself (a nameless immunologist regularly slays his students by recalling that 'the bursa is strictly for the birds').

All X-irradiated after birth	Peripheral blood lymphocyte count	Ig conc.	Antibody	Delayed skin reaction to tuberculin	Graft rejection
Intact	14 800	+ +	+ + +	+ +	+ +
Thymectomized	9 000	+ +	+	−	+
Bursectomized	13 200	−	−	+	+

Table 9.4. *Effect of neonatal bursectomy and thymectomy on the development of immunological competence in the chicken. (From Cooper M.D., Peterson R.D.A., South M.A. & Good R.A. (1966)* **J. Exp. Med.** *123, 75, with permission of the editors.)*

CHAPTER 9

The immunoglobulin gene superfamily of recognition molecules

All the molecules involved in antigen recognition which we have described at such (painful!) length in Chapter 3 are members of a gene superfamily related by sequence and presumably a common ancestry. All polypeptide members of this family which includes heavy and light Ig chains, T-cell receptor α and β chains, class I and class II peptides and β$_2$-microglobulin, are composed of one or more immunoglobulin homology units. Each unit is roughly 110 amino acids in length and is characterized by certain conserved residues around the two cysteines found in every domain and the alternating hydrophobic and hydrophilic amino acids which give rise to the familiar anti-parallel β-pleated strands with interspersed short variable lengths having a marked propensity to form reversed turns —the 'immunoglobulin fold' in short.

Attention has been drawn to a very important feature of the domain structure, namely the mutual complementarity which allows strong interdomain non-covalent interactions such as those between V$_H$ and V$_L$ and the two C$_H$3 regions which form the IgG pFc' fragment. Gene duplication and diversification can create mutual families of interacting molecules such as T-cell receptors with MHC, and IgA with the poly-Ig receptor (figure 9.18). On this basis, it is not surprising that the domain homology units are turning up in other surface molecules concerned in cell—cell interactions such as T8 and Ly2 which associate in some way with class I MHC, and T4 and L3T4 which help focus the helper cell onto target class II MHC. Once a structure like that proves to be successful, the forces of evolution make sure that it is widely exploited.

SUMMARY

Ontogeny

Multipotential stem cells from the bone marrow give rise to all the formed elements of the blood. The differentiation of T-cells occurs within the micro-environment of the thymus. Differentiation to immunocompetent T-cell subsets is accompanied by changes in the surface phenotype which can be recognized with monoclonal antibodies. T-cell receptor genes rearrange in the thymus, V$_\beta$ and V$_\gamma$ early in embryogenesis and V$_\alpha$ later when the ex-

151

Figure 9.18. *The immunoglobulin gene superfamily, a series of surface molecules involved in cell—cell recognition which all share a common structure, the* **immunoglobulin homology unit,** *suggesting evolution from a single primordial ancestral gene. (a) Multigene families involved in antigen recognition (the single copy β$_2$-microglobulin is included because of its association with class I). (b) Single copy genes. Thy 1 is present on T-cells and neurones. Poly-Ig transports IgA across mucosal membranes. N-CAM is an adhesion molecule binding neuronal cells together. Other molecules now included in this superfamily are α1B glycoprotein, a human plasma protein; neurocytoplasmic protein 3 (NP3), a brain-specific molecule; OX-2, of unknown function present on lymphocytes and neurones; and the T3 δ chain. (Reprinted by permission from* **Nature 323, 15,** *copyright © 1986, MacMillan Magazines Limited.)*

pression of V_γ mRNA falls to low levels. The thymus epithelial cells 'imprint' their MHC haplotype on the developing T-cells so they are restricted to the recognition of antigen in the context of that haplotype. Deoxyguanosine destroys thymic macrophages and interdigitating dendritic cells, and abrogates the ability of the thymus to induce self-tolerance in the developing T-cells.

B-cells differentiate in the fetal liver and then in the bone marrow to become immunocompetent B-cells after passing through pre-B and immature B-cell stages. Some class-switching can occur before contact with antigen as a result of micro-environmental factors. A minor population expresses the T-cell marker CD5 (T1), or in the mouse Ly1. The sequence of Ig variable gene rearrangements is DJ, VDJ then V-J_κ and, if unproductive, V-J_λ. If the rearrangement at any stage is unproductive, i.e. does not lead to an acceptable gene reading frame, the allele on the sister chromosome is rearranged. The mechanisms of allelic exclusion ensure that each lymphocyte is programmed for only one antibody. Responses to different antigens appear sequentially with age. Very early B-cells are very sensitive to negative signals from surface receptor cross-linking which shut off synthesis of surface Ig. A high proportion of the very first B-cells to mature are idiotype—anti-idiotype pairs suggesting that network interactions may be important at this stage. Maternal IgG crosses the placenta and pro-vides a high level of passive immunity at birth. The antigen-independent differentiation within primary lymphoid organs and antigen-driven maturation in secondary lymphoid organs are summarized in figure 9.19.

Lymphoproliferative disorders

Deregulation of the c-myc proto-oncogene is a characteristic feature of many B-cell tumours and keeps them in the cell cycle. This is associated with translocation of the c-myc gene to Ig heavy or light chain loci. Other B- and T-cell tumours show different translocations but always to a locus relating to an antigen receptor. A second signal is required for malignancy since mice transfected with μ-chain enhancer linked to c-myc have hyperplastic B-cells but do not produce tumours for 6–8 weeks and even then they are monoclonal. Different lymphoid malignancies show maturation arrest at characteristic stages in differentiation. Because the B-cell tumours express the phenotypic markers of their normal counterparts, it is now possible to make a diagnosis of lymphoid malignancy based on the origin of the tumour cell using the batteries of available monoclonal antibodies and modern immuno-enzymatic cytochemical tests. The features of the various B- and T-cell tumours are discussed. Immunodeficiency often occurs because the tumour cells inhibit the development of their normal cellular counterpart.

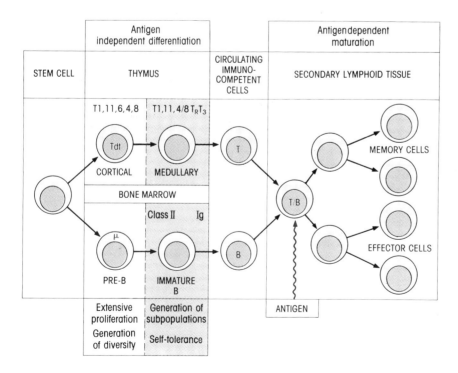

Figure 9.19. *Antigen-independent differentiation and antigen-dependent maturation of T- and B-cells. Thymocytes are also imprinted to recognize self-MHC-haplotype. Tdt = terminal deoxynucleotidyl transferase.*

CHAPTER 9

Phylogeny

Recognition of self is of fundamental importance for multicellular organisms, even lowly forms like sponges and earthworms. Invertebrates have humoral defence mechanisms and there is some evidence of inducible 'anti-some' production. B- and T-cell responses are well defined in the vertebrates and the evolution of these distinct lineages was accompanied by the development of separate sites for differentiation. The success of the immunoglobulin domain structure, possibly through its ability to give non-covalent mutual binding, has been exploited by evolution to produce the Ig gene superfamily of recognition molecules including Ig, T-cell receptors, MHC class I and II, β_2-microglobulin, T4, T8, the poly-Ig receptor and Thy 1.

Further reading

Horton J. (1985) Evolution of immunity. In *Immunology*. I.M. Roitt, J. Brostoff & D.K. Male (eds), p. 91. Gower Medical Publishing, London.

Kelly K. & Siebenlist U. (1986) Regulation and expression of c-myc in normal and malignant cells. *Ann. Rev. Immunol.*, **4**, 317.

Stein H. & Mason D.Y. (1985) Immunological analysis of tissue sections in diagnosis of lymphoma. In *Recent Advances in Haematology*, A.V. Hoffbrand (ed.), **4**, 127. Churchill Livingstone, UK.

Yancopoulos G.D. & Alt F.W. (1986) Regulation of the assembly and expression of variable region genes. *Ann. Rev. Immunol.*, **4**, 339.

153

IMMUNITY TO INFECTION
I – Adversarial Strategies

154   We are engaged in constant warfare with the microbes which surround us and the processes of mutation and evolution have tried to select micro-organisms which have evolved means of evading our defence mechanisms. In this chapter, we look at the varied, often ingenious, adversarial strategies which we and our enemies have developed over very long periods of time.

BACTERIA SUSCEPTIBLE TO KILLING BY PHAGOCYTOSIS

Bacterial strategies to avoid phagocytosis

The cell walls of bacteria are multifarious (figure 10.1) and in some cases are inherently resistant to a number of microbicidal agents, but a common mechanism by which virulent forms escape phagocytosis is by synthesis of an outer *capsule* which does not adhere readily to phagocytic cells. For example, as few as 10 encapsulated pneumococci can kill a mouse, but if the capsule is removed by treatment with hyaluronidase, 10 000 bacteria are required for the job.

Sometimes the capsule contains a molecule which actively *inhibits phagocytosis* when contact is made. Other bacteria secrete toxins which *kill the phagocytes* or enzymes which *impede* the normal operation of the *acute inflammatory response*.

Certain species which activate the alternative complement pathway manage to prevent lysis by *deviating* the site for generation of the *membrane attack complex* to a position distant from the bacterial surface. Presumably some organisms try to avoid undue provocation of phagocytic cells by adhering to and *colonizing* the *external mucosal surfaces* of the body.

The host counter-attack

The defence mechanisms exploit the specificity and variability of the antibody molecule. Antibodies can defeat these devious attempts to avoid engulfment by neutralizing the anti-phagocytic molecules and by binding to the surface of the organisms so 'opsonizing' them for ingestion by polymorphs and macrophages.

Toxin neutralization

Circulating antibodies act to neutralize the soluble anti-phagocytic molecules and other exotoxins (e.g. phospholipase C of *Clostridium welchii*) released by bacteria. Combination near the biologically active site of the toxin would stereochemically block reaction with the substrate, particularly if it were macromolecular; combination distant from the active site may also cause inhibition through allosteric conformational changes. In its complex with antibody, the toxin may be unable to diffuse away rapidly and will

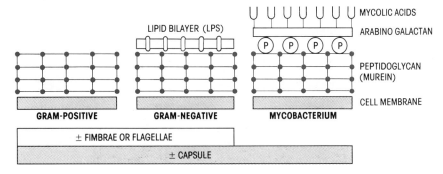

Figure 10.1. *The structure of bacterial cell walls. All types have an inner cell membrane and a peptidoglycan wall which can be cleaved by lysozyme and lysosomal enzymes. The outer lipid bilayer of Gram-negative bacteria which is susceptible to the action of complement or cationic proteins, sometimes contains lipopolysaccharide (LPS; also known as endotoxin;* composed of O-specific oligosaccharide side-chains attached to a basal core polysaccharide, itself linked to the mitogenic moiety, lipid A; 148 O antigen variants of **Escherichia coli** are known). The mycobacterial cell wall is highly resistant to breakdown. When present, capsules may protect the bacteria from phagocytosis.*

be susceptible to phagocytosis, especially if the complex can be increased in size by the action of naturally occurring autoantibodies to complexed IgG (anti-globulin factors) and C3b (immunoconglutinin).

Opsonization of bacteria

Encapsulated bacteria which resist phagocytosis become extremely attractive to polymorphs and macrophages when coated with antibody and their rate of clearance from the bloodstream is strikingly enhanced (figure 10.2). The less effective removal of coated bacteria in complement-depleted animals emphasizes the synergism between antibody and complement for opsonization which is mediated through specific high affinity receptors for IgG and C3b on the phagocyte surface (figure 10.3). It is clearly advantageous that the subclasses which bind strongly to these Fc receptors (e.g. IgG$_1$ and IgG$_3$ in the human) also fix complement well. Complexes containing C3b may show immune adherence to the CR1 receptors on primate red cells and rabbit platelets to provide aggregates which are transported to the liver for phagocytosis.

The CR1 receptors for C3b are also present on neutrophils, macrophages, B-cells and follicular dendritic cells in lymph nodes. The gene is linked in a cluster with C4b-binding protein and factor H, all of which subserve a regulatory function by binding to C3b or C4b to disassemble the C3/C5 convertases and act as cofactors for the proteolytic inactivation of C3b and C4b by factor I. CR2 receptors for C3d are present on B-cells, bind EB virus and may transduce accessory signals for B-cell activation (cf. p. 96). CR3 receptors on polymorphs, macrophages and NK cells all bind the inactivated form C3bi. Together with LFA-1 and CR4, whose function is uncertain, they form a family of two-chain proteins of which the β chain is always 95 kD molecular weight.

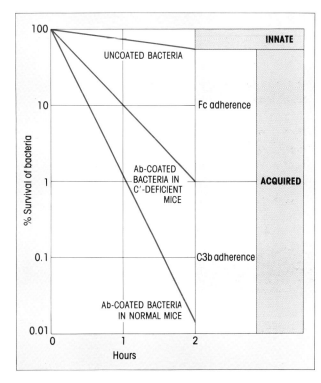

Figure 10.2. *Effect of opsonizing antibody and complement on rate of clearance of virulent bacteria from the blood. The uncoated bacteria are phagocytosed rather slowly (**innate immunity**) but on coating with antibody, adherence to phagocytes is increased many-fold (**acquired immunity**). The adherence is somewhat less effective in animals temporarily depleted of complement.*

Complexes containing C3 can be made larger and presumably more readily phagocytosed, by reaction with *immunoconglutinin*, which is an autoantibody to C3b just as rheumatoid factor is an autoantibody to IgG. It should not be confused with bovine *conglutinin* which is a non-antibody molecule which combines with the carbohydrate portion of C3b.

155

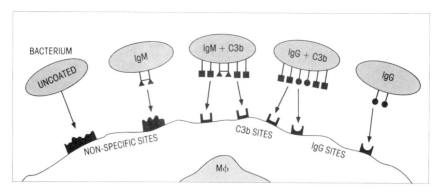

Figure 10.3. *Immunoglobulin and complement coats greatly increase the adherence of bacteria (and other antigens) to macrophages and polymorphs. Uncoated or IgM (▲—▲) coated bacteria adhere relatively weakly to non-specific sites but there are specific receptors for IgG (Fc) (●) and C3b (■, CR1 type) on the macrophage surface which considerably enhance the strength of binding. The augmenting effect of complement is due to the fact that two adjacent IgG molecules can fix many C3b molecules thereby increasing the number of links to the macrophage (cf. 'bonus' effect of multivalency; p. 61). Although IgM does not bind specifically to the macrophage, it promotes adherence through complement fixation.*

Some strains of Gram-negative bacteria which have a lipoprotein outer wall resembling mammalian surface membranes in structure are susceptible to the bactericidal action of fresh serum containing antibody. The antibody initiates the development of a complement-mediated lesion producing similar 'holes' to those caused by complement in mammalian cells (cf. figure 2.2); this is said to allow access of serum lysozyme to the inner peptidoglycan wall of the bacterium with eventual cell death. Activation of complement through union of antibody and bacterium will also generate the C3a and C5a anaphylatoxins leading to extensive transudation of serum components including more antibody, and to the chemotactic attraction of polymorphs to aid in phagocytosis as described earlier (cf. figure 2.17).

The secretory immune system protects the external mucosal surfaces

Adherence to the epithelial cells of the mucous membranes is essential for viral infection and bacterial colonization. IgA antibodies afford protection in the external body fluids, tears, saliva, nasal secretions and those bathing the surfaces of the intestine (so-called 'coproantibodies') and lung, by coating bacteria and viruses and preventing such adherence to mucosal surfaces. It might be anticipated that in order to fulfil this function, secretory IgA molecules would themselves have very little innate adhesiveness for cells, and certainly no high affinity Fc receptors for this Ig class have yet been described.

If an infectious agent succeeds in penetrating the IgA barrier, it comes up against the next line of defence of the secretory system (p. 87) which is manned by IgE. It is worth noting that most serum IgE arises from plasma cells in mucosal tissues and in the lymph nodes that drain them. Although present in low concentration, IgE is bound very firmly to the Fc receptors of the mast cell (p. 43) and contact with antigen leads to the release of mediators which effectively recruit agents of the immune response and generate a local acute inflammatory reaction. Thus histamine, by increasing vascular permeability, causes the transudation of IgG and complement into the area while chemotactic factors for neutrophils and eosinophils attract the effector cells needed to dispose of the infectious organism coated with specific IgG and C3b (figure 10.4). Where the opsonized organism is too large for phagocytosis, these cells can kill by an extracellular mechanism after attachment by their Fcγ receptors. This phenomenon, termed antibody-dependent cell-mediated cytotoxicity (ADCC) has been discussed earlier (p. 26) and there is evidence for its involvement in parasitic infections (p. 167). There are obvious parallels between the ways in which complement-derived anaphylatoxins and IgE utilize the mast cell to cause local amplification of the immune defences.

Some specific examples

First let us see how these considerations apply to the defence against infection by common organisms such as streptococci and staphylococci. β-Haemolytic streptococci were classified by Lancefield according to their carbohydrate antigen and the most important from the standpoint of human disease

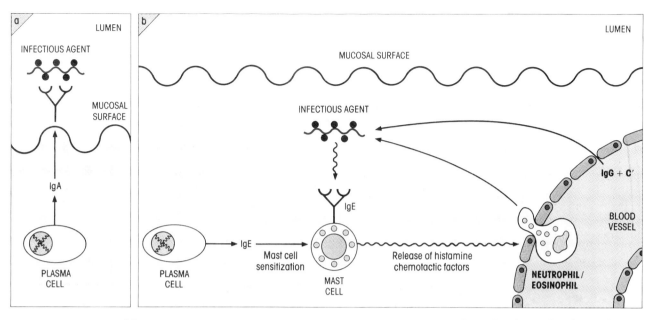

Figure 10.4. *Defence of the mucosal surfaces. IgA prevents adherence of organisms to the mucosa. IgE recruits agents of* *the immune response by firing the release of mediators from mast cells.*

are those belonging to group A. However, the most immunogenic surface component is the M-protein (variants of which form the basis of the Griffith typing). This protein inhibits phagocytosis and the protection afforded by antibodies to the M-component is attributable to the striking increase in phagocytosis which they induce. High-titred antibodies to the streptolysin O exotoxin (ASO) are indicative of recent streptococcal infection. The erythrogenic toxin elaborated by strains which give rise to scarlet fever is neutralized by antibody and the erythematous intradermal reaction to the injected toxin is only seen in individuals lacking antibody (Dick reaction). Antibody also neutralizes bacterial enzymes like hyaluronidase which act to spread the infection.

A growing body of evidence is tending to incriminate *Streptococcus mutans* as an important cause of dental caries. The organism has a constitutive enzyme, glucosyltransferase, able to convert sucrose to dextran which is utilized for adhesion to the tooth surface. Passive transfer of IgG, but not IgA or IgM, antibodies to *S. mutans* in monkeys conferred protection against caries. It is thought that IgG antibody and complement in the gingival crevicular fluid bathing the tooth opsonize the bacteria to facilitate phagocytosis and killing by polymorphonuclear leucocytes.

Virulent forms of staphylococci, of which *S. aureus* is perhaps the most common, resist phagocytosis. This may be due partly to capsule formation *in vivo*

and partly to the elaboration of factors such as a coagulase enzyme which could protect the bacterium by a barrier of fibrin. It has been suggested that the ability of a cell wall component, protein A, to combine with the Fc portion of IgG (other than subclass IgG3) is responsible for inhibition of phagocytosis by virulent strains, but IgG–protein A complexes fix complement and one study reports that protein A actually increases complement-mediated phagocytosis. We must return an open verdict on that issue. It seems to be accepted that *S. aureus* is readily phagocytosed in the presence of *adequate* amounts of antibody but a small proportion of the ingested bacteria survives and they are difficult organisms to eliminate completely. Where the infection is inadequately controlled, severe lesions may occur in the immunized host as a consequence of type IV delayed hypersensitivity reactions. Thus, staphylococci were found to be avirulent when injected into mice passively immunized with antibody but caused extensive tissue damage in animals previously given sensitized T-cells (Glynn).

Other examples where antibodies are required to overcome the inherently anti-phagocytic properties of bacterial capsules are seen in immunity to infection by pneumococci, meningococci and *Haemophilus influenzae*. *Bacillus anthrax* possesses an anti-phagocytic capsule composed of a gamma polypeptide of D-glutamic acid but although anti-capsular antibodies effectively promote uptake by polymorphs, the exotoxin is so potent that vaccines are inadequate unless they also stimulate anti-toxin immunity. In addition to releasing such lethal exotoxins, *Pseudomonas aeruginosa* also produces an elastase that inactivates C3a and C5a; as a result only minimal inflammatory responses are made.

The ploy of diverting complement activation to insensitive sites is seen rather well with different strains of Gram-negative organisms which vary in the number of O-specific oligosaccharide side-chains attached to the lipid-A-linked core polysaccharide of the endotoxin (cf. figure 10.1). Variants with long side-chains are relatively insensitive to killing by serum through the alternative complement pathway (p. 17); as the side-chains become shorter and shorter, the serum sensitivity increases. Although all variants activate the alternative pathway, only those with short or no side-chains allow the cytotoxic membrane attack complex to be inserted near to the outer lipid bilayer. On the other hand, antibodies focus the complex to a more vulnerable site.

The destruction of gonococci by serum containing antibody is dependent upon the formation of the membrane attack complex and rare individuals lacking C8 or C9 are susceptible to *Neisseria* infection. With respect to the infective process itself, IgA produced in the genital tract in response to *N. gonorrhoeae* inhibits the attachment of the organisms, through their pili, to mucosal cells, but seems unable to afford adequate protection against re-infection. This could be due to the existence of multiple cross-reacting serotypes but might also be a reflection of the ability of gonococcal protease to split IgA$_1$ dimers. Meningococci which frequently infect the nasopharynx, *Haemophilus influenzae* and *Strep. pneumoniae* have similar unfair proteases.

Cholera is caused by the colonization of the small intestine by *Vibrio cholerae* and the subsequent action of its enterotoxin. The B subunits of the toxin bind to specific GM1 monosialoganglioside receptors and translocate the A subunit across the membrane where it activates adenyl cyclase. The increased cAMP then causes fluid loss by inhibiting uptake of sodium chloride and stimulating active Cl$^-$ secretion by intestinal epithelial cells. Locally synthesized IgA antibodies against *V. cholerae* lipopolysaccharide and the toxin provide independent protection against cholera, the first by inhibiting bacterial adherence to the intestinal wall, the second by blocking attachment of the toxin to its receptor. In accord with this analysis is the epidemiological data showing that children who drink milk with high titres of IgA antibodies specific for either of these antigens are less likely to develop clinical cholera.

I thought it might be helpful to summarize the ways in which antibody can parry the different facets of bacterial invasion (figure 10.5).

BACTERIA WHICH GROW IN AN INTRACELLULAR HABITAT

Bacterial gambits

Some strains of bacteria such as the tubercle and leprosy bacilli, and listeria and brucella organisms, are able to live and continue their growth within the cytoplasm of macrophages after their uptake by phagocytosis. They defy the mighty macrophage by subverting the killing mechanisms in a variety of ways. Organisms such as *Mycobacterium tuberculosis* inhibit fusion of the lysosomes with the phagocytic vacuole containing the ingested bacterium (figure 10.6). By contrast, *M. leprae* is not bothered by fusion since its outer coat is fairly resistant to attack, while some rickettsias (and the protozoon *Trypanosoma cruzi*) slip out of their phagosome prison to lie happily free within the cytoplasm. *Legionella* are said to inhibit the respiratory burst confirming the view that if there is a mechanism available to inhibit, some micro-organisms will eventually find a way to do it.

Defence is by cell-mediated immunity (CMI)

In an elegant series of experiments, Mackaness has demonstrated the importance of CMI reactions for the killing of these intracellular parasites and the establishment of an immune state. Animals infected with moderate doses of *M. tuberculosis* overcome the infection and are immune to subsequent challenge with the bacillus. Surprisingly, if they are given an unrelated organism such as *Listeria monocytogenes at the same time* as the second infection with tubercle bacillus, they are resistant and can kill the listeria which have been engulfed by macrophages. Without the prior immunity to *M. tuberculosis* or the second challenge with this organism, the animal would have succumbed to listeria infection. In the same way, an animal immune to listeria can rapidly kill tubercle bacilli given at the same time as

158

Figure 10.5. *Antibody defences against bacterial invasion.*

Antibody to fimbrae lipoteichoic acids and some capsules	--->	Attachment		
Trigger complement through Gram – ve outer lipid bilayers	--->	Proliferation of organisms	<---	Block metabolic transport mechanisms, e.g. receptor for iron-chelating compounds
Antibody to M proteins and capsules. Opsonization via Fc and C3 receptors	--->	Avoidance of phagocytosis	<---	Neutralize immunorepellents
		Damage to host		
Antibody to toxins Neutralization	--->	Toxic / Invasive	<---	Neutralize spreading factors, e.g. hyaluronidase

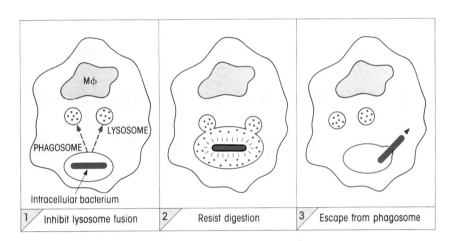

Figure 10.6. *Evasion of phagocytic death by intracellular bacteria.*

1. Inhibit lysosome fusion   2. Resist digestion   3. Escape from phagosome

a second infection with listeria (table 10.1). Thus the triggering of a specific secondary immune response to one organism may endow the animal with a simultaneous but transient non-specific resistance to unrelated microbes of similar growth habits.

This immunity—both specific and non-specific—can be transferred to a normal recipient with T-lymphocytes but not macrophages or serum from an immune animal (figure 10.7). In support of this view that the specific immunity is mediated by T-cells is the greater susceptibility to infection with tubercle and leprosy bacilli of mice in which the T-lymphocytes have been depressed by thymectomy plus anti-lymphocyte serum. In human leprosy, the disease presents as a spectrum ranging from the *tuberculoid* form with few viable organisms, to the *lepromatous* form characterized by an abundance of *M. leprae* within the macrophages. As Turk has

emphasized, the tuberculoid state is associated with an active T-lymphocyte system giving good antigen-specific transformation of lymphocytes and cell-mediated dermal hypersensitivity responses, although still not good enough to completely eradicate the bacilli. In the lepromatous form, there is poor T-cell reactivity and the paracortical areas in

Table 10.1. *Induction of specific and non-specific immunity by a CMI reaction.*

Primary infection	Tubercle bacillus		Nothing	Listeria
Challenge	Tubercle bacillus	Listeria	Tubercle bacillus	Tubercle bacillus	Tubercle bacillus
			+	+	+
			Listeria	Listeria	Listeria
Result	**Immunity**	Infection	**Immunity**	Infection	**Immunity**

INFECTION – ADVERSARIAL STRATEGIES

the lymph nodes are depleted of lymphocytes although there are numerous plasma cells which contribute to a high level of circulating antibody. Clearly CMI rather than humoral immunity is important for the control of the leprosy bacillus.

TB infection of donor	Transfer	Infect recipient with TB + listeria	Result
	Serum		**Infection**
	Macrophages		**Infection**
	Lymphocytes		**Immunity**

Figure 10.7. *Transfer of specific and non-specific immunity by lymphocytes from an immune animal. The syngeneic recipient of the lymphocytes resisted simultaneous challenge with tubercle and listeria organisms. The recipients were not immune to listeria given without the tubercle. The immunity was mediated by T-cells since lymphocytes lost their power to confer passive immunity on the recipients if treated with a cytotoxic anti-T cell serum plus complement prior to injection. Serum or macrophages were ineffective in transferring immunity (after Mackaness).*

Activated macrophages kill intracellular parasites

When monocytes first settle down in the tissue to become 'resident' macrophages they are essentially down-regulated with respect to expression of surface receptors and function. They can be activated in several stages (figure 10.8). Macrophages (Mφ) taken from sites of inflammation induced by complement or non-immunological stimuli such as thioglycollate, are considerably increased in size, acid hydrolase content, secretion of neutral proteinases and phagocytic function. If I may give one example, the C3b receptors on resident Mφ are not freely mobile in the membrane so cannot permit the 'zippering' process required for phagocytosis (p. 4); consequently, they bind but do not ingest C3b-coated red cells. Inflammatory Mφ, on the other hand, have C3 receptors which display considerable lateral mobility and the C3 opsonized erythrocytes are readily phagocytosed.

However, the ability to kill obligate intracellular microbes only comes when the cells are stimulated to a further stage of activation usually mediated by macrophage activating factor(s) such as IFNγ released from stimulated lymphokine-producing T-cells.

Striking changes on surface components accompany activation. In mouse macrophages there is an increase in class II MHC (dramatic), Fc receptors for IgG2b and binding sites for tumour cells; the mannose receptor, the F4/80 marker and IgG2a receptors all decline while the Mac-I component associated with the C3bi receptor remains unchanged. The activated macrophage is undeniably a remarkable and formidable cell, capable of secreting the 60-odd substances which are concerned in chronic inflammatory reactions (figure 10.9)—not the sort to meet in an alley on a dark night!

The mechanism of the Mackaness phenomenon now becomes clear. The specificity of the CMI lies at the level of the initial reaction of the primed T-cell with the challenge antigen which releases macrophage activating lymphokines; the non-specific immunity arises from the newly acquired ability of the activated macrophage to kill almost *any* organism it

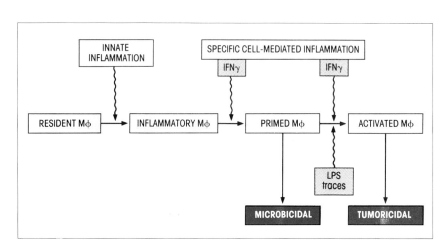

Figure 10.8. *Stages in the activation of macrophages (Mφ) for microbicidal and tumoricidal function.*

160

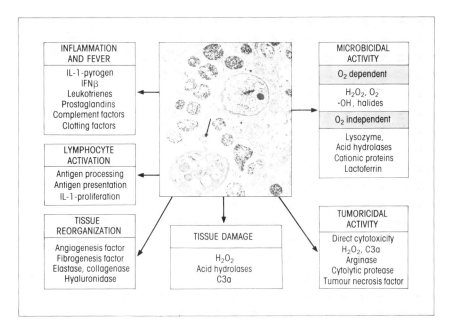

Figure 10.9. *The role of the activated macrophage in the initiation and mediation of chronic inflammation with concomitant tissue repair, and in the killing of microbes and tumour cells. It is possible that macrophages differentiate along distinct pathways to subserve these different functions.*

The electron micrograph shows a highly activated macrophage with many lysosomal structures which have been highlighted by the uptake of thorotrast; one (arrowed) is seen fusing with a phagosome containing the protozoon **Toxoplasma gondii** *(courtesy of Prof. C. Jones).*

has phagocytosed (figure 10.10). Similar phenomena have been induced in ordinary macrophage cultures treated with lymphokine preparations obtained by incubating sensitized T-cells with antigen.

Where the host has difficulty in effectively eliminating such organisms, the chronic CMI response to locally released antigen leads to the accumulation of densely packed macrophages which release fibrogenic factors and stimulate the formation of granulation tissue and ultimately fibrosis. The resulting structure, termed a granuloma, represents an attempt by the body to isolate a site of persistent infection.

IMMUNITY TO VIRAL INFECTION

Genetically controlled constitutional factors which render a host or certain of his cells non-permissive (i.e. resistant to takeover of their replicative machinery by virus) play a dominant role in influencing the vulnerability of a given individual to infection. Macrophages may readily take up viruses non-specifically and kill them. However, in some instances the macrophages allow replication and if the virus is capable of producing cytopathic effects in various organs, the infection may be lethal; with non-cytopathic agents such as lymphocytic choriomeningitis, Aleutian mink disease and equine in-

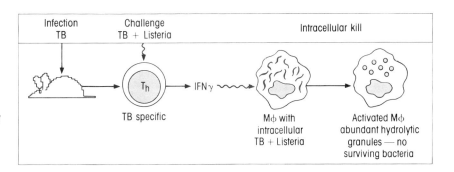

Figure 10.10. *The 'lymphokine connection': non-specific macrophage killing of intracellular bacteria triggered by a specific T-cell-mediated immunity reaction accounts for the Mackaness phenomenon.*

INFECTION — ADVERSARIAL STRATEGIES

fectious anaemia viruses, a persistent infection will result.

Antigenic drift and shift

In the course of their constant duel with the immune system, viruses are continually changing the structure of their surface antigens. They do so by processes termed 'antigenic drift' and 'antigenic shift', the nature of which may be made more apparent by consideration of different influenza strains. The surface of the influenza virus contains a haemagglutinin by which it adheres to cells prior to infection, and a neuraminidase which releases newly formed virus from the surface sialic acid of the infected cell; of these the haemagglutinin is the more important for the establishment of protective immunity. Minor changes in antigenicity of the haemagglutinin occur through point mutations in the viral genome (drift) but major changes arise through wholesale swapping of genetic material with reservoirs of different viruses in other animal hosts (shift). When alterations in the haemagglutinin are sufficient to render previous immunity ineffective, new influenza epidemics break out (figure 10.11).

Over the last 50 years epidemics have been associated with the emergence by antigenic shift of the A/PR8 strain in 1933 with the structure H_0N_1 (the official nomenclature assigns numbers to each haemagglutinin and neuraminidase major variant), A/FM1 in 1947 (H_1N_1), A/Singapore in 1957 (H_2N_2) and A/Hong Kong in 1968 (H_3N_2); note that each new epidemic was associated with a fundamental change in the haemagglutinin.

Protection by serum antibody

The antibody molecule can neutralize viruses by a variety of means. It may stereochemically inhibit combination with the receptor site on cells, thereby preventing penetration and subsequent intracellular multiplication, the protective effect of antibodies to influenza viral haemagglutinin providing a good example. Similarly, antibodies to the measles haemagglutinin prevent entry into the cell but spread of virus from cell to cell is stopped by antibodies to the fusion antigen. Antibody may destroy a virus particle directly through activation of the classical complement pathway or produce aggregation, enhanced phagocytosis and intracellular death by mechanisms already discussed.

Relatively low concentrations of circulating antibody can be effective and one is familiar with the protection afforded by poliomyelitis antibodies, and by human γ-globulin given prophylactically to individuals exposed to measles. The most clear-cut protection is seen in diseases with long incubation times where the virus has to travel through the bloodstream before it reaches the tissue which it finally infects. For example, in poliomyelitis the virus gains access to the body via the gastro-intestinal tract and eventually passes through the circulation to reach the brain cells which become infected. Within the blood, the virus is neutralized by quite low levels of specific antibody while the prolonged period before the virus infects the brain allows time for a secondary immune response in a primed host.

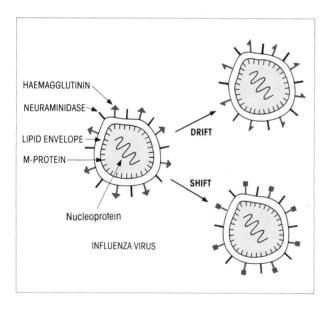

HAEMAGGLUTININ

NEURAMINIDASE

LIPID ENVELOPE

M-PROTEIN

Nucleoprotein

INFLUENZA VIRUS

DRIFT

SHIFT

Figure 10.11. *Antigenic drift and shift in influenza virus. The changes in haemagglutinin structure caused by drift may be small enough to allow protection by immunity to earlier strains. This may not happen with radical changes in the antigen associated with antigenic shift and so new virus epidemics break out.*

Local factors

With other viral diseases, such as influenza and the common cold, there is a short incubation time related to the fact that the final target organ for the virus is the same as the portal of entry and no intermediate stage involving passage through the body occurs. There is little time for a primary antibody response to be mounted and in all likelihood the rapid production of interferon is the most significant mechanism used to counter the viral infection. Experimental studies certainly indicate that after an early peak of interferon production, there is a rapid fall in the titre of live virus in the lungs of mice infected with influenza (figure 10.12). Antibody, as assessed by the *serum* titre, seems to arrive on the scene much too late to be of value in aiding recovery. However, recent investigations have shown that antibody levels may be elevated in the *local* fluids bathing the infected surfaces, e.g. nasal mucosa and lung, despite low serum titres and it is the production of anti-viral antibody (most prominently IgA) by locally deployed immunologically primed cells which may prove to be of great importance for the *prevention* of subsequent infection. Unfortunately, in so far as the common cold is concerned, a subsequent infection is likely to involve an antigenically unrelated virus so that general immunity to colds is difficult to achieve.

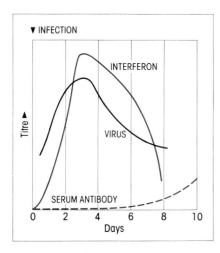

Figure 10.12. *Appearance of interferon and serum antibody in relation to recovery from influenza virus infection of the lungs of mice (from Isaacs A. (1961)* **New Scientist 11, 81).**

Cell-mediated immunity gets to the intracellular virus

We emphasized the general point in Chapter 2 that to a first approximation, antibody dealt with extracellular infective agents and cell-mediated immunity with intracellular ones. The same holds true for viruses which try to shelter from antibody in an intracellular habitat. Local or systemic antibodies can block the spread of cytolytic viruses which are released from the host cell they have just killed, but alone they are usually inadequate to control those viruses which modify the antigens of the cell membrane and bud off from the surface as infectious particles because they are also capable of spreading to adjacent cells without becoming exposed to antibody (figure 10.13). Included in this group are: oncorna (= oncogenic RNA virus, e.g. murine leukaemogenic), orthomyxo (influenza), paramyxo (mumps, measles), toga (dengue), rhabdo (rabies), arena (lymphocytic choriomeningitis), adeno, herpes (simplex, varicella zoster, cytomegalo, Epstein—Barr, Marek's disease), pox (vaccinia), papova (SV40, polyoma) and rubella viruses. The importance of cell-mediated immunity for recovery from infection with these agents is underlined by the inability of children with primary T-cell immunodeficiency to cope with such viruses, whereas patients with Ig deficiency but intact cell-mediated immunity are not troubled in this way.

T-lymphocytes from a sensitized host are directly cytotoxic to cells infected with viruses from this group, the new surface antigens on the target cells being recognized by specific receptors on the aggressor lymphocytes. Cytotoxic T-cells are less strain-specific, i.e. show broader cross-reaction, than antibody and, strikingly, of course are haplotype specific, i.e. they do not attack cells infected with the same virus but carrying different class I major histocompatibility antigens (cf. figure 4.13). They can usually be detected in the peripheral blood lymphocytes of individuals who have recovered from infection with influenza, cytomegalovirus or Epstein—Barr virus by re-exposure *in vitro* to appropriately infected cells. In the case of cytomegalovirus, for example, the targets are cells with the 'early antigen' on their surface expressed within 6 hours of infection. In fact, provided the surface antigens are expressed before the virus has replicated, as is usually the case, it is clearly advantageous for the cytotoxic cell to strike as soon as the viral antigen appears. That cytolytic T-cells may be important in viral infection in the human is suggested by studies on volunteers showing that high levels of cytotoxic activity before challenge with live influenza correlated with low or absent shedding of virus.

After a natural infection, both antibody and cytotoxic T-cells are generated and subsequent protection is long lived. By contrast, injection of killed influenza produces antibodies but no cytotoxic T-cells and protection is only short term. There have

163

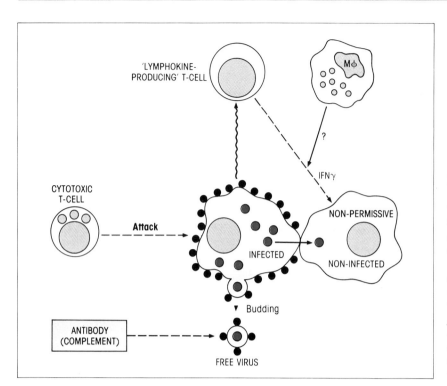

Figure 10.13. *Control of infection by 'budding' viruses. Cytotoxic T-cells kill virally infected targets directly after recognition of new surface antigen. Interaction with a separate subpopulation of T-cells releases lymphokines which attract macrophages and prime contiguous cells with interferon to make them resistant to viral infection. Free virus released by budding from the cell surface is neutralized by antibody (which is usually thymus dependent pointing to yet another contribution by the T-cell to viral immunity).*

also been some studies showing that influenza-specific cytotoxic T-cell clones can reduce lung virus titres in infected mice. Curiously, peptide fragments of the viral nucleoprotein make cells into good targets for cytotoxic T-cells which develop spontaneously during influenza infection (cf. figure 4.15).

If some viruses do escape this mechanism and manage to sidle laterally into an adjacent cell, CMI still has another card up its sleeve because T-helpers stimulated by the viral antigen can release the lymphokine IFNγ which will render the contiguous cells non-permissive for the replication of any virus acquired by intercellular transfer (figure 10.13). It may also increase the non-specific cytotoxicity of NK cells (p. 13) for infected cells. This generation of 'immune interferon' (IFNγ) in response to non-nucleic acid viral components provides a valuable back-up mechanism when dealing with viruses which are intrinsically poor stimulators of interferon synthesis.

The neutralization of free virus particles by antibody is relatively straightforward but the interaction with infected cells is rather more complex. Access to the surface antigens by T-cells would be denied were they blocked by coating with antibody. None the less, these antibodies should be able to initiate antibody-dependent cell-mediated cytotoxicity (ADCC; p. 200) and this has been reported with herpes, vaccinia and mumps-infected target cells while Oldstone has described the complement-mediated killing of measles-infected cells by F(ab')$_2$ antibody fragments via the alternative pathway. Antibody may play a different tune, however, since in the case of measles-infected cells, although 10^6 antibody molecules per cell permit complement-mediated cytotoxicity, 10^5 molecules do not kill but cause capping and shedding of surface antigen (cf. p. 141) leaving the cell resistant to attack by any immunological mechanism.

IMMUNITY TO PARASITIC INFECTIONS

The diverse organisms responsible for the major parasitic diseases are listed in figure 10.14. The numbers affected are truly horrifying and the sum of misery they engender is too large to comprehend. To be successful, a parasite must avoid wholesale killing of the human host and yet at the same time escape destruction by the immune system. In practice, each type of parasite is virtually a world unto itself in the complexity of the mechanisms by which this is achieved.

PARASITES RESPONSIBLE	DISEASE

PROTOZOA

Plasmodium vivax P. falciparum P. ovale P. malariae	Malaria
Leishmania tropica L. donovani L. brazillensis	Leishmaniasis — Tropical sore, Kala azar, Espundia
Trypanosoma cruzi	Chagas disease
T. rhodesiense T. gambiense	Sleeping sickness

HELMINTHS

TREMATODES (flukes)

| Schistosoma mansoni
S. haematobium
S. japonicum | Schistosomiasis |

NEMATODES (roundworms)

Trichinella spiralis	Trichinosis
Strongyloides duodenale Necator americanus	Hookworm
Wucheria bancrofti Onchocerca volvulus, etc.	Filariasis

Millions of people infected (log scale) — 0, 1, 10, 100, 1000

Figure 10.14. *The major parasites in man and the sheer enormity of the numbers of people infected.*

165

The host responses

A wide variety of defensive mechanisms are deployed by the host but the rough generalization may be made that a humoral response develops when the organisms invade the bloodstream (malaria, trypanosomiasis) whereas parasites which grow within the tissues (e.g. cutaneous leishmaniasis) usually elicit cell-mediated immunity (table 10.2).

Humoral immunity

Antibodies of the right specificity present in adequate concentrations and affinity are effective in providing protection against blood-borne parasites such as *Trypanosoma brucei* and the sporozoite and merozoite stages of malaria. Thus individuals receiving IgG from solidly immune adults in malaria endemic areas are themselves protected against infection, the effector mechanisms being opsonization and phagocytosis, and complement-dependent lysis.

A marked feature of the immune reaction to helminthic infections such as *Trichinella spiralis* in man and *Nippostrongylus brasiliensis* in the rat is the high level of IgE antibody produced. In man, serum levels of IgE can rise from normal values of around 100 ng/ml to as high as 10 000 ng/ml. This exceptional increase has encouraged the view that IgE represents an important line of defence. One can see that antigen-specific triggering of IgE-coated

PARASITE	TRYPANOSOMA BRUCEI	PLASMODIUM	TRYPANOSOMA CRUZI	LEISHMANIA
HABITAT	Free in blood	Inside red cell	Inside macrophage	Inside macrophage
ANTIBODY				
Importance	+ + + +	+ + +	+ +	+
Mechanism	Lysis with complement. Opsonizes for phagocytosis	Blocks invasion. Opsonizes for phagocytosis	Limits spread in acute infection	Limits spread
Means of evasion	Antigenic variation	Intracellular habitat	Intracellular habitat	Intracellular habitat
CELL MEDIATED				
Importance	–	+ (?)	+ + + (Chronic phase)	+ + + +
Mechanism	–	Direct and lymphokine mediated macrophage activation	Macrophage activation by lymphokines and killing by metabolites of O_2	

Table 10.2. *The relative importance of antibody and cell-mediated responses in protozoal infections.*

mast cells would lead to exudation of serum proteins containing high concentrations of protective antibodies in all the major Ig classes and the release of eosinophil chemotactic factor. It is relevant to note that schistosomules, the early immature form of the schistosome, have been killed in cultures containing both specific IgG and eosinophils, which induce a form of antibody-dependent cell-mediated cytotoxicity by binding through their Fcγ receptors to the IgG-coated organism (figure 10.15); after 12 hours or so, the major basic protein forming the electron-dense core of the eosinophilic granules is released on to the parasite and brings about its destruction. Further evidence for an involvement of this cell comes from the experiment in which the protection afforded by passive transfer of antiserum *in vivo* was blocked by pretreatment of the recipient with an anti-eosinophil serum. It has recently been found that eosinophils can also kill IgE-coated schistosomules but the mechanism is different because activation of the IgE (Fcε) receptors now triggers release of platelet activating factors and the eosinophil peroxidase. This dichotomy in Fcγ and Fcε receptor pathways is also evident from reports that IgE but not IgG can mediate schistosome killing by macrophages or platelets. There is no telling what will happen next.

Cell-mediated immunity

Aside from infections of cattle with the protozoon *Theilaria parva* which modifies the antigenic composition of the cells it parasitizes, no prominent defensive role for cytotoxic T-cells has been apparent. Lymphokine-producing T-cells, on the other hand, are of special importance for the activation of macrophages to kill intracellular organisms such as *Toxoplasma gondii*, *Trypanosoma cruzi* and *Leishmania* spp. which normally subvert the macrophage microbicidal mechanisms (see below). The whole effect can be witnessed *in vitro* when interferon is added to cultures of macrophages supporting the intracellular growth of *Leishmania donovani* and other similar organisms. Although lymphokine-producing cells are a vital component in defence, their balance with other cells is important. Thus, certain strains of mice are susceptible to infection with *L. major*. If their L3T4 cells are partially reduced by injection of monoclonal antibody *in vivo*, 80% become resistant, whereas an excess of an L3T4 lymphokine-producing clone specific for the organism exacerbated disease. An optimal balance of L3T4 and Ly2 cells seems essential in some way.

Eliminating worm infestations of the gut is a more tricky operation and the combined forces of

Figure 10.15. *Electron micrograph showing an eosinophil (E) attached to the surface of a schistosomulum (S) in the presence of specific antibody. The cell develops large vacuoles (V) which appear to release their contents on to the parasite (× 16 500). (Courtesy of Drs D.J. McLaren & C.D. Mackenzie.)*

cellular and humoral immunity are required to expel the unwanted guest. One of the models studied is the response to *Nippostrongylus brasiliensis*; transfer studies in rats (Ogilvie) have shown that, although antibody produces some damage to the worms, T-cells from *immune* donors are required for vigorous expulsion which is probably achieved through lymphokine activation of intestinal goblet cells (figure 10.16).

Evasive strategies by the parasite

Resistance to effector mechanisms

We have already mentioned the way in which different protozoal parasites hide away from the effects of antibody by using the interior of a macrophage as a sanctuary. To do this they must block the normal microbicidal mechanisms and they use similar methods to those deployed by intracellular obligate and facultative bacteria (cf. p. 158). *Toxoplasma gondii* inhibits phagosome—lysosome fusion by lining up host cell mitochondria along the phagosome membrane. *Trypanosoma cruzi* escapes from the confines of the phagosome into the cytoplasm while *Leishmania* parasites are surrounded by an electron-dense material which probably protects them from the oxidative burst which can nevertheless still kill them if the macrophages are appropriately activated.

Avoiding antigen recognition by the host

Some parasites *disguise* themselves to look like the host. This can be achieved by molecular mimicry as instanced by cross-reactivity between *Ascaris* antigens and human collagen. Another way is to cover the surface with host protein. Schistosomes are very good at that; the adult worm takes up host red-cell glycoproteins, MHC molecules and IgG and lives happily in the mesenteric vessels of the host, despite the fact that the blood which bathes it contains antibodies which can prevent reinfection.

Another very crafty ruse, rather akin to moving the goal posts in football, is *antigenic variation* in which the parasites escape from the cytocidal action of humoral antibody on their cycling blood forms by the ingenious trick of altering their antigenic constitution. Figure 10.17 illustrates how the trypanosome continues to infect the host, even after fully protective antibodies appear, by switching to the expression of a new antigenic variant which these antibodies cannot inactivate; as antibodies to the new antigens are synthesized, the parasite escapes again by changing to yet a further variant and so on. The same phenomenon has been observed with *Plasmodium* spp. and this may explain why, in hyperendemic areas, children are subjected to repeated attacks of malaria for their first few years and are then solidly immune to further infection. Immunity must presumably be developed against all the antigenic variants before full protection can be attained, and indeed it is known that ·

168

Figure 10.16. *The expulsion of nematode worms from the gut. The parasite is first damaged by IgG antibody passing into the gut lumen possibly as a consequence of IgE-mediated inflammation and possibly aided by accessory ADCC cells.*

Lymphokines released by antigen-specific triggering of T-cells stimulate proliferation of goblet cells and secretion of materials which coat the damaged worm and facilitate its expulsion from the body.

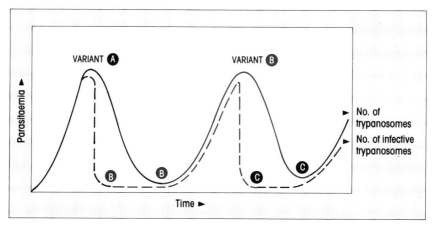

Figure 10.17. *Antigenic variation during chronic trypanosome infection. As antibody to the initial variant A is formed, the blood trypanosomes become complexed prior to phagocytosis and are no longer infective, leaving a small number of viable parasites which have acquired a new antigenic constitution. This new variant (B) now multiplies until it, too, is neutralized by the primary antibody response*

and is succeeded by variant C (after A.R. Gray, see further reading list). At any time, only one of the variant surface glycoproteins (VSG) is expressed and covers the surface of the protozoon to the exclusion of all other antigens. Nearly 9% of the genome is devoted to generation of VSGs. Switching occurs by insertion of a duplicate gene into a new genomic location.

CHAPTER 10

IgG from individuals with solid immunity can effectively terminate malaria infections in young children.

Of course, antigenic variation poses a big problem for vaccine development and a number of investigators in the malaria field have turned their attention to the invariant antigens of the sporozoite which is the form with which the host is first infected; this rapidly goes to the liver to emerge later as a merozoite which infects the red cells. The sporozoite has a characteristic antigen with multiple tetrapeptide repeats. *Plasmodium falciparum*, for example, has 37 repeats of the tetrapeptide asparagylalanylasparagylproline (NANP). Field trials of vaccines with polymers of NANP and similar tetrapeptides from other species are in progress. Because the sporozoite only takes 30 minutes to reach the liver, the antibody has to act fast so that inactivation is limited by diffusion events and hence dependent on the concentration of antibody molecules. The destruction of blood stage malaria by reactive oxygen intermediates has maintained interest in forms of therapy such as BCG and *Corynebacterium parvum* injection which non-specifically stimulate their production.

Deviation of the host immune response

Immunosuppression has been found in most of the parasite infections studied. During infection by *T. brucei*, for example, antibody and cell-mediated immunity is only 5–10% of the normal value while T-suppressor activity is prominent.

The ability of certain helminths to activate IgE producing B-cells polyclonally is good for the parasite and correspondingly not so good for the host, since a high concentration of irrelevant IgE binding to a mast cell will crowd out the parasite-specific IgE molecules and diminish the possibility of triggering the mast cell by specific antigen to initiate a protective defensive reaction.

Immunopathology

Where parasites persist chronically in the face of an immune response, the interaction with foreign antigen frequently produces tissue damaging reactions. One example is the immune-complex-induced nephrotic syndrome of Nigerian children associated with quartan malaria. Another is the liver damage resulting from T-cell-mediated granuloma formation around schistosome eggs (cf. figure 12.8). It

has even been argued that the delayed-type hypersensitivity reaction helps the eggs to escape from the intestinal blood capillaries into the gut lumen to continue the cycle outside the body, although others hold that it leads to eventual destruction of the eggs with resolution of the chronic inflammation.

Cross-reaction between parasite and self may give rise to autoimmunity and this has been proposed as the basis for the cardiomyopathy in Chagas' disease. It is also pertinent that the non-specific immunosuppression which is so widespread in parasitic diseases, tends to increase susceptibility to bacterial and viral infections and, in this context, the association between Burkitt's lymphoma and malaria has been ascribed to an inadequate host response to the Epstein–Barr virus.

SUMMARY

Immunity to infection involves a constant battle between the host defences and the mutant microbes trying to evolve evasive strategies. *Bacteria* try to avoid phagocytosis by surrounding themselves with capsules, secreting exotoxins which kill phagocytes or impede inflammatory reactions, deviating complement to inoffensive sites or by colonizing relatively inaccessible locations. Antibody combats these tricks by neutralizing the toxins, making complement deposition more even on the bacterial surface, and overcoming the anti-phagocytic nature of the capsules by opsonizing them with Ig and C3b.

The secretory immune system protects the external mucosal surfaces. IgA inhibits adherence of bacteria. IgE bound to mast cells can initiate the influx of protective IgG, complement and polymorphs to the site by a miniature acute inflammatory response.

Intracellular bacteria such as tubercle and leprosy bacilli grow within macrophages. They defy killing mechanisms by inhibiting lysosome fusion, by having strong outer coats and by escaping from the phagosome into the cytoplasm. They are killed by cell-mediated immunity: specifically sensitized lymphokine-producing T-helpers release γ-interferon on contact with infected macrophages which powerfully activates the formation of reactive oxygen intermediates (ROI) and other microbicidal mechanisms.

Viruses try to avoid the immune system by changes in the antigenicity of their surface antigens. Point mutations bring about minor changes (antigenic drift) but radical changes leading to endemics can result from wholesale swapping of

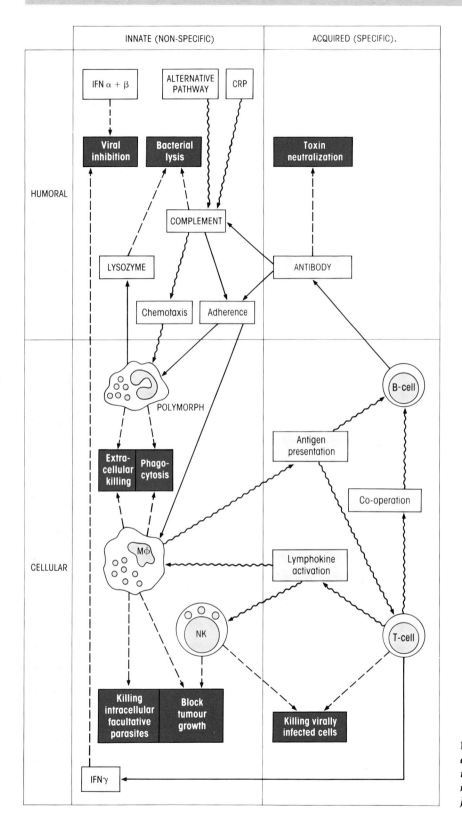

Figure 10.18. *Simplified scheme to emphasize the interactions between innate and acquired immunity mechanisms. (Developed from Playfair J.H.L. (1974)* **Brit. Med. Bull.** *30, 24.)*

genetic material with different viruses in other animal hosts (antigenic shift).

Antibody neutralizes free virus and is particularly effective when the virus has to travel through the bloodstream before reaching its final target. Where the target is the same as the portal of entry, e.g. the lungs, interferon is dominant in recovery from infection. Antibody is important in preventing reinfection. 'Budding' viruses which can invade lateral cells without becoming exposed to antibody are combatted by cell-mediated immunity. Infected cells express a virally related antigen on their surface a short time after entry of the virus and rapid killing of the cell by cytotoxic T-cells prevents viral multiplication which depends upon the replicative machinery of the intact host cell. T-helpers producing γ-interferon bathe the contiguous cells and prevent them from becoming infected by lateral spread of virus.

Diseases involving *protozoal parasites* and *helminths* affect hundreds of millions of people. Antibodies are usually effective against the blood-borne forms. IgE production is notoriously increased in worm infestations and can lead to mast-cell-mediated influx of Ig and eosinophils; schistosomes coated with IgG or IgE are killed by adherent eosinophils through extracellular mechanisms involving release of cationic proteins and peroxidase. Organisms such as *Leishmania* spp., *Trypanosoma cruzi* and *Toxoplasma gondii* hide from antibodies inside macrophages and use the same strategies as intracellular parasitic bacteria to survive, and like them are killed when the macrophages are activated by lymphokines produced during cell-mediated immune responses. Expulsion of intestinal worms requires the coordinated action of antibody and the release of mucin by lymphokine-stimulated goblet cells.

Some parasites avoid recognition by disguising themselves as the host either through molecular mimicry or by absorbing host proteins to their surface. Other organisms such as *Trypanosoma brucei* and various malarial species have the extraordinary ability to cover their surface with a domi-nant antigen which is changed by genetic switch mechanisms to a different molecule as antibody is formed to the first variant. Most parasites also tend to produce non-specific suppression of host responses.

Chronic persistence of parasite antigen in the face of an immune response often produces tissue-damaging immunopathological reactions such as immune complex nephrotic syndrome, liver granulomata and autoimmune lesions of the heart. Generalized immunosuppression increases susceptibility to bacterial and viral infections.

As the features of the response to infection are analysed, we see more clearly how the specific acquired response operates to amplify and enhance innate immune mechanisms; the interactions are summarized in figure 10.18.

Further reading

Baron S. (ed.) (1986) *Medical Microbiology*, 2nd edn. Addison-Wesley Publishers, Menlo Park, California, USA.
Capron A.R.G. (ed.) (1982) Immunoparasitology. In *Clinics in Immunology & Allergy*. Vol.2(3). W.B. Saunders, London.
Gray A.R. (1969) Antigenic variation in trypanosomes. *Bull. World Health Organisation,* **41**, 805.
Ivanyi L. (ed.) (1986) *Immunological Aspects of Oral Disease*. MTP Press, Lancaster, UK.
Mims C.A. & White D.O. (1984) *Viral Pathogenesis and Immunology*. Blackwell Scientific Publications, Oxford. (One of the best accounts of the interaction between virus and host.)
Mitchel G.F. (1987) Cellular and molecular aspects of host–parasite relationships. In *Progress in Immunology* **VI**. Cinader B. & Miller R.G. (eds). Academic Press, Orlando, USA.
Underdown B.J. & Schiff J.M. (1986) IgA: strategic defense initiative at the mucosal surface. *Ann. Rev. Immunol.,* **4**, 389.

171

IMMUNITY TO INFECTION

II – Prophylaxis and Immunodeficiency

172 The control of infection is approached from several directions. One method of breaking the chain of infection has been achieved in the UK with rabies and psittacosis by controlling the importation of dogs and parrots respectively. Improvements in public health—water supply, sewage systems, education in personal hygiene—prevent the spread of cholera and many other diseases. And of course when other measures fail we can fall back on the induction of immunity.

PASSIVELY ACQUIRED IMMUNITY

Temporary protection against infection can be established by giving preformed antibody from another individual of the same or a different species. As the acquired antibodies are utilized by combination with antigen or catabolized in the normal way, this potection is gradually lost.

Homologous antibodies

Maternal

In the first few months of life while the baby's own lymphoid system is slowly getting under way, protection is afforded by maternally derived antibodies acquired by placental transfer and by intestinal absorption of colostral immunoglobulins. The major

immunoglobulin in milk is secretory IgA and this is not absorbed by the baby but remains in the intestine to protect the mucosal surfaces. In this respect it is quite striking that the sIgA antibodies are directed against bacterial and viral antigens often present in the intestine, and it is presumed that IgA-producing cells, responding to gut antigens, migrate and colonize breast tissue (as part of the MALT immune system; p. 86) where the antibodies they produce appear in the milk.

γ-Globulin

Preparations of pooled human adult γ-globulin are of value to modify the effects of chicken pox or measles, particularly in individuals with defective immune responses such as premature infants, children with primary immunodeficiency or protein malnutrition or patients on steroid treatment. Contacts with cases of infectious hepatitis and smallpox may also be afforded protection by γ-globulin, especially when in the latter case the material is derived from the serum of individuals vaccinated some weeks previously. Human anti-tetanus immunoglobulin is preferable to horse anti-toxin which can cause serum reactions.

Isolated γ-globulin preparations tend to form small aggregates spontaneously and these can lead to severe anaphylactic reactions when administered intravenously on account of their ability to aggregate platelets and to activate complement and generate C3a and C5a anaphylatoxins. For this reason the material is always injected intramuscularly. Preparations free of aggregates would be welcome as would separate pools with raised antibody titres to selected organisms such as vaccinia, *Herpes zoster*, tetanus and perhaps rubella. This need will ultimately be satisfied when it becomes possible to produce human monoclonal antibodies on demand.

Heterologous antibodies

Horse globulins containing anti-tetanus and anti-diphtheria toxins have been extensively employed prophylactically, but at the present time the practice is more restricted because of the complication of serum sickness developing in response to the foreign protein. This is more likely to occur in subjects already sensitized by previous contact with horse globulin; thus individuals who have been given horse anti-tetanus (e.g. for immediate protection after receiving a wound out in the open) are later advised to undergo a course of active immunization to obviate the need for further injections of horse protein in any subsequent emergency.

VACCINATION

In the case of tetanus, active immunization is of benefit to the individual but not to the community since it will not eliminate the organism which is formed in the faeces of domestic animals and persists in the soil as highly resistant spores. Where a disease depends on human transmission, immunity in just a proportion of the population can help the whole community if it leads to a fall in the reproduction rate (i.e. the number of further cases produced by each infected individual) to less than one; under these circumstances the disease will die out, witness for example the disappearance of diphtheria from communities in which around 75% of the children have been immunized (figure 11.1). In contrast, focal outbreaks of poliomyelitis have occurred in communities which object to immunization on religious grounds.

The objective of vaccination is to provide effective immunity by establishing adequate levels of antibody and a primed population of cells which can rapidly expand on renewed contact with antigen. The first contact with antigen during vaccination obviously should not be injurious and the manoeuvre is to avoid the pathogenic effect while maintaining protective antigens.

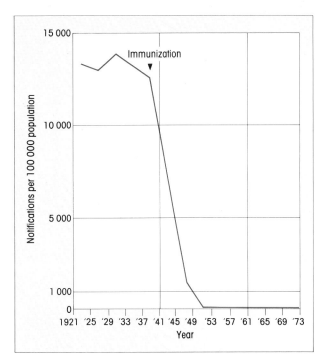

Figure 11.1. *Notification of diphtheria in England and Wales per 100 000 population showing dramatic fall after immunization. (Reproduced from* **Immunisation** *by G. Dick, 1978, Update Books; with kind permission of author and publishers.)*

173

Killed organisms as vaccines

The simplest way to destroy the ability of microbes to cause disease yet maintain their antigenic constitution is to prevent their replication by killing in an appropriate manner. Parasitic worms and, to a lesser extent, protozoa are extremely difficult to grow up in bulk to manufacture killed vaccines. This problem does not arise for many bacteria and viruses and, in these cases, the inactivated micro-organisms have generally provided safe antigens for immunization. Examples are typhoid (in combination with the relatively ineffective paratyphoid A and B), cholera and killed poliomyelitis (Salk) vaccines. The success of the Salk vaccine was slightly marred by a small rise in the incidence of deaths from poliomyelitis in 1960–61 (figure 11.2) but this has now been attributed to poor antigenicity of one of the three different strains of virus used and present-day vaccines are far more potent. Care has to be taken to ensure that important protective antigens are not destroyed in the inactivation process. During the production of an early killed measles vaccine, the fusion antigen which permits cellular

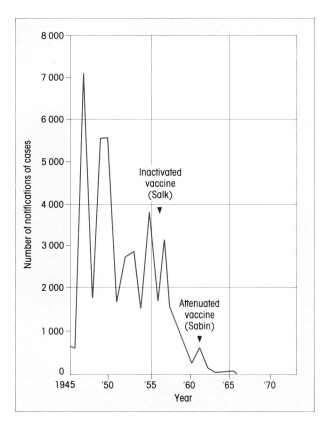

Figure 11.2. *Notifications of paralytic poliomyelitis in England and Wales showing the beneficial effects of community immunization with killed and live vaccines. (Reproduced from* Immunisation *by G. Dick, 1978, Update Books; with kind permission of author and publishers.)*

spread of virus was inactivated; as a result, incomplete immunity was produced and this left the individual susceptible to the development of immunopathological complications on subsequent natural infection. The dangers of incomplete immunity are especially worrying in areas where measles is endemic and the immune response is relatively enfeebled due to protein malnutrition. Since the widespread correction of this dietary deficiency is unlikely in the near future, it is worth considering whether non-specific stimulation by immunopotentiating drugs or thymus hormones at the time of vaccination might provide a feasible solution.

This idea of supplementing a deficient adaptive immune response with some synergistic treatment has surfaced in other contexts. Thus, the antibiotic polymyxin B is too toxic for normal use; however, if certain end groups are removed, the molecule loses its toxicity but still retains its ability to disturb the outer wall of Gram-negative bacteria thereby allowing potentially lytic antibodies and complement to reach previously inaccessible bacterial inner membranes. Another curious phenomenon which might

be exploited is the finding that the amoeba *Entamoeba histolytica*, which is resistant to lysis by antibody and complement, shows greatly increased susceptibility if treated with an otherwise non-toxic protein inhibitor.

Live attenuated organisms have many advantages as vaccines

The objective of attenuation is to produce a modified organism which mimics the natural behaviour of the original microbe without causing significant disease. In many instances the immunity conferred by killed vaccines, even when given with adjuvant (see below), is often inferior to that resulting from infection with live organisms. This must be partly because the replication of the living microbes confronts the host with a larger and more sustained dose of antigen and that, with budding viruses, infected cells are required for the establishment of good cytotoxic T-cell memory. Another significant advantage of using live organisms is that the immune response takes place largely at the site of the natural infection. This is well illustrated by the nasopharyngeal IgA response to immunization with polio vaccine. In contrast with the ineffectiveness of parenteral injection of killed vaccine, intranasal administration evoked a good local antibody response; but whereas this declined over a period of 2 months or so, per oral immunization with *live attenuated* virus established a persistently high IgA antibody level (figure 11.3).

Classical methods of attenuation

The objective of attenuation, that of producing an organism which causes only a very mild form of the natural disease, can be equally well attained by using strains which are virulent for another species, but avirulent in man. The best example of this was Jenner's remarkable demonstration that cowpox would protect against smallpox. Since then, a global effort by the World Health Organization combining extensive vaccination and selective epidemiological control methods, has eradicated the human disease.

Attenuation itself can be achieved by modifying the conditions under which an organism grows. Pasteur first achieved the production of live but non-virulent forms of chicken cholera bacillus and anthrax by such artifices as culture at higher temperatures and under anaerobic conditions, and was able to confer immunity by infection with the attenuated organisms. A virulent strain of *Mycobacterium tuberculosis* became attenuated by chance in 1908 when Calmette and Guérin at the Institut Pasteur, Lille, added bile to the culture medium in an attempt to achieve dispersed growth. After 13 years of culture in bile-containing medium, the strain remained attenuated and was used successfully to vaccinate children against tuberculosis. The same organism, BCG (Bacille, Calmette, Guérin), is widely used today for immunization of tuberculin-negative individuals; it may also bestow a reasonable degree of protection against *Mycobacterium leprae* but the circumstances in which this can be achieved have not been fully identified. Attenuation by cold adaptation of influenza and other respiratory viruses seems hopeful; the organism can grow at the lower temperatures (32−34°C) of the upper respiratory tract, but fails to produce clinical disease because of its inability to replicate in the lower respiratory tract (37°C).

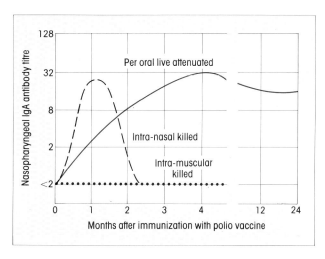

Figure 11.3 *Local IgA response to polio vaccine. Local secretory antibody synthesis is confined to the specific anatomical sites which have been directly stimulated by contact with antigen. (Data from Ogra P.L. et al. (1975) In* **Viral Immunology and Immunopathology,** *p. 67. Notkins A.L. (ed.). Academic Press, New York.)*

Attenuation by recombinant DNA technology

Genetic recombination is being used to develop various attenuated strains of viruses such as influenza with lower virulence for man and some with an increased multiplication rate in eggs (enabling newly endemic strains of influenza to be adapted for rapid vaccine production). The potential is clearly quite enormous. A new approach termed 'infection-permissive immunization', util-

izes parenteral administration of a recombinant virus which bears the relevant neuraminidase but an irrelevant haemaglutinin: the partial immunity so produced still permits natural infection but prevents the development of disease, and it is anticipated that this process will establish an effective resistance to subsequent contact with the virus.

Viral vectors for other genes

An ingenious trick is to use a virus as a 'piggy-back' for genes from another virus that cannot be grown successfully, or which is inherently dangerous. Large DNA viruses such as vaccinia can act as carriers for one or many foreign genes while retaining infectivity for animals and cultured cells, and the proteins encoded by these genes are appropriately expressed with respect to glycosylation and secretion by the infected cells. An example of a construct in which vaccinia is a vector for an inserted foreign gene is described in figure 11.4.

A wide variety of genes has been expressed by vaccinia virus vectors and it has been demonstrated that the products of genes coding for viral envelope proteins such as influenza virus haemagglutinin, vesicular stomatis virus glycoprotein, HIV-I gp120 and herpes simplex virus glycoprotein D, could be correctly processed and inserted into the plasma membrane of infected cells. Hepatitis surface antigen (HBsAg) was secreted from recombinant vaccinia virus infected cells as the characteristic 22 nm particles. It is an impressive approach and chimpanzees have been protected against the clinical effects of hepatitis B virus, while mice inoculated with the influenza haemagglutinin recombinant generated cytotoxic T-cells and were protected against influenza infection.

There is some worry about the infrequent but serious complications of smallpox vaccination although some initial animal experiments suggest that thymidine kinase negative recombinants may not be so virulent. For veterinary use, of course, there is no problem.

Constraints on the use of attenuated vaccines

Attenuated vaccines for poliomyelitis (Sabin), measles and rubella have gained general acceptance. None the less, with certain vaccines there is a very small, but still real, risk of developing complications such as the encephalitis which can occur following measles immunization; note, however, that the natural infection carries a far greater risk of

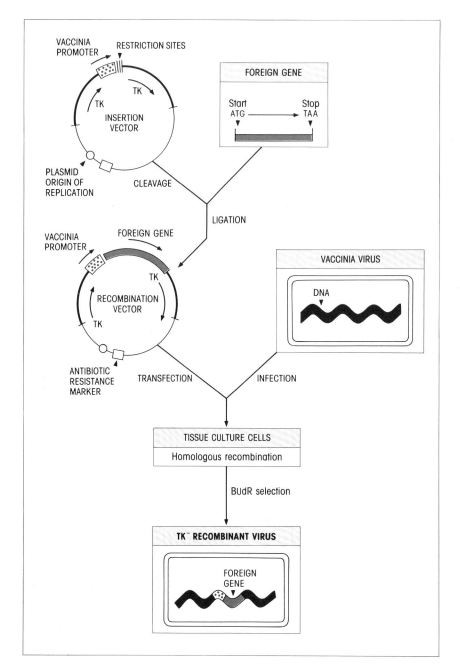

Figure 11.4. *Construction of vaccinia virus recombinants that express a foreign gene. The gene in question, say encoding hepatitis surface antigen (HBsAg), is first inserted into an appropriate vector so that it is adjacent to a vaccinia promoter and flanking vaccinia DNA sequences (in this case thymidine kinase—TK) which determines the site of recombination with the virus. The plasmid is replicated and then used to transfect cells that are simultaneously infected with vaccinia. Homologous recombination inserts the promoter plus foreign gene into the viral genome and the resulting TK⁻ recombinant is selected by picking viral plaques resistant to 5-bromodeoxyuridine (BUdR). TK is not essential for viral growth. (Reproduced from B. Moss (1985)* **Immunology Today 6, 243, with permission.)**

encephalitis (*c.* 1:2000)! With live viral vaccines there is a possibility that the nucleic acid might be incorporated into the host's genome or that there may be reversion to a virulent form, although this will be unlikely if the attenuated strains contain several mutations. Another disadvantage of attenuated strains is the difficulty and expense of maintaining appropriate cold storage facilities especially in out-of-the-way places. In diseases such as viral hepatitis and cancer, the dangers associated with live vaccines would make their use unthinkable. Generally speaking, the risk of complication must be balanced against the expected chance of contracting the disease with its own complications. Where this is minimal some may prefer to avoid general vaccination and to rely upon a crash course backed up if necessary by passive immunization in the localities around isolated outbreaks of infectious disease.

It is important to recognize those children with immunodeficiency before injection of live organisms; a child with impaired T-cell reactivity can become overwhelmed by BCG and die. Perhaps this is only a sick story, but it is said that in one particular country there are no adults with T-cell deficiency. The reason? All children had been immunized with live BCG as part of a community health programme(!). The extent to which children with partial deficiencies are at risk has yet to be assessed. It is also inadvisable to give live vaccines to patients being treated with steroids, immunosuppressive drugs or radiotherapy or who have malignant conditions such as lymphoma and leukaemia; pregnant mothers must also be included here because of the vulnerability of the fetus.

The deviating influence of maternally derived IgG antibody has been discussed in an earlier chapter. Injection of preformed (monoclonal) IgM antibody at the time of immunization with a malaria vaccine seemed to overcome this problem in young mice, but it remains to be seen whether this can be developed into a practical strategy. Preliminary results suggest that infants of 4–6 months can be seroconverted by inhaled aerosol measles vaccine which presumably evades the maternal antibody; this will have singular relevance in endemic measles areas where almost split-second timing is required with conventional immunization as passively acquired antibody wanes.

Vaccines containing individual protective antigens

A whole parasite or bacterium usually contains many antigens which are not concerned in the protective response of the host but may give rise to problems by suppressing the response to protective antigens or by provoking hypersensitivity as we saw in the last chapter. Vaccination with the isolated protective antigens may avoid these complications and identification of these antigens then opens up the possibility of producing them synthetically

in circumstances where bulk growth of the organism is impractical or isolation of the individual components too expensive.

Identification of protective antigens is greatly facilitated if one has an experimental model. If protection is antibody-mediated, one can try out different monoclonal antibodies and use the successful ones to pull out the antigen. Where antigenic variation is a major factor, desperate attempts are being made to identify some element of constancy which could provide a basis for vaccination, again using monoclonal antibodies with their ability to recognize a single specificity in a highly complex mixture. If protection is based primarily on T-cell activity, the approach would then be through the identification of individual T-cell clones capable of passively transferring protection.

The use of purified components

Bacterial exotoxins such as those produced by diphtheria and tetanus bacilli have long been used as immunogens. First, they must of course be detoxified and this is achieved by formaldehyde treatment which fortunately does not destroy the major immunogenic determinants (figure 11.5). Immunization with the *toxoid* will therefore provoke the formation of protective antibodies which neutralize the toxin by stereochemically blocking the active site and encourage removal by phagocytic cells. The toxoid is generally given after adsorption to aluminium hydroxide which acts as an adjuvant and produces higher antibody titres. In the case of cholera, a vaccine which combines the B subunit of cholera toxin with killed vibrios is reported to stimulate gut mucosal antibody formation when given orally, the response being said to equal that seen after clinical cholera. Purified pneumococcal and meningococcal polysaccharide vaccines will probably require coupling to some immunogenic carrier protein since they fail to stimulate T-helpers or induce adequate memory.

Antigens can be synthesized through gene cloning

Recombinant DNA technology enables us to make genes encoding part or the whole of a protein peptide chain almost at will, and express them in an appropriate vector. We have already ruminated upon vaccinia virus recombinants but very often we wish to utilize the gene product on its own to be incorporated into an adjuvant. As we understand it, the product secreted by yeast cells expressing the

HBsAg gene is immunogenic and likely to be available soon as a commercial vaccine. Gene cloning is economical and the potential is vast. A rather cunning way to improve the performance of a relatively weak immunogen is to stitch the gene segment encoding the hydrophobic membrane region of IgM onto the C-terminus of the antigen gene so giving the molecule an anchor to hold it in the membranes, particularly of dendritic cells and macrophages, where presumably it will be very effectively presented to antigen-specific lymphocytes. One restriction to gene cloning is that carbohydrate antigens cannot be synthesized directly by recombinant DNA technology although preliminary attempts to clone the cohort of genes which encode the cascade of synthetic enzymes needed to produce complex carbohydrates are under way.

Figure 11.5. *Modification of toxin to harmless toxoid without losing many of the antigenic determinants. Thus antibodies to the toxoid will react well with the original toxin.*

Antigens can be mimicked by synthetic peptides

Small peptide sequences corresponding with important epitopes on a microbial antigen can be synthesized readily and economically; long ones are too expensive to manufacture. Naturally, the peptide must be linked to a T-dependent carrier and incorporated into an adjuvant for immunogenicity, the latter in some examples being achieved by direct coupling to muramyl dipeptide (MDP; see below). One might predict that although the synthetic peptide has the correct linear *sequence* of amino acids, its random structure would make it a poor model for the *conformation* of the parent antigen. Curiously this does not always seem to be a serious drawback. The 'loop' peptide of diphtheria toxin, when internally disulphide linked, evokes a good neutralizing response. The same is true for a short peptide derived from the foot and mouth

virus-specific protein (VP1). A peptide sequence from polio virus VP1 induced poor neutralizing antibody but did prime the recipient for a good response to the whole organism. It may be that short peptides do not always have the conformation to stimulate adequate B-cell responses, but conceivably they could prime antigen-specific T-cells which recognize the primary sequence rather than the tertiary configuration of a protein; if the primed T-cells enable the host to mount an adequate protective response on subsequent exposure to natural infection, this could prove to be a useful prophylactic strategy.

Having said this, the evidence is mounting that the majority of protein determinants are discontinuous, i.e. involve amino acid residues far apart in the primary sequence but brought close to each other by peptide folding (cf. p. 56). In such cases, peptides which represent linear sequences of the primary structure will, at best, only mimic part of a determinant. Defining a discontinuous determinant by X-ray crystallography and site-related mutagenesis is going to take a long time and by computer analysis, perhaps even longer.

Idiotypes can be exploited for vaccines

The attempt to produce molecules which act as substitute or 'surrogate' epitopes may be of considerable importance for parasite vaccines if one wishes to separate determinants on an individual antigen that stimulate T-helpers from those which activate T-suppressors. As we have discussed, one problem with peptides as surrogate determinants is the difficulty in triggering lymphocyte receptors which recognize conformational determinants characteristic for the native rather than the unfolded protein antigen. One solution is to produce anti-idiotypes which act as 'internal images' of the determinant and therefore possess an acceptable conformation at the outset.

If the reader trundles back to figure 8.6, it will be seen that there are two main categories of anti-idiotype: Ab2α which recognize cross-reacting, presumably regulatory, idiotypes and Ab2β which are thought to behave as internal images of the antigenic determinant. In those instances where the major Id is mostly associated with a given specificity (e.g. murine T15 Id is largely present on antibodies to phosphoryl choline), then Ab2α anti-Ids could provide useful potential vaccines but, in general, the Ab2β are capable of stimulating a wider range of lymphocytes (figure 11.6). Although the internal image anti-idiotypes concerned with the majority of microbial antigens are probably rather poorly represented in the B-cell repertoire, they can be pulled out by monoclonal antibody technology and grown up in substantial amounts using the approach described in figure 11.7.

Comparison of a monoclonal anti-Id internal image surrogate for HBsAg protective *a* determinant, with a peptide composed of residues 139–147 of HBsAg also meant to mimic the *a* determinant, very reassuringly showed mutual interference in competing for antibodies to HBsAg (figure 11.8). Interestingly, the anti-Id had a higher affinity for HBsAg antisera but reacted with a smaller proportion of the available antibodies than the peptide. This suggests that the anti-Id has a better fixed conformation but is restricted in the number of contact residues available for binding to the spectrum

of antibodies in a polyclonal serum. This implies that a cocktail of monoclonal anti-Ids mimicking any given epitope would be needed for effective immunization. As a general point, it is also preferable to target immunization against more than one epitope because a single epitope can alter by mutation during the course of an infection; furthermore, a lone epitope is more likely to show up Ir gene deficiency (cf. p. 126) in an outbred population giving rise to inadequate immunity in these individuals, although if the surrogate epitope is presented on a carrier this would not pose a problem. It should be stressed that vaccines based on peptides or anti-Ids are still in a very experimental stage although both types of agent have been reported to protect chimpanzees against hepatitis B infection.

The overall strategies for vaccination are summarized in figure 11.9.

Figure 11.6. *The theoretical reactivity of anti-idiotypes to cross-reacting regulatory idiotypes (Ab2α), or those which behave as internal images of the antigen (Ab2β), with lymphocyte receptors. The final response will reflect the range of receptors switched on by anti-Id. (a) If the major Id is present on most receptors with the required specificity, a large proportion of the cells switched on by Ab2α will react with antigen. (b) If the major Id is present on receptors with many different specificities, only a small proportion of the cells switched on by Ab2α will react with antigen. (c) In most cases receptors reacting with the same epitope display a variety of idiotypes. Because Ab2β resembles the epitope on the antigen, many cells switched on by the anti-Id should react with antigen.*

180

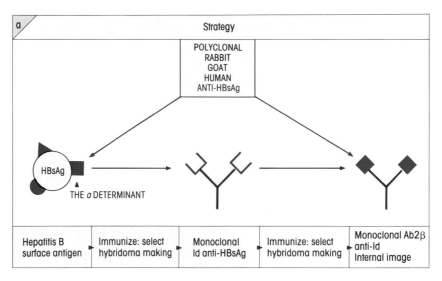

a	Strategy

POLYCLONAL
RABBIT
GOAT
HUMAN
ANTI-HBsAg

HBsAg

THE *a* DETERMINANT

Hepatitis B surface antigen	Immunize: select hybridoma making	Monoclonal Id anti-HBsAg	Immunize: select hybridoma making	Monoclonal Ab2β anti-Id Internal image

b	Identification of internal image anti-Id

Hybridoma cells making internal image anti-Id stained with **prevaccination** human serum plus fluorescent anti-human Ig	The same cells treated with **post HBsAg vaccination human** serum showing positive cytoplasmic staining
NEGATIVE CONTROL	**POSITIVE FOR INTERNAL IMAGE**

Figure 11.7. *Production of monoclonal anti-idiotype behaving as an internal image of the protective a determinant of hepatitis B surface antigen (HBsAg). A monoclonal anti-HBsAg is used to generate a range of anti-Id hybridomas; the internal image clones are selected by their ability to behave like the original antigen in reacting with a variety of polyclonal anti-HBsAg from different species. For simplicity the Ab2β is shown as identical in shape with the antigen epitope, but this need not be so; it has to be capable of substituting for the antigen to provide a sufficient number of contact points with the antibody and theoretically does not need to look exactly like the antigen; indeed when Ab2β anti-Ids mimic carbohydrate antigens or acetylcholine and other hormone agonists, they obviously cannot be structurally identical. (See Roitt I.M. et al. (1985)* **Immunology Today 6, 265,** *for a more detailed analysis.) (a) Strategy. (b) Identification of internal image anti-Id (based on Thanavala Y.M. et al. (1985)* **Immunology 55, 197).**

Adjuvants

For practical and economic reasons, prophylactic immunization should involve the minimum number of injections and the least amount of antigen. We have referred to the undoubted advantages of replicating attenuated organisms in this respect but non-living organisms frequently require an adjuvant which by definition is a substance incorporated into or injected simultaneously with antigen which potentiates the immune response (Latin *adjuvare*—to help). The mode of action of adjuvants may be considered under several headings:

CHAPTER 11

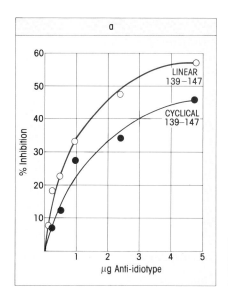

Figure 11.8. *Comparison of reactions of anti-HBsAg with monoclonal internal image anti-idiotype and peptide surrogates for HBsAg a determinant. (a) Inhibition of binding of monoclonal anti-HBsAg to the linear and cyclic peptide* *representing HBsAg residues 139–147 by anti-Id. (b) Affinities and combining capacities of polyclonal anti-HBs for HBsAg peptides and monoclonal anti-Id (from Thanavala Y.M. et al. (1986)* J. Exp. Med. 164, 227).

b				
Antigen	Anti-HBs antiserum			
	Human convalescent pool		Rabbit	
	Antibody-combining sites (pmol per 10 μl serum)	K	Antibody-combining sites	K
Cyclical 139–147	97	7.2×10^7	110	3.3×10^7
Linear 139–147	119	8.0×10^6	106	9.0×10^6
2F10 anti-idiotype	7.7	1.4×10^8	7.2	9.0×10^8
4D4 anti-idiotype	—	—	6.7	2.0×10^8
2E7 anti-idiotype	5.4	5.8×10^8	12.1	3.5×10^8
3H1 anti-idiotype	—	—	—	—

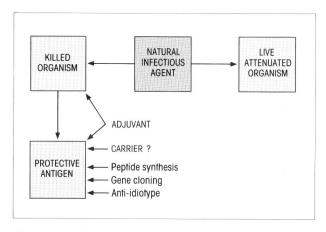

Figure 11.9. *Strategies for vaccination.*

Depot effects

Free antigen usually disperses rapidly from the local tissues draining the injection site and an important function of the so-called repository adjuvants is to counteract this by providing a long-lived reservoir of antigen, either at an extracellular location or within macrophages. The most common adjuvants of this type used in man are aluminium compounds (phosphate and hydroxide) and Freund's incomplete adjuvant (in which the antigen is incorporated in the aqueous phase of a stabilized water in paraffin oil emulsion). Both types increase the antibody response but the emulsions tend to produce higher and far more sustained antibody levels with a broadening of the response to include more of the epitopes in the antigen preparation. Because of the life-long persistence of oil in the tissues and the occasional production of sterile abscesses, and the unpalatable fact that paraffin oil produces tumours in mice, attention has been focused on the replacement of incomplete Freund's with different types of oils such as squalene or biodegradable peanut oil. It is claimed that antibody titres are comparable to those obtained with Freund's and that no long-term adverse effects in man have yet been encountered.

Macrophage activation

Under the influence of the repository adjuvants, macrophages form granulomata which provide sites for interaction with antibody-forming cells. The maintenance by the depot of consistent antigen concentrations, particularly on the macrophage surface, ensures that as antigen-sensitive cells divide within the granuloma, their progeny are highly likely to be further stimulated by antigen. Virtually all adjuvants stimulate macrophages, the majority probably through direct action, but complete Freund's adjuvant appears to act on the macrophage through the T-cell (cf. p. 103; it will be recalled that complete Freund's is made from the incomplete adjuvant by addition of killed mycobacterium, or more recently the water soluble muramyl dipeptide, MDP, isolated from its active components). The activated macrophages are thought to act by improving immunogenicity through an increase in the amount of antigen on their surface and the efficiency of its presentation to lymphocytes, by the provision of accessory signals to direct lymphocytes towards an immune response rather than tolerance, and by the secretion of soluble stimulatory factors (e.g. interleukin-1) which influence the proliferation of lymphocytes.

Specific effects on lymphocytes

The immunopotentiating and other effects of the mycobacterial component in complete Freund are so striking that their use in man is not normally countenanced; enhancement of T-cell function is seen in helper activity, delayed type hypersensitivity and the production of autoimmune disease. In man, BCG is a potent stimulator of T- and B-cells and macrophages. Levamisole boosts delayed hypersensitivity and isoprinosine is said to overcome the IL-2 defect in autoimmune MRL mice bearing the lymphoproliferative (lpr) gene while polyanions such as poly A:U, and the fungal polysaccharide lentinan, promote T-helper cells. Pertussis toxin, an exotoxin from *Bordetella pertussis*, potentiates cell-mediated immunity partly through its ability to alter recirculation of T-lymphocytes. By contrast, bacterial lipopolysaccharide and polyanions such as dextran sulphate are B-cell mitogens with a preferential effect on Bμ cells.

Although the role of modulatory leucocyte mediators such as transfer factor and interferon in these interactions is unclear, it is of interest that poly-lysine-stabilized poly-I:C, which produces good interferon levels in primates, is said to be an effective adjuvant for immunization to influenza virus.

Anti-tumour action

This will be discussed in Chapter 12 but one may summarize by saying that the major effect is mediated through cytotoxic and cytostatic actions of activated macrophages on tumours, with the stimulation of specific T-cell immunity to the tumour antigens as a further possibility.

New vehicles for antigen delivery

Recent interest has centred on the use of small lipid membrane vesicles (*liposomes*) as agents for the presentation of antigen to the immune system. It may be that the liposome acts as a storage vacuole within the macrophage or perhaps fuses with the macrophage membrane to provide a suitably immunogenic complex. Proteins anchored in the lipid membrane by hydrophobic means give augmented cell-mediated immunity. One envisages the possibility of selecting the type of lymphocyte activated by incorporating accessory signalling agents into the liposome membrane, e.g. MDP derivatives, polyanions or levamisole to stimulate T-cells, components of ascaris or *Bordetella pertussis* to exaggerate IgE production, T-cell soluble factors for the triggering of Bγ cells, C3b for homing to lymph node follicles and so on.

Another innovation is the ISCOM (immuno-stimulating complex), a matrix of a glycoside derived from the bark of a South American tree *Saponari-aquiloya molina*. Viral proteins attached to the micellar form of the glycoside through hydrophobic interactions are highly immunogenic and allow immune responses to structures which are poorly exposed in the virus particle. We should also be keeping an eye open for advances in controlled delivery of antigens using water soluble glasses.

PRIMARY IMMUNODEFICIENCY STATES IN THE HUMAN

In accord with the dictum that 'most things that can go wrong, do so', a multiplicity of immunodeficiency states in man have been recognized. These are classified in table 11.1 together with some of the most clear-cut (and correspondingly rare) examples. We have earlier stressed the manner in which the interplay of complement, antibody and phagocytic cells constitutes the basis of a tripartite defence mechanism against pyogenic (pus-forming) infections with bacteria which require prior opsonization before phagocytosis. It is not surprising then, that deficiency in any one of these factors may predispose the individual to repeated infections of this type. Patients with T-cell deficiency of course present a markedly different pattern of infection, being susceptible to those viruses and moulds which are normally eradicated by cell-mediated immunity.

A relatively high incidence of malignancies, and of autoantibodies with or without autoimmune

Deficiency	Example	Immune response		Infection	Treatment
		Humoral	Cellular		
Complement	C3 deficiency	Normal	Normal	Pyogenic bacteria	Antibiotics
Myeloid cell	Chronic granulomatous disease	Normal	Normal	Catalase-positive bacteria	Antibiotics
B-cell	Infantile sex-linked α-γ-globulinaemia (Bruton)	↓	Normal	Pyogenic bacteria *Pneumocystis carinii*	γ-Globulin
T-cell	Thymic hypoplasia (DiGeorge)	↓	↓	Certain viruses *Candida*	Thymus graft
Stem cell	Severe combined deficiency (Swiss-type)	↓	↓	All the above	Bone marrow graft

Table 11.1. *Classification of immunodeficiency states with examples.*

disease, has been documented in patients with immunodeficiency but the reason for this association is not yet clear, although failure of T-cell regulation or inability to control key viral infections are among the suggestions canvassed.

Deficiencies of innate immune mechanisms

Phagocytic cell defects

In chronic granulomatous disease the monocytes and polymorphs fail to produce reactive oxygen intermediates due to a defect in the cytochrome b_{-245} normally activated by phagocytosis. Many bacteria oblige by generating H_2O_2 through their own metabolic processes, but if they are catalase positive, the peroxide is destroyed and the bacteria will survive. Thus polymorphs from these patients readily take up catalase positive staphylococci in the presence of antibody and complement but fail to kill them intracellularly. In Chediak—Higashi disease (what a lovely name!), the lysosomes are structurally and functionally abnormal and the patients suffer from pyogenic infections which can be fatal. Among other rare conditions, myeloperoxidase deficiency is associated with susceptibility to systemic candidiasis, while a defective polymorph response to chemotactic stimuli characterizes the lazy leucocyte syndrome.

Complement system deficiencies

Defects in control proteins

The importance of complement in defence against infections is emphasized by the occurrence of re-

peated life-threatening infection with pyogenic bacteria in a patient lacking factor I, the C3b inactivator. Because of his inability to destroy C3b there is continual activation of the alternative pathway through the feedback loop leading to very low C3 and factor B levels with normal, C1, 4 and 2.

Red blood cells are bombarded daily with 1000 molecules of C3b generated through the formation of fluid phase alternative pathway C3 convertase from the spontaneous hydrolysis of the internal thioester of C3. There are three regulatory components on the red cell surface to deal with this. The CRI binds and breaks down C3b with the help of factor I. Decay accelerating factor (DAF) breaks down the C3 convertase complex. There is also an inhibitor of the formation of the C5—9 membrane attack complex. If the latter two regulators are deficient, serious lysis of the red cells occurs, a condition known as paroxysmal nocturnal haemoglobinuria (PNH).

An inhibitor of active C1 is grossly lacking in *hereditary angioedema* and this can lead to recurring episodes of acute circumscribed non-inflammatory oedema mediated by a vasoactive C2 fragment (figure 11.10). The patients are heterozygotes and synthesize small amounts of the inhibitor which can be raised to useful levels by administration of the synthetic anabolic steroid danazol or, in critical cases, of the purified inhibitor itself. ε-Aminocaproic acid, which blocks the plasmin-induced liberation of the C2 kinin, provides an alternative treatment.

Deficiency of components of the complement pathway

Failure to generate the classical C3-convertase through deficiencies in C1r, C4 and C2 has been reported in a small number of cases associated with

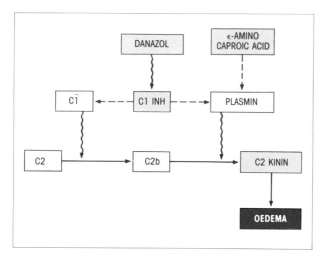

Figure 11.10. *C1 inhibitor deficiency and angioedema. C1 inhibitor stoichiometrically inhibits C̄1, plasmin, kallikrein and activated Hageman factor and deficiency leads to formation of the vasoactive C2 kinin by the mechanism shown. The synthesis of C1 inhibitor can be boosted by methyl-testosterone or preferably the less masculinizing synthetic steroid, Danazol; alternatively, attacks can be controlled by giving ε-aminocaproic acid to inhibit the plasmin.*

184

an unusually high incidence of SLE-like syndromes (cf. p. 198) perhaps due to a decreased ability to mount an adequate host response to infection with a putative aetiological agent or to eliminate antigen—antibody complexes effectively (cf. p. 207). Permanent deficiencies in C5, C6, C7, C8 and C9 have all been described in man, yet in virtually every case the individuals are healthy and not particularly prone to infection apart from an increased susceptibility to disseminated *Neisseria gonorrhoeae* and *N. meningitidis*. Thus full operation of the terminal complement system does not appear to be essential for survival and adequate protection must be largely afforded by opsonizing antibodies and the immune adherence mechanism.

B-cell deficiency

In Bruton's congenital a-γ-globulinaemia the production of immunoglobulin in affected males is grossly depressed and there are few lymphoid follicles or plasma cells in lymph node biopsies. The children are subject to repeated infection by pyogenic bacteria—*Staphylococcus aureus*, *Streptococcus pyogenes* and *pneumoniae*, *Neisseria meningitidis*,

Haemophilus influenzae—and by a rare protozoon, *Pneumocystis carinii*, which produces a strange form of pneumonia. Cell-mediated immune responses are normal and viral infections such as measles and smallpox are readily brought under control. Therapy involves the repeated administration of human γ-globulin to maintain adequate concentrations of circulating immunoglobulin.

IgA deficiency is encountered with relative frequency and these patients often have detectable antibodies to IgA. It is uncertain whether these antibodies prevented development of the IgA system or whether lack of tolerance resulting from an absent IgA system allowed the body to make antibodies to exogenous determinants immunologically related to IgA.

The most common form of immunodeficiency, late onset hypogammaglobulinaemia (also known as common, variable immunodeficiency), is characterized by recurrent pyogenic infections and probably includes many entities. The marrow contains normal numbers of immature B-cells, but a third of the patients lack circulating B-cells with surface Ig and, of the remainder, half have subnormal numbers. Where present they are unable to differentiate to plasma cells in some cases or to secrete antibody in others. T-cells are, however, also affected; each lymphocyte has a low surface 5-nucleotidase, the T_M cells lack the characteristic non-specific esterase spot, around 30% have poor responses to the polyclonal T-cell activator phytohaemagglutinin (PHA) and a small proportion have T-cells of phenotype T8⁺, MHC class II⁺ with marked suppressor activity for B-cells. An excess of such cells, revealed by their ability to suppress pokeweed-driven immunoglobulin synthesis by HLA-identical normal lymphocytes, is a feature of the chronic graft-vs-host disease which follows allogeneic bone marrow transplantation in man.

Transient hypogammaglobulinaemia of infancy, characterized by recurrent respiratory infections, is associated with low IgG levels which often return somewhat abruptly to normal by 4 years of age. There is a deficiency in the number of circulating lymphocytes and in their ability to generate help for Ig production by B-cells activated by pokeweed mitogen, but this becomes normal as the disease resolves spontaneously.

Immunoglobulin deficiency occurs naturally in human infants as the maternal IgG level wanes and may become a serious problem in very premature babies.

T-cell deficiency

The DiGeorge and Nezelof syndromes are characterized by a failure of the thymus to develop properly from the third and fourth pharyngeal pouches during embryogenesis (DiGeorge children also lack parathyroids and have severe cardiovascular abnormalities). Consequently, stem cells cannot differentiate to become T-lymphocytes and the 'thymus dependent' areas in lymphoid tissue are sparsely populated; in contrast lymphoid follicles are seen but even these are poorly developed (figure 11.11). Cell-mediated immune responses are undetectable and although the infants can deal with common bacterial infections they may be overwhelmed by vaccinia or measles, or by BCG if given by mistake. •Humoral antibodies can be elicited but the response is subnormal, presumably reflecting the need for the cooperative involvement of T-cells. (The similarity of this condition to neonatal thymectomy and of B-cell deficiency to neonatal bursectomy in the chicken should not go unmentioned.) Treatment by grafting neonatal thymus leads to restoration of immunocompetence but unless graft and donor are well matched, the thymus is ultimately rejected by the ungrateful host cells it has helped to

maturity; in any event, some matching between the major histocompatibility antigens on the non-lymphocytic thymus cells and peripheral cells is essential for the proper functioning of the T-lymphocytes (p. 137).

Complete absence of the thymus is pretty rare and more often one is dealing with a 'partial DiGeorge' in which the T-cells may rise from 6% at birth to around 30% of the total circulating lymphocytes by the end of the first year; antibody responses are adequate. Selective T-cell depression can arise from deficiency in the enzyme, purine nucleoside phosphorylase. The poor T-cell responses make these patients especially susceptible to infection with varicella and vaccinia viruses but, despite having less than 10% circulating T-cells, they have normal B-cell immunity suggesting that T−B collaboration can operate at much lower T-cell levels in the human than in the mouse.

Cell-mediated immunity is depressed in immunodeficient patients with ataxia telangiectasia or with thrombocytopenia and eczema (Wiskott−Aldrich syndrome) and it is of great interest that in both conditions about 10% of the patients so far studied have died of malignancies of the lymphoid system or of epithelial tumours. Wiskott−Aldrich is associated with a low IgM and poor antibody responses to many polysaccharides; evidence that a

185

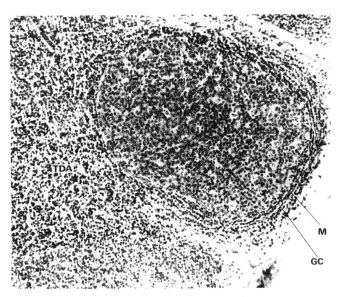

Figure 11.11. *Lymph node cortex. (a) From patient with Di George syndrome showing depleted thymus-dependent area (TDA) and small primary follicles (PF); (b) from normal subject: the populated T-cell area and the well-developed* *secondary follicle with its mantle of small lymphocytes (M) and pale staining germinal centre (GC) provide a marked contrast. (DiGeorge material kindly supplied by Dr D. Webster; photograph by Mr C.J. Sym.)*

INFECTION – PROPHYLAXIS AND IMMUNODEFICIENCY

vital defect in macrophage presentation of antigen underlies the disorder has been presented. The concomitant lack of IgE with IgA may be partly responsible for the greater susceptibility to upper respiratory infections in ataxia telangiectasia as compared with individuals deficient in IgA alone. Treatment by injection of transfer factor has been attempted and some success reported.

Isolated cases of T-cell deficiency have been described where the serum contains a lymphocytotoxic antibody which presumably must be selective for T- rather than B-lymphocytes.

T-cells from some patients with mucocutaneous candidiasis are unable to produce MIF when stimulated *in vitro* and it is conceivable that other selective failures of lymphokine synthesis may be uncovered.

Stem-cell deficiency

Without proper differentiation of the common lymphoid stem cell, both T- and B-lymphocytes will fail to develop and there will be a severe combined immunodeficiency of cellular and humoral responses. Normal immune function can be established in the children by grafting with histocompatible bone marrow from a sibling. Cells from other donors too readily initiate a potentially lethal graft-vs-host reaction (cf. p. 217) even when reasonably well matched, unless steps are first taken to rid the graft of any immunocompetent T-lymphocytes. Some patients lack the enzyme adenosine deaminase which affects both B- and T-cells but predominantly the latter. Half the patients do well on transfusions of normal red cells containing the enzyme whereas others with a longer-standing more severe deficiency which might have affected the thymus epithelium, also require treatment with thymic extracts (thymosin).

The rapidly fatal variant of severe combined immunodeficiency associated with lack of myeloid cell precursors is termed reticular dysgenesis. An attempt has been made to summarize the cellular basis of the various deficiency states in figure 11.12.

Recognition of immunodeficiencies

Defects in immunoglobulins can be assessed by quantitative estimations; levels of 2 g/l arbitrarily define the practical lower limit of normal. The humoral immune response can be examined by first screening the serum for natural antibodies (A and B

isohaemagglutinins, hetero-antibody to sheep red cells, bactericidins against *E. coli*) and then attempting to induce active immunization with diphtheria, tetanus, pertussis and killed poliomyelitis—but no live vaccines.

Patients with T-cell deficiency will be hypo- or unreactive in skin tests to such antigens as tuberculin, *Candida*, tricophytin, streptokinase/streptodornase and mumps. Active skin sensitization with dinitrochlorobenzene may be undertaken. The reactivity of peripheral blood mononuclear cells to phytohaemagglutinin is a good indicator of T-lymphocyte reactivity as is also the one-way mixed lymphocyte reaction (see Chapter 13). Enumeration of T-cells is most readily achieved by counting the number of cells forming spontaneous rosettes with sheep erythrocytes (figure 2.5e) or staining with a T3 monoclonal antibody (cf. figure 2.5c).

In vitro tests for complement and for the bactericidal and other functions of polymorphs are available while the reduction of nitroblue tetrazolium (NBT) provides a measure of the oxidative enzymes associated with active phagocytosis.

SECONDARY IMMUNODEFICIENCY

Immune responsiveness can be depressed nonspecifically by many factors. Cell-mediated immunity in particular may be impaired in a state of malnutrition even of the degree which may be encountered in urban areas of the more affluent regions of the world. Iron deficiency is particularly important in this respect.

Viral infections are not infrequently immunosuppressive, and in the case of measles in man, Newcastle disease in chickens and rinderpest in cattle, this has been attributed to a direct cytotoxic effect of virus on the lymphoid cells. In lepromatous leprosy and malarial infection there is evidence for a constraint on immune responsiveness imposed by distortion of the normal lymphoid traffic pathways and, additionally, in the latter instance, macrophage function appears to be aberrant. Plasma factors from patients with secondary syphilis which block phytohaemagglutinin transformation of lymphocytes from normal subjects could be responsible for the general reduction in CMI seen in this disease.

Many agents such as X-rays, cytotoxic drugs and corticosteroids, although often used in a non-immunological context, can none the less have dire

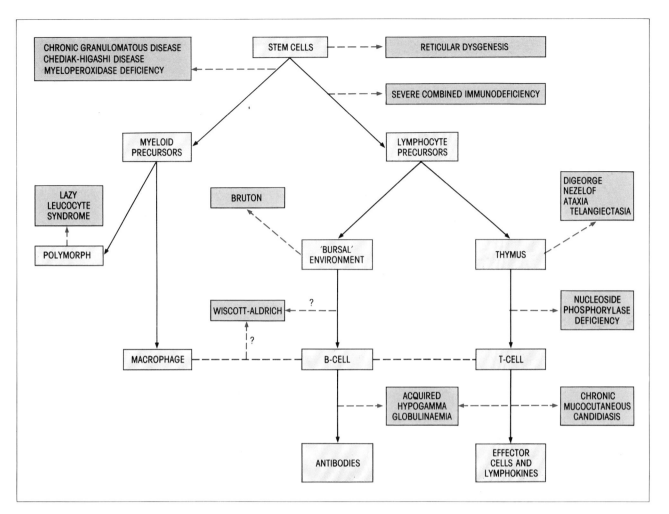

Figure 11.12. *The cellular basis of immunodeficiency states. The arrow indicates the cell type or differentiation process which is defective.*

effects on the immune system (p. 224). B-lymphoproliferative disorders like chronic lymphatic leukaemia, myeloma and Waldenström's macroglobulinaemia are associated with varying degrees of hypo-γ-globulinaemia and impaired antibody responses. Their common infections with pyogenic bacteria contrast with the situation in Hodgkin's disease where the patients display all the hallmarks of defective cell-mediated immunity—susceptibility to tubercle bacillus, *Brucella*, *Cryptococcus* and herpes zoster virus.

Acquired immunodeficiency syndrome (AIDS)

AIDS is a particularly unpleasant fatal disease which is beginning to look as though it will achieve endemic proportions and has thereby caused widespread alarm (and knowledge of immunology) amongst the public. In parts of Africa where the incidence is alarming, transmission is largely by heterosexual contact, but in the remainder of the world, the majority of cases so far have occurred in male homosexuals with other groups at risk including intravenous drug abusers, haemophiliacs receiving factor VIII derived from pooled plasma and infants of sexually promiscuous or drug-addicted mothers. None the less, the number of infected heterosexuals is steadily increasing. A mortality rate of 80% within 2 years accounts for the severity of the disease. Death is usually due to pulmonary infection, but serious complications involving the nervous system are appearing in about 30% of cases. In essence, there is a sudden onset of immunodeficiency associated with opportunistic infections involving, most commonly, *Pneumocystis carinii*, but also cytomegalovirus (figure 11.13), EB and herpes simplex viruses, fungi such as *Candida*, *Aspergillus* and *Cryptococcus*, and the protozoon *Toxoplasma*: additionally, there is exceptional susceptibility for Kaposi's sarcoma. There is also an AIDS-related complex characterized by fever, weight loss and lymphadenopathy.

AIDS results from infection by a human immunodeficiency virus (HIV)

Transmission of the disease is through infection with blood or semen containing the LAV/HTLV-III virus which has been isolated from various body fluids of AIDS patients (LAV = lymphadenopathy associated virus; HTLV-III = human T-lymphotrophic virus; because of failure to agree nomenclature, it is now likely to be called HIV-I). HTLV-III was so named because of its resemblence to the oncogenic virus HTLV-I (and its relative HTLV-II) which is closely linked to the production of a T-cell leukaemia of high prevalence in Japan. Whereas HTLV-I induces lymphoproliferation, LAV/HTLV-III is a member of the lentivirus group which cause destruction of the cells they infect; these include a simian TLV isolated from the African green monkey and thought by some to provide a possible gene pool from which the AIDS virus might have arisen, the visna virus responsible for cns and lung lesions in sheep, and viruses which cause equine infectious anaemia and caprine arthritis. All are RNA retroviruses which utilize a reverse transcriptase to convert their genetic RNA into the corresponding DNA which is integrated into the host cell. HIV-I is a budding virus whose genome has been characterized and its structure established (figure 11.14).

The AIDS infection depletes helper-T-cells

The T4 (CD4) molecule on helper–inducer T-cells is the surface receptor which enables the AIDS virus to bind to and infect lymphocytes. This results in a drastic and often complete destruction of the helper-cell population with a corresponding fall in the peripheral blood T4 count (figure 11.15), and a drop in the T4 : T8 ratio since T8 cells are largely unaffected.

How this comes about is not as obvious as one would imagine. Although HIV-I is cytopathic for T-cells, only 1 in 10^4 to 1 in 10^5 of the surviving peripheral T4 cells in AIDS patients are positive for the viral genome. Suggested mechanisms include deletion of a critical subpopulation required for survival of the whole T4 set, or production of a substance with lymphotoxic properties; autoantibodies to lymphocytes appear in a high percentage of AIDS patients but there is no evidence that they are cytotoxic. The consequences for cell-mediated immune responses as exemplified by the depressed delayed-type skin reactivity to common antigens (figure 11.16) and the failure to produce cytomegalovirus-specific cytotoxic T-cells, are quite devastating and leave the patient wide open to diseases caused by normally non-pathogenic (i.e. opportunistic) agents such as *Pneumocystis carinii* and cytomegalovirus.

Figure 11.13. *Viral pneumonia due to cytomegalovirus; radiograph showing extensive diffuse pneumonitis in both lung fields, characteristic of viral infection. (Reproduced from **Infectious Diseases Illustrated**, Lambert H.P. and Farrar W.E. (eds) (1982) p.2.2. W.B. Saunders and Gower Medical Publishing, with permission.)*

188

Figure 11.14. *Characteristics of the HIV-I(LAV/HTLV-III) AIDS virus. (a) HIV-I genome. LTR = long terminal repeats concerned in regulation of viral expression; TAT = trans-acting activator essential for viral replication and expression. (b) HIV-I structure. (c) Electron micrograph of CBL-1 isolate of human immunodeficiency virus type I (HIV-I), isolated from patient with lymphoma. Mature and budding virus particles can be seen at the surface of CCRF-CEM human leukaemia cells that are used for HIV-I propagation. Colloidal gold particles indicate binding of human serum antibodies from an AIDS patient. (× 121 500.) (Courtesy of D. Robertson & R. A. Weiss.)*

AIDS patients also have hypergammaglobulinae-mia and large numbers of B-cells which spontane-ously secrete Ig in culture suggesting that they are polyclonally stimulated; this would make them re-fractory to immunization with new antigens or to triggering stimuli from anti-IgM. The polyclonal activation might be a result of the ability of AIDS virus to infect follicular dendritic cells, or of the

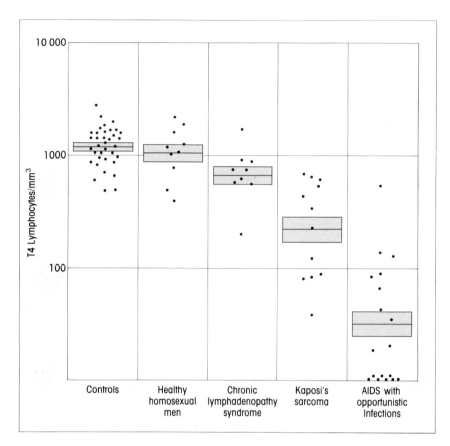

Figure 11.15. *Absolute levels of circulating CD4 (T4) positive lymphocytes in patients with AIDS, Kaposi's sarcoma and chronic lymphadenopathy syndrome. Each point represents an individual patient. (From Lane H.C. et al. (1985)* **Amer. J. Med.** *78, 417–22.)*

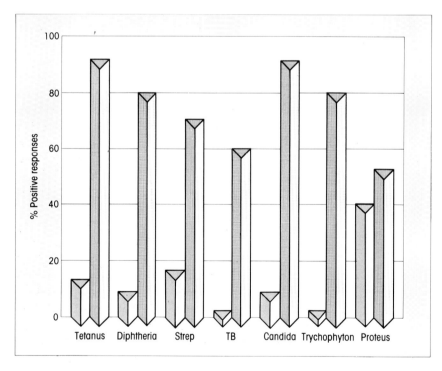

Figure 11.16. *Skin test reactivity to common microbial antigens among AIDS patients (□; n=20) and controls (□; n=10). Other studies with more advanced patients have reported completely negative skin tests. (Reproduced from Lane H.C. & Fauci A.S. (1985)* **Ann. Rev. Immunol.** *3, 477, with permission.)*

production of some T-cell factor, or stimulation by viruses such as EBV and cytomegalovirus which cannot be controlled by the ailing T-cells.

Diagnosis of AIDS

An individual with opportunistic infections, lymphopenia, low T4 but relatively normal T8 in the peripheral blood, raised IgG and IgA levels and poor skin tests to common recall antigens may well have AIDS particularly if they come from a group at risk. Confirmation comes from lymph node biopsy, and the demonstration of viral antibodies by enzyme-linked immunosorbent assay (ELISA) or by 'immunoblotting' (cf. pp. 76 and 79). Positive isolation of HIV-I is it—finito.

The control of AIDS

After inadvertent transfusion of infected plasma, the first antibodies to appear are directed to the p110 envelope glycoprotein; antibodies to core proteins p25 and 18 may be seen later. Most antibodies are non-neutralizing in that they fail to prevent infection of susceptible cells in culture, and in the rare instances when they are neutralizing, the titres are disappointingly low. If the molecule concerned in binding to the T4 on the helper cells is fashioned after MHC class II which also recognizes T4, it may be difficult if not impossible to produce an immune response to it because of self-tolerance. Furthermore, the p110 gene seems rather jumpy with respect to mutation. Thus it is not certain that finding a suitable vaccine is going to be that easy.

Immunological reconstitution with matched bone marrow only gives transient improvement. Trials are underway with recombinant immunostimulators, IL-2 and IFNγ. The reverse transcriptase enzyme ought to be a good target for anti-viral therapy with drugs like suramin and ribavarin.

A change in social behaviour patterns must make a difference to the spread of AIDS. Some religious fanatics hail the disease as God's answer to declining morals but that does seem rather hard on the haemophiliacs. However, it does look as though for the time being we should be 'good boys and girls'.

SUMMARY

Passive immunity can be acquired by maternal antibodies or from homologous pooled γ-globulin. Horse antisera are more restricted because of the danger of serum sickness. Active immunization provides a protective state through contact with a harmless form of the disease organism. Killed bacteria and viruses are easy to obtain and have been used widely. However, in many cases live attenuated organisms have the advantages that by replication they provide the host with a bigger antigen challenge and by behaving as the natural infecting agent, the most useful type of response in the appropriate location in the body is achieved. Live viruses such as vaccinia can be used as a piggyback for immunizing with genes from other viruses which are more difficult to grow or are inherently dangerous. Attenuated vaccines run the risk of reverting to the virulent form. They must *never* be used with immunocompromised hosts.

Whole organisms have a multiplicity of antigens some of which are not protective, may induce hypersensitivity or might even be frankly immunosuppressive. It makes sense in these cases to use purified components and there is greatly increased use of recombinant DNA technology to produce these antigens. There is great interest in the possibility of using either synthetic peptides or monoclonal internal image anti-idiotypes as vaccines. These have the advantage that they mimic single antigenic determinants and may avoid induction of T-suppression or even of autoimmunity when certain whole antigens are employed. Both approaches are still in the experimental stage so far as large-scale immunization of human populations is concerned.

Adjuvants work by producing depots of antigen, and by activating macrophages; they sometimes have direct effects on lymphocytes. New methods of delivery include linking the antigen to small lipid membrane vesicles (liposomes) or a special glycoside matrix (ISCOM).

Primary immunodeficiency states in the human occur, albeit somewhat rarely, as a result of a defect in almost any stage of differentiation in the whole immune system. Defects in phagocytic cells, the complement pathways or the B-cell system lead in particular to infection with bacteria which are disposed of by opsonization and phagocytosis. Patients with T-cell deficiencies are susceptible to viruses and moulds which are normally eradicated by cell-mediated immunity.

Immunodeficiency may arise as a secondary consequence of malnutrition, lymphoproliferative disorders, agents such as X-rays and cytotoxic drugs and viral infections. The most notorious of these involves the LAV/HTLV-III (now called HIV-I) retrovirus which causes the acquired immunodeficiency syndrome (AIDS) in which attack by the virus on CD4 (T4) helper T-cells destroys the ability to give a cell-mediated immune response and leaves the patient open to infection with opportunist organisms such as *Pneumocystis carinii* and cytomegalovirus which can kill. Poor to non-existent neutralizing antibodies to the AIDS virus are made during an infection.

Further reading

Bell R. & Torrigiani G. (eds) (1986) *Progress Towards Better Vaccines.* Oxford University Press, Oxford.

Chandra R.K. (ed.) (1983) *Primary and Secondary Immunodeficiency Disorders.* Churchill Livingstone, Edinburgh, UK.

Dick G. (1986) *Practical Immunization.* MTP Press, Lancaster, UK.

Gallo R.C. & Chayt K.J. (1987) Human T-lymphotropic virus type III. *Hematologic Pathol.,* **1**, 1.

Gluckman J.C., Klatzmann D. & Montagnier L. (1986) Lymphadenopathy-associated virus infection and AIDS. *Ann. Rev. Immunol.,* **4**, 97.

Porter R. & Whelan J. (eds) (1986) Synthetic Peptides as Antigens. *Ciba Foundation Symposium,* **119**. Wiley, Chichester, UK.

Roitt I.M. (ed.) (1984) New Trends in Vaccines. In *Immune Intervention,* **1**. Academic Press, London.

Warren H.S., Vogel F.R. & Chedid L.A. (1986) Current status of immunological adjuvants. *Ann. Rev. Immunol.,* **4**, 369.

Wells J.V. & Nelson D.S. (eds) (1986) *Clinical Immunology Illustrated.* Williams & Wilkins, Sydney.

WHO/IUIS Report (1982) Appropriate uses of human Ig in clinical practice. *Bull. World Health Organisation,* **60**, 43.

HYPERSENSITIVITY

An inappropriate immune response can lead to tissue damage

When an individual has been immunologically primed, further contact with antigen leads to secondary boosting of the immune response. However, the reaction may be excessive and lead to gross tissue damage (*hypersensitivity*) if the antigen is present in relatively large amounts or if the humoral and cellular immune state is at a heightened level. It should be emphasized that the mechanisms underlying these inappropriate reactions are those normally employed by the body in combating infection as discussed in Chapter 10. We speak of *hypersensitivity reactions* and a state of *hypersensitivity*. Coombs and Gell defined four types of hypersensitivity, to which can be added a fifth, viz. 'stimulatory', which they mention. Types I, II, III and V depend on the interaction of antigen with humoral antibody and tend to be called 'immediate' type reactions although some are more immediate than others! Type IV involves receptors bound to the lymphocyte surface and because of the longer time course this has in the past been referred to as 'delayed-type sensitivity'.

TYPE I—ANAPHYLACTIC HYPERSENSITIVITY

The phenomenon of anaphylaxis

A single injection of 1 mg of an antigen such as egg albumin into a guinea-pig has no obvious effect. However, if the injection is repeated two to three weeks later, the sensitized animal reacts very dramatically with the symptoms of generalized anaphylaxis; almost immediately the guinea-pig begins to wheeze and within a few minutes dies from asphyxia. Examination shows intense constriction of the bronchioles and bronchi and generally there is (i) contraction of smooth muscle and (ii) dilatation of capillaries. Similar reactions can occur in human subjects and have been observed following wasp and bee stings or injections of penicillin in appropriately sensitive individuals. In many instances only a timely intravenous injection of adrenaline to counter the smooth muscle contraction and capillary dilatation can prevent death.

Sir Henry Dale recognized that histamine mimics the systemic changes of anaphylaxis and furthermore that the uterus from a sensitized guinea-pig releases histamine and contracts on exposure to antigen (Schultz–Dale technique). Serum from such an animal can passively sensitize the uterus from a normal guinea-pig so that it, too, will contract on addition of the specific antigen. Contraction is associated with an explosive degranulation of the mast cells (figure 1.13) which is responsible for the release of histamine and a number of other mediators (figure 1.14). Passive transfer of anaphylactic sensitivity can be observed locally in the skin using Ovary's *passive cutaneous anaphylaxis* (PCA) technique; high dilutions of guinea-pig serum containing anaphylactic antibodies may be injected into the skin of a normal animal and following the intravenous injection of antigen with a dye such as Evans' Blue, the anaphylactic reaction in the skin will lead to release of vasoactive amines and hence a local 'blueing'.

Cross-linking of IgE receptors triggers mast cells

Two main types of mast cell have been recognized, exemplified in the rat by those in the intestinal mucosa and those in the peritoneum and other connective tissue sites. They differ in a number of respects, for example in the type of protease and proteoglycan in their granules, and in the proliferative response of the mucosal mast cell to the T-cell lymphokine IL-3. However, both types display a high affinity receptor for the $C\varepsilon2 : C\varepsilon3$ junction region of IgE Fc, a property shared with their circulating counterpart, the basophil. The strength of binding to the mast cell is evident from the retention of IgE antibodies at a site of intradermal injection for several weeks; IgG4 in the human also binds to the mast cell receptor but more weakly and disperses from the injection site within a day or so. It has long been established that the anaphylactic antibodies in the human are mainly of the IgE class.

The IgE receptor has been purified from a rat basophilic leukaemia line and has the structure shown in figure 12.1. Cross-linking of IgE antibodies bound to a mast cell by a divalent hapten will trigger mediator release; trimers are more effective and tetramers even more so. Degranulation is also induced when the IgE is cross-linked with anti-IgE but univalent (Fab) anti-IgE is inactive. That the critical event is the cross-linking of the receptors themselves is clearly shown by the ability of antibodies raised against the receptor to trigger the mast cell (figure 12.2).

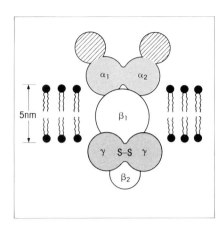

Figure 12.1. *Diagram of receptor for IgE. The α chain binds IgE. Its carbohydrate portion is shaded. The β chain traverses the membrane and the two covalently linked γ chains are facing the cytoplasm. (Reproduced from Metzger H. et al. (1986)* **Ann. Rev. Immunol. 4, 419,** *with permission.* © *1986 by Annual Reviews Inc.)*

Bridging of receptors is rapidly followed by the breakdown of phosphatidyl inositol to inositol triphosphate (IP3), the generation of diacylglycerol and an increase in intracytoplasmic free calcium (figure 12.3). Since inhibitors of methyltransferases and serine esterases inhibit all these events and mediator release, it is assumed that activation of these enzymes by receptor bridging is the initial event. Phospholipase c activation generates both IP3 (cf. activation of B-cells, p. 94), which mobilizes intracellular Ca^{2+}, and diacylglycerol which in turn activates protein kinase c. The biochemical cascade produces membrane-active 'fusogens' such as lysophosphatidic acid which may facilitate granular membrane fusion and degranulation, and the series of arachidonic acid metabolites formed by the cyclo-oxygenase and lipoxygenase pathways (cf. figure

Figure 12.2. *Cross-linking of IgE receptors either by divalent hapten or antibody to the receptors themselves leads to mast cell degranulation.*

194

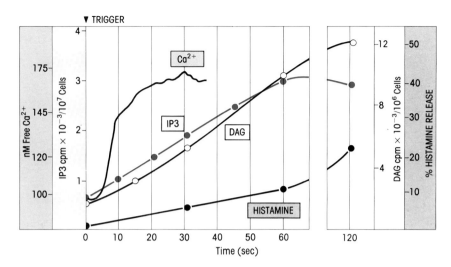

▼ TRIGGER

Figure 12.3. *Mast cell triggering: time course of changes in cytoplasmic Ca²⁺, formation of diacylglycerol (DAG) and inositol triphosphate (IP3) and release of histamine from IL-3 dependent mouse mast cell line PT-18 sensitized with monoclonal IgE anti-DNP (dinitrophenyl) and triggered with* a multivalent DNP-human serum albumin conjugate. *(Combined data taken from Ishizaka T., White J.R. & Saito H. (1986)* In **Progress in Immunology VI**, *p.870, Cinader B. and Miller R.G. (eds). Academic Press, with permission.)*

1.14). To recapitulate, the preformed mediators released from the granules include histamine, heparin, eosinophil and neutrophil chemotactic factors, and platelet activating factor, while leukotrienes B4, C4 and D4, prostaglandins and thromboxanes are all newly synthesized. The role of cyclic AMP is uncertain: receptor bridging produces a short-lived rise in cAMP but a preformed high level of cAMP inhibits receptor-induced degranulation.

Under normal circumstances, these mediators help to orchestrate the development of a defensive acute inflammatory reaction (and in this context let us not forget that C3a and C5a can also trigger mast cells although not through IgE receptors). When there is a massive release of these mediators under abnormal conditions as in atopic disease, their bronchoconstrictive and vasodilatory effects predominate and become distinctly threatening.

Atopic allergy

Nearly 10% of the population suffer to a greater or lesser degree with allergies involving localized anaphylactic reactions to extrinsic allergens such as grass pollens, animal danders, the faeces from mites in house dust (figure 12.4) and so on. Contact of the allergen with cell-bound IgE in the bronchial tree, the nasal mucosa and the conjunctival tissues releases mediators of anaphylaxis and produces the symptoms of asthma or hay fever as the case may be (figure 12.5).

Awareness of the importance of sensitization to food allergens in the gut has increased dramatically. Contact of the food with specific IgE on mast cells in the gastro-intestinal tract may produce local reactions such as diarrhoea and vomiting or may allow the allergen to enter the body by causing a change in gut permeability through mediator release; the allergen may complex with antibodies and cause

Figure 12.4. *House dust mite—a major cause of allergic disease. The electron micrograph shows the rather nasty looking mite graced by the name* **Dermatophagoides pteryonyssinus** *and faecal pellets on the bottom left which is the major source of allergen. The biconcave pollen grains (top left) shown for comparison indicate the size of particle which can become airborne and reach the lungs. The mite itself is much too large for that. (Reproduced by courtesy of Dr E. Tovey.)*

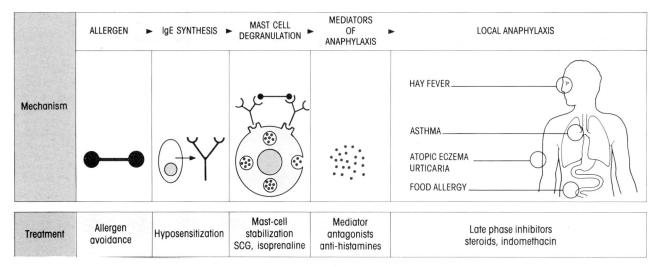

Mechanism	ALLERGEN ►	IgE SYNTHESIS ►	MAST CELL DEGRANULATION ►	MEDIATORS OF ANAPHYLAXIS ►	LOCAL ANAPHYLAXIS

Mechanism row illustration with: HAY FEVER, ASTHMA, ATOPIC ECZEMA URTICARIA, FOOD ALLERGY

Treatment	Allergen avoidance	Hyposensitization	Mast-cell stabilization SCG, isoprenaline	Mediator antagonists anti-histamines	Late phase inhibitors steroids, indomethacin

Figure 12.5. *Atopic allergies: sites of local anaphylaxis and possible therapies.*

distal lesions by depositing in the joints, for example, or it may diffuse freely to other sensitized sites such as skin (figure 12.8b) or lungs where it will cause a further local anaphylactic reaction. Thus eating strawberries may produce urticarial reactions and egg may precipitate an asthmatic attack in appropriately sensitized individuals. The role of the sensitized gut acting as a 'gate' to allow entry of allergens is strongly suggested by experiments in which oral sodium cromoglycate, a mast cell stabilizer, prevents subsequent asthma after ingestion of the provoking food (figure 12.6).

There is a strong familial predisposition to the development of atopic allergy (figure 12.7a) but although this is linked to inheritance of a given HLA haplotype within any one family, no association with specific HLA types has so far come to light. One factor seems to be the overall ability to synthesize the IgE isotype, the higher the level of IgE in the blood the greater the likelihood of becoming atopic (figure 12.7b). Curiously, it is said that patients with allergy are less likely than their non-atopic counterparts to develop tumours.

Clinical tests for allergy

Sensitivity is normally assessed by the response to intradermal challenge with antigen. The release of histamine and other mediators rapidly produces a wheal and erythema (figure 12.8a), maximal within 30 minutes and then subsiding. The responsible IgE antibodies can be demonstrated by passive cutaneous anaphylaxis by testing the ability of patient's serum to passively sensitize the skin of normal

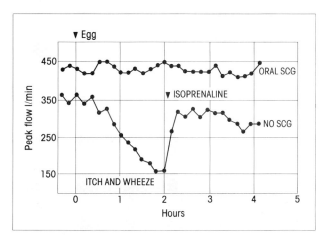

Figure 12.6. *The role of gut sensitivity in the development of asthma to food allergens. A patient challenged by feeding with egg developed asthma within hours as shown here by the depressed lung function test of measuring peak air flow; the symptoms at the end organ stage were counteracted by isoprenaline. However, oral sodium cromoglycate (SCG) which prevents antigen-specific mast cell triggering, also prevented the onset of asthma after oral challenge with egg. Note that SCG taken orally has no effect on the response of an asthmatic to inhaled allergen. (From Brostoff J. (1986) In* Food Allergy, *p.441, Brostoff J. and Challacombe S.J. (eds), Baillière Tindall, reproduced with permission.)*

humans (Praüsnitz–Kustner or 'P–K' test) or preferably of monkeys. This passive sensitization of human skin can be blocked most effectively by prior injection of a myeloma of IgE rather than of any other class. The interpretation is that the specialized sites on the skin mast cells become fully saturated by binding to the Fc regions of the IgE myeloma

CHAPTER 12

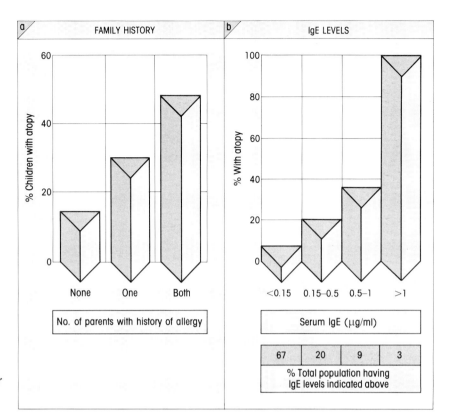

Figure 12.7. *Risk factors in allergy: (a) family history; (b) IgE levels—the higher the serum IgE concentration, the greater the chance of developing atopy.*

197

a FAMILY HISTORY

% Children with atopy (y-axis: 0, 20, 40, 60)

None — One — Both

No. of parents with history of allergy

b IgE LEVELS

% With atopy (y-axis: 0, 20, 40, 60, 80, 100)

<0.15 — 0.15–0.5 — 0.5–1 — >1

Serum IgE (μg/ml)

67	20	9	3

% Total population having IgE levels indicated above

---

globulin which blocks the subsequent attachment of specific IgE antibodies.

There is an increasing recognition that immediate wheal and flare reactions may be followed by a late phase reaction (cf. figure 12.8a) which sometimes lasts for 24 hours; it is characterized by a dense cellular infiltrate and is more oedematous than the early reaction. The weight of opinion is that this is partially mediated by a high molecular weight neutrophil chemotactic factor released from the mast cell. These late phase reactions can also be seen following challenge of the nasal mucosa and bronchi of allergic subjects and may be of major importance in the development of chronic asthma. In this respect, it is worthy of note that the major basic protein of the eosinophil granule, which is present in high levels in the sputum of asthma patients, has been shown to cause damage to bronchial epithelium in organ culture which mimics that seen in bronchial asthma.

The correlation between skin prick test responses and the radioallergosorbent test (RAST, p. 78) for allergen-specific serum IgE is fairly good. In some instances, intranasal challenge with allergen may provoke a response even when both these tests are negative, probably as a result of local synthesis of IgE antibodies.

Therapy

If one considers the sequence of reactions from initial exposure to allergen right through to the production of atopic disease, it can be seen that several points in the chain provide legitimate targets for therapy (figure 12.5). Avoidance of contact with *potential* allergens is often impractical although, to give one example, feeding infants cow's milk at too early an age is discouraged. After sensitization, avoidance where possible is obviously worthwhile but the reluctance of some parents to dispose of the family cat to stop little Algernon's wheezing is sometimes quite surprising.

Attempts to desensitize patients immunologically by repeated treatment with allergen have at least the merit of a long history and in a significant but as yet unpredictable proportion of patients can lead to worthwhile improvement. It has generally been assumed that the purpose of these inoculations was to boost the synthesis of 'blocking' IgG antibody whose function was to divert the allergen from contact with tissue-bound IgE. This would be of unquestioned value were the increase in protective antibody (? particularly IgA) to occur locally at the sites vulnerable to allergen exposure. However, if T-lymphocyte cooperation is important for IgE synthesis, the beneficial effects of antigen injection

Figure 12.8 facing page and above. *Hypersensitivity reactions.*

Type I *(a) Skin prick tests with grass pollen allergen in a patient with typical summer hay fever. Skin tests were performed 5 hours (left) and 20 minutes (right) before the photograph was taken. The tests on the right show a typical end point titration of a type I immediate wheal and flare reaction. The late phase skin reaction (left) can be clearly seen at 5 hours especially where a large immediate response has preceded it. Figures for allergen dilution are given. (b) An atopic eczema reaction on the back of a knee of a child allergic to rice and eggs.*

Type III *(c) Facial appearance in systemic lupus erythematosus (SLE). Lesions of recent onset are symmetrical, red and oedematous. They are often most pronounced on the areas of the face which receive most light exposure, i.e. the upper cheeks and bridge of the nose, and the prominences of the forehead. (d) Vasculitic lesions in SLE. Small purpuric macules are seen. (e) Erythema nodosum leprosum, forearm. The patient has lepromatous leprosy with superimposed erythema nodosum leprosum. These acutely inflamed nodules were extremely tender and the patient was pyrexial. (f) Polyarteritis nodosa, ankle and foot. Livedo reticularis with chronic painful ulceration is sometimes seen in this disease. (g) Histology of acute inflammatory reaction in polyarteritis nodosa associated with immune complex formation with hepatitis B surface (HBs) antigen. A vessel showing thrombus (Thr) formation and fibrinoid necrosis (FN) is surrounded by a mixed inflammatory infiltrate, largely polymorphs. (h) High power view of acute*

inflammatory response in loose connective tissue of patient with polyarteritis nodosa—polymorphs (PMN) are prominent. (i) Immunofluorescence studies of immune complexes in the renal artery of a patient with chronic hepatitis B infection stained with fluoresceinated anti-hepatitis B antigen (left) and rhodaminated anti-IgM (right). The presence of both antigen and antibody in the intima and media of the arterial wall indicate the deposition of the complexes at this site. IgG and C3 deposits are also detectable with the same distribution.

Type IV *(j) Mantoux test showing cell-mediated hypersensitivity reaction to tuberculin, characterized by induration and erythema. (k) Type IV contact hypersensitivity reaction to nickel caused by the clasp of a necklace. (l) Chronic type IV inflammatory lesion in tuberculous lung showing caseous necrosis (CN), epithelioid cells (E), giant cells (G) and mononuclear inflammatory cells (M). (m) Perivascular lymphocytic infiltrates (PL) and blister (Bl) formation characterize a contact sensitivity reaction of the skin. (n) High power view to show the lymphocytic nature of the infiltrate in a contact hypersensitivity reaction. (o) Delayed-type hypersensitivity lesion of mononuclear inflammatory cells (M) around schistosome egg (SE) within the liver parenchyma (LP). ((a), (b) and (j) kindly provided by Dr J. Brostoff, (c), (d), (e) and (f) by Dr G. Levene, (g), (h), (m) and (n) by Prof. N. Woolf, (i) by Prof. A. Nowoslowski, (l) by Dr R. Barnetson and (o) by Dr M. Doenhoff; (k) reproduced from Brit. Soc. Immunol. teaching slides with permission of the Society and Dermatology Department, London Hospital.)*

may also be mediated through induction of tolerant or even suppressor T-cells. There was initial promise in the observation that IgE-producing cells or their precursors could be switched off with comparative ease by haptens coupled to thymus-independent carriers such as poly-D-Glu.Lys. or isologous IgG, or by substitution of the allergen by polyethylene glycol. Better results must ultimately be attainable when we understand the rationale of 'hyposensitization' through the use of purified allergens, assessment of T-cell reactivity and quantitative measurement of specific IgG, IgA and IgE antibodies in individuals undergoing treatment. The affinity of these antibodies and their availability at local sites of allergen challenge such as the nasal mucosa are factors which cannot be ignored.

At the drug level, much relief has been obtained with agents such as isoprenaline and sodium cromoglycate which bind to different receptors on the mast cell surface and make it resistant to triggering. The symptoms of allergy are largely but not always controllable by anti-histamines, particularly when one is dealing with late phase reactions for which recourse to steroids may be necessary.

TYPE II—ANTIBODY-DEPENDENT CYTOTOXIC HYPERSENSITIVITY

Where an antigen is present on the surface of a cell, combination with antibody will encourage the demise of that cell by promoting contact with phagocytes either by reduction in surface charge, by opsonic adherence directly through the Fc, or by immune adherence through bound C3. Cell death may also occur through activation of the full complement system up to C8 and C9 producing direct membrane damage. Although in the case of haemolytic antibodies, the generation of a single active complement site is enough to cause erythrocyte lysis, other cells appear to have repair mechanisms and it is likely that several complement sites need to be recruited in order to overwhelm the cell's defences.

The operation of a quite distinct cytotoxic mechanism derives from the finding that target cells coated with low concentrations of IgG antibody can be killed 'non-specifically' through an extracellular non-phagocytic mechanism involving non-sensitized lymphoreticular cells which bind to the target by their specific receptors for the $C\gamma2$ and $C\gamma3$ domains of IgG Fc (figure 12.9). It should be noted that this so-called antibody-dependent cell-mediated cytotoxicity (ADCC) may be exhibited by both phagocytic and non-phagocytic myeloid cells (polymorphs and monocytes) and by large granular lymphocytes with Fc receptors dubbed 'K-cells' which are almost certainly identical with the natural killer (NK) cells (p. 13). Contact between the effector and target cells is essential and activity is inhibited by cytochalasin B which interferes with cell movement, and aggregated IgG which binds firmly to the Fc receptors and blocks their ability to interact with antibody on the surface of the target.

So far, ADCC has been studied exclusively as a phenomenon *in vitro*; to give examples, human K-cells have been shown to be strikingly unpleasant

Figure 12.9. *Killing of antibody-coated target by antibody-dependent cell-mediated cytotoxicity (ADCC). The surface receptors for Ig Fc region bind the effector cell to the target which is then killed by an extracellular mechanism. Several different cell types may display ADCC activity. (a) Diagram* *of effector and target cells. (b) Electron micrograph of attack on antibody-coated chick red cell by a mouse large granular lymphocyte showing close apposition of effector and target and vacuolation in the cytoplasm of the latter (courtesy of P. Penfold).*

to chicken red cells coated with rabbit antibody and schistosomules coated with either IgG or IgE can be killed by eosinophils (cf. figure 10.15). Whether ADCC is merely a curiosity of the laboratory test-tube or plays a positive role *in vivo* remains an open question. Functionally, this extracellular cytotoxic mechanism would be expected to be of significance where the target is too large for ingestion by phago-cytosis, e.g. large parasites and solid tumours. It could also act as a back-up system for T-cell killing when antibody production might otherwise lead to protection of the target from attack by T-cells through blocking of the surface antigens; the evolution of ADCC mechanisms would ensure that the antibody-coated target was still vulnerable.

The mechanisms leading to cell death in type II hypersensitivity are summarized in figure 12.10.

Type II reactions between members of the same species (isoimmune)

Transfusion reactions

Of the many different polymorphic constituents of the human red cell membrane, ABO blood groups form the dominant system. The antigenic groups A and B are derived from H substance (figure 12.11) by the action of glycosyl transferases encoded by A or B genes respectively. Individuals with both genes (group AB) have the two antigens on their red cells while those lacking these genes (group O) synthe-size H substance only. Antibodies to A or to B occur when the antigen is absent from the red cell surface;

thus a person of blood group A will possess anti-B and so on. These *isohaemagglutinins* are usually IgM and are thought to arise through immunization against antigens of the gut flora which are similar to the blood group substances so that the antibodies formed cross-react with the appropriate red cell type. If an individual is blood group A, he will be tolerant to antigens closely similar to A and will only form cross-reacting antibodies capable of ag-glutinating B red cells; similarly an O individual will make anti-A and anti-B (table 12.1). On trans-fusion, mismatched red cells will be coated by the isohaemagglutinins and cause severe reactions.

Rhesus incompatibility

The rhesus (Rh) blood groups form the other major antigenic system, the RhD antigen being of the most consequence for isoimmune reactions. A mother with an RhD negative blood group (i.e. dd geno-type) can readily be sensitized by red cells from a baby carrying RhD antigens (DD or Dd genotype). This occurs most often at the birth of the first child when a placental bleed can release a large number of the baby's erythrocytes into the mother. The antibodies formed are predominantly of the IgG class and are able to cross the placenta in any subsequent pregnancy. Reaction with the D-anti-gen on the fetal red cells leads to their destruction through opsonic adherence giving haemolytic dis-ease of the newborn (figure 12.12).

These anti-D antibodies fail to agglutinate RhD+ red cells *in vitro* ('incomplete antibodies') because the low density of antigenic sites does not allow sufficient antibody bridges to be formed between

Figure 12.10. *Type II—antibody-dependent cytotoxic hypersensitivity. Antibodies directed against cell surface antigens cause cell death not only by C-dependent lysis but also by adherence reactions leading to phagocytosis or through non-phagocytic extracellular killing by certain lymphoreticular cells (antibody-dependent cell-mediated cytotoxicity).*

GROUP A
A SUBSTANCE

A GENE

GROUP O
H SUBSTANCE

OLIGOSACCHARIDE

CERAMIDE
CELL MEMBRANE

B GENE

GROUP B
B SUBSTANCE

Figure 12.11. *The ABO system. The allelic genes A and B code for transferases which add either N-acetylgalactosamine or galactose respectively to H substance. The oligosaccharide is anchored to the cell membrane by coupling to a sphingomyelin called ceramide. 85% of the population secrete blood group substances in the saliva where the oligosaccharides are present as soluble polypeptide conjugates formed under the action of a secretor (se) gene.*

the negatively charged erythrocytes to overcome the electrostatic repulsive forces. Erythrocytes coated with anti-D can be made to agglutinate by addition of albumin or of an anti-immunoglobulin serum (Coombs' reagent; figure 12.13).

If a mother has natural isohaemagglutinins which can react with any fetal erythrocytes reaching her circulation, sensitization to the D antigens is less likely due to 'deviation' of the red cells away from the antigen-sensitive cells. For example, a group O RhD−ve mother with a group A RhD+ve baby would destroy any fetal erythrocytes with her anti-A before they could immunize to produce anti-D. In an extension of this principle, RhD−ve mothers are now treated prophylactically with small amounts of avid IgG anti-D at the time of birth of the first child, and this greatly reduces the risk of sensitization. Another success for immunology.

Organ transplants

A long-standing homograft which has withstood the first onslaught of the cell-mediated reaction can evoke humoral antibodies in the host directed against surface transplantation antigens on the graft. These may be directly cytotoxic or cause adherence

Table 12.1. *ABO blood groups and serum antibodies.*

BLOOD GROUP (PHENOTYPE)	GENOTYPE	ANTIGEN	SERUM ANTIBODY
A	AA, AO	A	ANTI-B
B	BB, BO	B	ANTI-A
AB	AB	A and B	NONE
O	OO	H	ANTI-A ANTI-B

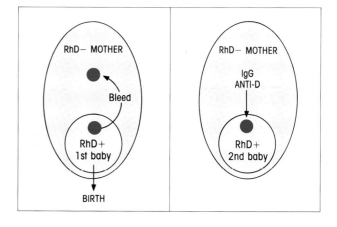

Figure 12.12. *Haemolytic disease of the newborn due to rhesus incompatibility.*

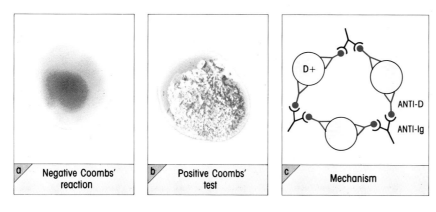

Figure 12.13. *The Coombs' test for antibody-coated red cells used for detecting rhesus-antibodies and in the diagnosis of autoimmune haemolytic anaemia (cf. table 14.2, Note 5, p.240). (Photographs courtesy of Dr A. Cooke.)*

202

of phagocytic cells or 'non-specific' attack by K-cells. They may also lead to platelet adherence when they combine with antigens on the surface of the vascular endothelium (figure 13.7, p. 220). Hyper-acute rejection is mediated by preformed antibodies in the graft recipient.

Autoimmune type II hypersensitivity reactions

Autoantibodies to the patient's own red cells are produced in autoimmune haemolytic anaemia. Red cells coated with these antibodies have a shortened half-life largely through their adherence to phago-cytic cells. Similar mechanisms account for the anaemia in patients with cold haemagglutinin disease who have monoclonal anti-I after infection with *Mycoplasma pneumoniae*, and in some cases of paroxysmal cold haemoglobinuria associated with the actively lytic Donath–Landsteiner antibodies of specificity anti-blood group P.

The sera of patients with Hashimoto's thyroiditis contain antibodies which in the presence of complement are directly cytotoxic for isolated human thyroid cells in culture. In Goodpasture's syndrome (included here for convenience), antibodies to kidney glomerular basement membrane are present. Biopsies show these antibodies together with complement components bound to the basement membranes where the action of the full complement system leads to serious damage (figure 12.14a). I suppose one could also include the stripping of acetylcholine receptors from the muscle end-plate by autoantibodies in myasthenia gravis as a further example of type II hypersensitivity.

Type II drug reactions

This is complicated. Drugs may become coupled to body components and thereby undergo conversion from a hapten to a full antigen which will sensitize certain individuals (we don't know which). If IgE antibodies are produced, anaphylactic reactions can result. In some circumstances, particularly with topically applied ointments, cell-mediated hyper-sensitivity may be induced. In other cases where coupling to serum proteins occurs, the possibility of type III complex-mediated reactions may arise. In the present context we are concerned with those instances where the drug appears to form an anti-genic complex with the surface of a formed element

of the blood and evokes the production of antibodies which are cytotoxic for the cell–drug complex. When the drug is withdrawn, the sensitivity is no longer evident. Examples of this mechanism have been seen in the *haemolytic anaemia* sometimes associated with continued administration of chlorpromazine or phenacetin, in the *agranulocytosis* associated with the taking of amidopyrine or of quinidine, and the now classic situation of *thrombocytopenic purpura* which may be produced by Sedormid, a sedative of yesteryear. In the latter case, freshly drawn serum from the patient will lyse platelets in the presence, but not in the absence, of Sedormid; inactivation of complement by preheating the serum at 56°C for 30 minutes abrogates this effect.

TYPE III—IMMUNE-COMPLEX-MEDIATED HYPERSENSITIVITY

The body may be exposed to an excess of antigen over a protracted period in a number of circum-stances, persistent infection with a microbial organ-ism, autoimmunity to self-components and repeated contact with environmental agents. The union of such antigens and antibodies to form an insoluble complex at fixed sites within the body may well give rise to acute inflammatory reactions (figure 12.15). If complement is fixed, anaphylatoxins will be released as split products of C3 and C5 and these will cause release of mast cell mediators with vascu-lar permeability changes. The chemotactic factors also produced will lead to an influx of polymorpho-nuclear leucocytes which begin the phagocytosis of the immune complexes; this in turn results in the extracellular release of the polymorph granule con-tents, particularly when the complex is deposited on a basement membrane and cannot be phagocy-tosed (so-called 'frustrated phagocytosis'). The pro-teolytic enzymes (including neutral proteinases and collagenase), kinin-forming enzymes and polycat-ionic proteins which are released will of course damage local tissues and intensify the inflamma-tory responses. Further damage may be mediated by reactive lysis in which activated C5,6,7 becomes adventitiously attached to the surface of nearby cells and binds C8,9. Under appropriate conditions, platelets may be aggregated with two consequences: they provide yet a further source of vasoactive amines and may also form microthrombi which can lead to local ischaemia. (The discerning reader will appreciate the need for the system of inhibitors present in the body.) Insoluble complexes taken up

203

(a)

(b)

Figure 12.14. *Glomerulonephritis: (a) due to linear deposition of antibody to glomerular basement membrane here visualized by staining the human kidney biopsy with a fluorescent anti-IgG (courtesy of Dr F.J. Dixon) and (b) due to deposition of antigen−antibody complexes which can be seen as discrete masses lining the glomerular basement membrane following immunofluorescent staining with anti-IgG; patches of blue autofluorescence are present in the extraglomerular tissue (arrowed) (courtesy of Dr D. Doniach). Similar patterns to these are obtained with a fluorescent anti-C3.*

by macrophages cannot readily be digested and provide a persistent activating stimulus (figure 12.15).

The outcome of the formation of immune complexes *in vivo* depends not only on the absolute amounts of antigen and antibody, which determine the intensity of the reaction, but also on their *relative* proportions which govern the nature of the complexes (cf. precipitin curve, p. 70) and hence their distribution within the body. Between *antibody excess* and *mild antigen excess*, the complexes are rapidly precipitated and tend to be localized to the site of introduction of antigen, whereas in *moderate* to *gross antigen excess*, soluble complexes are formed.

The fate of these complexes is bound up closely with the operation of the classical complement pathway. Fixation of complement inhibits the precipitation of immune complexes by covalent attachment of C3b which prevents the Fc−Fc interactions required to form large insoluble aggregates (figure 12.16). These small complexes containing C3b bind by immune adherence to CR1 complement receptors on the human erythrocyte and are transported to fixed macrophages in the liver where they are safely inactivated. If there are defects in this system, for example deficiencies in classical pathway components (cf. p. 15; figure 12.16) or perhaps if the system is overloaded, then the immune complexes are free in the plasma and widespread disease

Figure 12.15. *Type III immune-complex-mediated hypersensitivity.*

involving deposition in the kidneys, joints and skin may result.

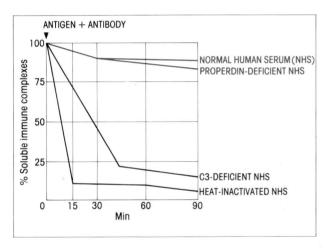

Figure 12.16. *Complement inhibits the formation of insoluble complexes as antigen and antibody combine. Serum deficient in C3 or in which complement had been inactivated by heating, failed to block the formation of precipitating complexes. Deficiency of the alternative pathway component properdin had no effect. (Data from Schifferli J.A., Ng Y.C. & Peters D.K. (1986)* N. Engl. J. Med. 315, 488, *reproduced with permission from the* New England Journal of Medicine.*)*

Inflammatory lesions due to locally formed complexes

The Arthus reaction

Maurice Arthus found that injection of soluble antigen intradermally into hyperimmunized rabbits with high levels of precipitating antibody, produced an erythematous and oedematous reaction reaching a peak at 3–8 hours and then usually re-

solving. The lesion was characterized by an intense infiltration with polymorphonuclear leucocytes (cf. figure 12.8h). The injected antigen precipitates with antibody often within the venule, too fast for the classical complement system to prevent it; subsequently the complex binds complement and, using fluorescent reagents, antigen, immunoglobulin and complement components can all be demonstrated in this lesion (figure 12.8i). Anaphylatoxin is soon generated and causes mast cell degranulation. Local intravascular complexes will also cause platelet aggregation and vasoactive amine release and, as a result, erythema and oedema increase. The formation of chemotactic factors leads to the influx of polymorphs. The Arthus reaction can be blocked by depletion of complement or of the neutrophil polymorphs (by nitrogen mustard or specific anti-polymorph sera).

Reactions to inhaled antigens

Intrapulmonary Arthus-type reactions to exogenous inhaled antigen appear to be responsible for a number of hypersensitivity disorders in man. The severe respiratory difficulties associated with farmer's lung occur within 6–8 hours of exposure to the dust from mouldy hay. The patients are found to be sensitized to thermophilic actinomycetes which grow in the mouldy hay, and extracts of these organisms give precipitin reactions with the subject's serum and Arthus reactions on intradermal injection. Inhalation of bacterial spores present in dust from the hay introduces antigen into the lungs and a complex-mediated hypersensitivity reaction occurs. Similar situations arise in pigeon-fancier's disease where the antigen is probably serum protein present in the dust from dried faeces, in rat handlers sensitized to rat serum proteins excreted

205

in the urine (figure 12.17) and in many other quaintly named cases of extrinsic allergic alveolitis resulting from continual inhalation of organic particles, e.g. cheese washer's disease (*Penicillium casei* spores), furrier's lung (fox fur proteins) and maple bark stripper's disease (spores of *Cryptostroma*). Evidence that an immediate anaphylactic type I response may sometimes be of importance for the initiation of an Arthus reaction comes from the study of patients with allergic bronchopulmonary aspergillosis who have high levels of IgE and precipitating IgG antibodies to *Aspergillus* species.

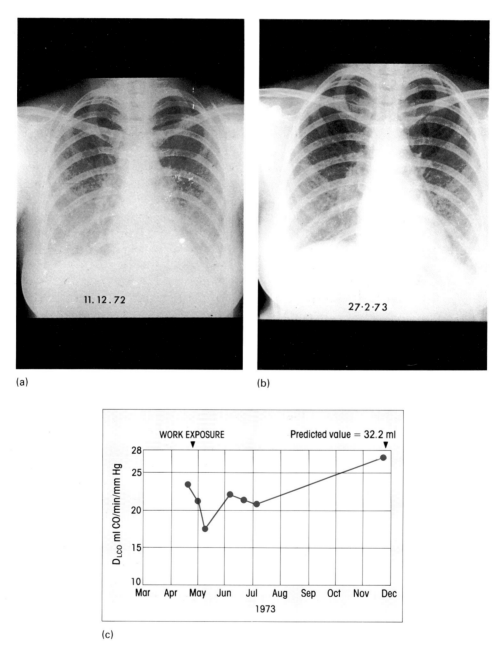

(a)   (b)

(c)

Figure 12.17. *Extrinsic allergic alveolitis due to rat serum proteins in a research assistant handling rats (type III hypersensitivity). Typical systemic and pulmonary reactions on inhalation and positive prick tests were elicited by rat serum proteins; precipitins against serum proteins in rat urine were present in the patient's serum. (a) Bilateral micronodular shadowing during acute episode. (b) Marked clearing within 11 days after cessation of exposure to rats. (c) Temporary fall in pulmonary gas exchange measured by DL_{CO} (gas transfer, single breath) following a 3-day exposure to rats at work (arrowed). (From Carroll K.B., Pepys J., Longbottom J.L., Hughes D.T.D. & Benson H.G. (1975) Clin. Allergy 5, 443; figures by courtesy of Prof. J. Pepys.)*

Reactions to internal antigens

Type III reactions are often provoked by the local release of antigen from infectious organisms within the body; for example, living filarial worms such as *Wuchereria bancrofti* are relatively harmless, but the dead parasite found in lymphatic vessels initiates an inflammatory reaction thought to be responsible for obstruction of lymph flow and the ensuing, rather monstrous, elephantiasis. Chemotherapy may cause an abrupt release of microbial antigens in individuals with high antibody levels, producing quite dramatic immune complex-mediated reactions such as erythema nodosum leprosum in the skin of dapsone-treated lepromatous leprosy patients (figure 12.8e) and the Jarisch–Herxheimer reaction in syphilitics on penicillin.

An interesting variant of the Arthus reaction is seen in rheumatoid arthritis where complexes are formed locally in the joint due to the production of self-associating IgG anti-IgG by synovial plasma cells (cf. p. 262).

It has also been recognized that complexes could be generated at a local site by a quite different mechanism involving non-specific adherence of an antigen to tissue structures followed by the binding of soluble antibody—in other words, the antigen becomes fixed in the tissue *before* not *after* combining with antibody. Although it is not clear to what extent this mechanism operates in patients with immune complex disease, let me describe the experimental observation on which it is based. After injection with bacterial endotoxin, mice release DNA into their circulation which binds specifically to the collagen in the basement membrane of the glomerular capillaries: infusion of anti-DNA now gives rise to antigen–antibody complexes in the kidney.

Disease resulting from circulating complexes

Serum sickness

Injection of relatively large doses of foreign serum (e.g. horse anti-diphtheria) used to be employed for various therapeutic purposes. It was not uncommon for a condition known as 'serum sickness' to arise some eight days after the injection. A rise in temperature, swollen lymph nodes, a generalized urticarial rash and painful swollen joints associated with a low serum complement and transient albuminuria could be encountered. These result from the deposition of soluble antigen–antibody complexes formed in antigen excess.

Some individuals begin to synthesize antibodies against the foreign protein—usually horse globulin. Since the antigen is still present in gross excess at that time, circulating soluble complexes of composition Ag_2Ab, Ag_3Ab_2, Ag_4Ab_3, etc. will be formed (cf. precipitin curve, figures 5.1 and 5.2). To be pathogenic, the complexes have to be of the right size—too big and they are snapped up smartly by the macrophages of the reticuloendothelial system, too small (<19S) and they fail to induce an inflammatory reaction. Even when they are the right size, it seems that they will only localize in vessel walls if there is a change in vascular permeability. This may come about through release of 5-hydrotryptamine (5HT) from platelets reacting with larger complexes or through an IgE or complement-mediated degranulation of basophils and mast cells to produce histamine, leukotrienes and platelet activating factor. The effect on the capillaries is to cause separation of the endothelial cells and exposure of the basement membrane to which the appropriately sized complexes attach, the skin, joints, kidneys and heart being particularly affected. As antibody synthesis increases, antigen is cleared and the patient normally recovers.

Immune complex glomerulonephritis

The deposition of complexes is a dynamic affair and long-lasting disease is only seen when the antigen is persistent as in chronic infections and auto-immune diseases. Experimentally, Dixon produced chronic glomerular lesions by repeated administration of foreign proteins to rabbits. Not all animals showed the lesion and perhaps only those genetically capable of producing low affinity antibody (Soothill & Steward) or antibodies to a restricted number of determinants (Christian) formed soluble complexes in the right size range. The smallest complexes reach the epithelial side but progressively larger complexes are retained in or on the endothelial side of the glomerular basement membrane (figure 12.18). They build up as 'lumpy' granules staining for antigen, immunoglobulin and complement (C3) by immunofluorescence (figure 12.14b) and appear as large amorphous masses in the electron microscope (cf. figure 15.5).

Many cases of glomerulonephritis are associated with circulating complexes and biopsies give a

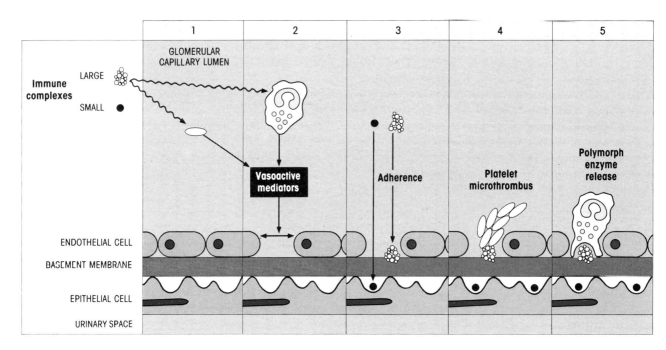

Figure 12.18. *Deposition of immune complexes in the kidney glomerulus. (1) Complexes induce release of vasoactive mediators from basophils and platelets which cause (2) separation of endothelial cells, (3) attachment of larger complexes to exposed basement membrane, smaller complexes passing through to epithelial side, (4) complexes induce platelet aggregation, (5) chemotactically attracted neutrophils release granule contents in 'frustrated phagocytosis' to damage basement membrane. Complex deposition is favoured in the glomerular capillary because it is a major filtration site and has a high hydrodynamic pressure. Deposition is greatly reduced in animals depleted of platelets or treated with vasoactive amine antagonists.*

fluorescent staining pattern similar to that of figure 12.14b which depicts DNA/anti-DNA/complement deposits in the kidney of a patient with systemic lupus erythematosus (cf. p. 258). Well known is the disease which can follow infection with certain strains of so-called 'nephritogenic' streptococci and the nephrotic syndrome of Nigerian children associated with quartan malaria where complexes with antigens of the infecting organism have been implicated. Immune complex nephritis can arise in the course of chronic viral infections; for example, mice infected with lymphocytic choriomeningitis virus develop a glomerulonephritis associated with circulating complexes of virus and antibody. This may well represent a model for many cases of glomerulonephritis in man.

Deposition of complexes at other sites

The choroid plexus being a major filtration site is also favoured for immune complex deposition and this could account for the frequency of central nervous disorders in systemic lupus. Neurologically affected patients tend to have depressed C4 in the cerebrospinal fluid (c.s.f.) and at post-mortem, SLE patients with neurological disturbances and high titre anti-DNA were shown to have scattered deposits of immunoglobulin and DNA in the choroid plexus. Subacute sclerosing panencephalitis is associated with a high c.s.f. to serum ratio of measles antibody, and deposits containing Ig and measles Ag may be found in neural tissue.

The vasculitic skin rashes which are a major feature of serum sickness are also characteristic of systemic and discoid lupus erythematosus (figure 12.8c and d) and biopsies of the lesions reveal amorphous deposits of Ig and C3 at the basement membrane of the dermal–epidermal junction.

The necrotizing arteritis produced in rabbits by experimental serum sickness closely resembles the histology of polyarteritis nodosa (figure 12.8g and h) and it has recently been reported that in some of these patients (figure 12.8f), immune complexes containing the HBs antigen of hepatitis B virus are present in the lesions (figure 12.8i). Another example is the haemorrhagic shock syndrome found with some frequency in South-East Asia during a second infection with a dengue virus. There are four types of virus, and antibodies to one type produced during a first infection may not neutralize a second strain but rather facilitate its entry into, and replication within, human monocytes by attachment of the complex to Fc receptors. The enhanced production of virus leads to immune complex formation and a massive intravascular activation of the classical complement pathway. In some instances drugs such as penicillin become antigenic after conjugation with body proteins and form complexes which mediate hypersensitivity reactions.

It should be said that persistence of circulating complexes does not invariably lead to type III hypersensitivity (e.g. in many cancer patients and in individuals with idiotype−anti-idiotype reactions). Perhaps in these cases the complexes lack the ability to initiate the changes required for complex deposition, but some hold the view that complexes detected in the serum may sometimes be artefacts released from their *in vivo* attachment to the erythrocyte CR1 receptors by the action of factor I during processing of the blood.

Detection of immune complex formation

Tissue-bound complexes are usually visualized by the immunofluorescent staining of biopsies with conjugated anti-immunoglobulins and anti-C3 (cf. figure 12.14b).

Many techniques for detecting circulating complexes have been described and because of variations in the size, complement-fixing ability and Ig class of different complexes, it is useful to apply more than one method. Bearing in mind the caveat concerning the possibility of artefacts just mentioned, in our laboratory we tend to prefer:
1 precipitation of complexed IgG from serum at concentrations of polyethylene glycol which do not bring down significant amounts of IgG monomer, followed by estimation of IgG in the precipitate by single radial diffusion or laser nephelometry, and
2 binding of C3b-containing complexes to beads coated with conglutinin (cf. p. 155) and estimation of the bound Ig with enzyme-labelled anti-Ig.

Other major techniques include (i) estimation of the binding of ^{125}I-Clq to complexes by co-precipitation with polyethylene glycol, (ii) inhibition by complexes of rheumatoid factor-induced aggregation of IgG-coated particles, and (iii) detection with radio-labelled anti-Ig of serum complexes capable of binding to bovine conglutinin or to the C3b (and to a lesser extent the Fc) receptors on the Raji cell line. Sera from patients with immune complex disease often form a cryoprecipitate when allowed to stand at 4°C. Measurement of serum C3 and its conversion product C3c are sometimes useful.

Treatment

The avoidance of exogenous inhaled antigens inducing type III reactions is obvious. Elimination of micro-organisms associated with immune complex disease by chemotherapy may provoke a further reaction due to copious release of antigen. Suppression of the accessory factors thought to be necessary for deposition of complexes would seem logical; for example, the development of serum sickness is prevented by histamine and 5HT antagonists. Disodium cromoglycate, heparin and salicylates are often used, the latter being an effective platelet stabilizer as well as a potent anti-inflammatory agent. Corticosteroids are particularly powerful inhibitors of inflammation and are immunosuppressive. In many cases, particularly those involving autoimmunity, conventional immunosuppressive agents may be justified. Where type III hypersensitivity is thought to arise from an inadequate immune response, the more aggressive approach of immunopotentiation to boost avidity is being advocated, but that is a path that will be trodden gently.

TYPE IV—CELL-MEDIATED (DELAYED-TYPE) HYPERSENSITIVITY

This form of hypersensitivity is encountered in many allergic reactions to bacteria, viruses and fungi, in the contact dermatitis resulting from sensitization to certain simple chemicals and in the rejection of transplanted tissues. Perhaps the best known example is the Mantoux reaction obtained by injection of tuberculin into the skin of an individual in whom previous infection with the mycobacterium had induced a state of cell-mediated immunity (CMI). The reaction is characterized by erythema and induration (figure 12.8j) which appears only after several hours (hence the term 'delayed') and reaches a maximum at 24−48 hours, thereafter subsiding. Histologically the earliest phase of the reaction is seen as a perivascular cuffing with mononuclear cells followed by a more extensive exudation of mono- and polymorphonuclear cells. The latter soon migrate out of the lesion leaving behind a predominantly mononuclear cell infiltrate consisting of

209

lymphocytes and cells of the monocyte—macrophage series (figure 12.8l). This contrasts with the essentially 'polymorph' character of the Arthus reaction (figure 12.8h).

Comparable reactions to soluble proteins are obtained when sensitization is induced by incorporation of the antigen into complete Freund's adjuvant (p. 181). In some but not all cases, if animals are primed with antigen alone or in incomplete Freund's adjuvant (which lacks the mycobacteria), the delayed hypersensitivity state is of shorter duration and the dermal response more transient. This is known as 'Jones—Mote' sensitivity but has recently been termed *cutaneous basophil hypersensitivity* on account of the high proportion of basophils infiltrating the skin lesion.

The cellular basis of type IV hypersensitivity

Unlike the other forms of hypersensitivity which we have discussed, delayed-type reactivity cannot be transferred from a sensitized to a non-sensitized individual with serum antibody; lymphoid cells, in particular the T-lymphocytes, are required. Transfer has been achieved in the human using viable white blood cells and, interestingly, by a low molecular weight material extracted from them (Lawrence's transfer factor). The nature of this substance is, however, a mystery. The extracts contain a variety of factors which appear capable of stimulating pre-committed T-cells mediating delayed hypersensitivity, but whether there is also an informational molecule conferring antigen-specific reactivity is still a highly contentious issue.

It cannot be stressed too often that the hypersensitivity lesion results from an exaggerated interaction between antigen and the *normal* cell-mediated immune mechanisms (cf. p. 110). Following earlier priming, memory T-cells recognize the antigen together with class II MHC molecules on a macrophage and are stimulated into blast cell transformation and proliferation. The stimulated T-cells release a number of soluble factors which function as mediators of the ensuing hypersensitivity response particularly by attracting and activating macrophages; they also help cytotoxic T-cell precursors to become killer cells which can cause tissue damage (figure 12.19).

Tissue damage produced by type IV reactions

Infections

The development of a state of cell-mediated hypersensitivity to bacterial products is probably responsible for the lesions associated with bacterial allergy such as the cavitation, caseation and general toxaemia seen in human tuberculosis and the granulomatous skin lesions found in patients with the

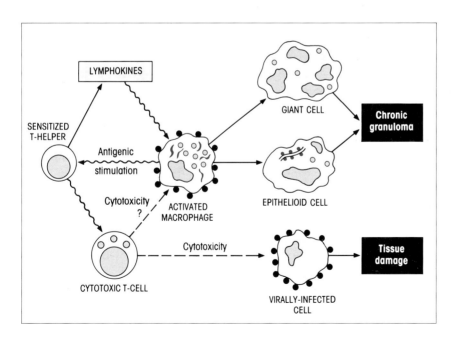

Figure 12.19. *The cellular basis of type IV hypersensitivity.*

borderline form of leprosy. When the battle between the replicating bacteria and the body defences fails to be resolved in favour of the host, persisting antigen provokes a chronic local delayed hypersensitivity reaction. Continual release of lymphokines from sensitized T-lymphocytes leads to the accumulation of large numbers of macrophages, many of which give rise to arrays of epithelioid cells, while others fuse to form giant cells. Macrophages bearing bacterial antigen on their surface may become targets for killer T-cells and be destroyed. Further tissue damage will occur as a result of indiscriminate cytotoxicity by lymphokine-activated macrophages (and NK cells?) and perhaps lymphotoxin itself. Morphologically, this combination of cell types with proliferating lymphocytes and fibroblasts associated with areas of fibrosis and necrosis is termed a *chronic granuloma* and represents an attempt by the body to wall-off a site of persistent infection (figure 12.8l; figure 12.19). It should be noted that granulomas can also arise from the persistence of indigestible antigen—antibody complexes or inorganic materials such as talc within macrophages, although non-immunological granulomas may be distinguished by the absence of lymphocytes.

The skin rashes in smallpox and measles and the lesions of herpes simplex may be largely attributed to delayed-type allergic reactions with extensive damage to virally infected cells by cytotoxic T-lymphocytes. Cell-mediated hypersensitivity has also been demonstrated in the fungal diseases, candidiasis, dermatomycosis, coccidioidomycosis and histoplasmosis, and in the parasitic diseases, leishmaniasis and schistosomiasis where the pathology has been attributed to a reaction against soluble enzymes derived from the eggs which lodge in the liver capillaries (figure 12.8o).

Sarcoidosis is a disease of unknown aetiology affecting lymphoid tissue and involving the formation of chronic granulomas. Delayed-type hypersensitivity is depressed and the patients are anergic on skin testing with tuberculin; curiously they give positive responses if cortisone is injected together with the antigen and it has been suggested that cortisone-sensitive T suppressors might be responsible for the anergy. The patients develop a granulomatous reaction a few weeks after intradermal injection of spleen extract from another sarcoid patient—the Kweim reaction.

Contact dermatitis

The epidermal route of inoculation tends to favour the development of a T-cell response through processing by Ia-rich dendritic Langerhans' cells (cf. figure 2.5i) which migrate to the lymph nodes and present antigen to T-lymphocytes. Thus, delayed-type reactions in the skin are often produced by foreign materials capable of binding to body constituents, possibly surface molecules of the Langerhans' cell, to form new antigens. The reaction is characterized by a mononuclear cell infiltrate peaking at 12–15 hours, accompanied by oedema of the epidermis with microvesicle formation (figure 12.8m and n). Contact hypersensitivity can occur in people who become sensitized while working with chemicals such as picryl chloride and chromates, or who repeatedly come into contact with the substance urushiol from the poison ivy plant. *p*-Phenylene diamine in certain hair dyes, neomycin in topically applied ointments, and nickel salts formed from articles such as nickel jewellery clasps (figure 12.8k), can provoke similar reactions.

Other examples

Delayed hypersensitivity contributes significantly to the prolonged reactions which result from insect bites. The possible implication of homograft rejection by cytotoxic T-cells as a mechanism for the control of cancer cells is discussed in Chapter 13. The contribution made by cell-mediated hypersensitivity reactions to different autoimmune diseases is still rather uncertain (cf. p. 264).

TYPE V—STIMULATORY HYPERSENSITIVITY

Many cells receive instruction by agents such as hormones through surface receptors which specifically bind the external agent presumably through complementarity of structure. This combination may lead to allosteric changes in configuration of the receptor or of adjacent molecules which become activated and transmit a signal to the cell interior. For example, when thyroid stimulating hormone (TSH) of pituitary origin binds to the thyroid cell receptors, there appears to be an activation of adenyl cyclase in the membrane which generates cyclic-AMP from ATP and this 'second messenger' acts to stimulate activity in the thyroid cell. The thyroid

211

stimulating antibody present in the sera of thyrotoxic patients (cf. p. 255) is an autoantibody directed against an antigen on the thyroid surface which stimulates the cell and produces the same changes as TSH, similarly utilizing the cyclic-AMP pathway. It is likely that the antibody combines with a site on the TSH receptor or an adjacent molecule to produce the changes required for adenyl cyclase activation. The situation is analogous to lymphocyte stimulation; B-lymphocytes with immunoglobulin surface receptors can be stimulated by changes induced through the receptor molecules either by binding of specific antigen or by an antibody to the immunoglobulin (even anti-Fc) as shown in figure 12.20. Intriguingly, there are indications that cimetidine-resistant duodenal ulcer patients may have stimulatory antibodies directed to H2 histamine receptors.

Other experimental examples of stimulation by antibodies to cell surface antigens may be cited: the transformation of human T-lymphocytes by monoclonal antibodies to the T3 antigen; the production of cell division in thyroid cells by 'growth' autoantibodies; the induction of pinocytosis by anti-macrophage serum; and the mitogenic effect of antibodies to sea-urchin eggs. It is worthy of note that although antibodies to enzymes directed against determinants near to the active site can exert a blocking effect, combination with more distant determinants can sometimes bring about allosteric conformational changes which are associated with a considerable increase in enzymic activity as has been described for certain variants of penicillinase and β-galactosidase.

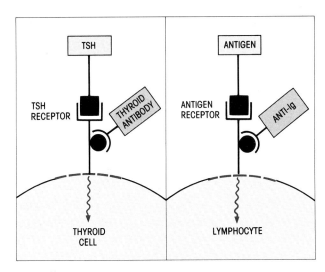

Figure 12.20. *Stimulation of thyroid cell and of lymphocyte by physiological agent or by antibody both of which cause comparable membrane changes leading to cell activation by reacting with surface receptors.*

'INNATE' HYPERSENSITIVITY REACTIONS

Excessive activation of the alternative complement pathway can lead to tissue-damaging hypersensitivity reactions such as disseminated intravascular coagulation. A good model for this is the Shwartzmann reaction produced in rabbits by intravascular endotoxin. This activates the alternative pathway so that the endotoxin becomes coated with C3b and sticks to platelets by immune adherence; the C5,6,7 complexes generated cause platelet destruction by reactive lysis with release of clotting factors. Although in man, C3b adherence reactions involve red cells and leucocytes rather than platelets, somewhat similar mechanisms associated with intense complement consumption underlie the disseminated intravascular coagulation seen in human patients with Gram-negative septicaemia or dengue haemorrhagic shock produced by a substantial viraemia occurring in the second infection of individuals with high titre antibodies.

The reader's attention has already been drawn to the unusual susceptibility of the erythrocytes to lysis in paroxysomal nocturnal haemoglobinuria resulting from deficiency in C3b control proteins on the red cell surface (p. 183). Undue C3 consumption is associated with mesangiocapillary glomerulonephritis and partial lipodystrophy in patients with the so-called C3 nephritic factor which appears to be an IgG autoantibody capable of activating the alternative pathway by combining with and stabilizing the C3bBb convertase.

SUMMARY

The normal effector mechanisms for cell-mediated and humoral immunity are dependent upon the activation of T- and B-cells respectively. Excessive stimulation of these effector mechanisms by antigen in a sensitized host can lead to tissue damage and we speak of hypersensitivity reactions of which five main types can be distinguished.

Type I—anaphylactic hypersensitivity

This depends upon the reaction of antigen with specific IgE antibody bound through its Fc to the mast cell, leading to release from the granules of mediators including histamine, leukotrienes and platelet activating factor, plus eosinophil and neutrophil chemotactic factors. Hay fever and extrinsic asthma represent the most common atopic allergic disorders. The offending antigen is identified by intradermal prick tests giving immediate wheal and erythema reactions or by provocation testing. Late-stage cellular reactions may be important for the development of chronic bronchial asthma. There is a strong familial disposition; the tendency to produce high levels of IgE is an important contributing factor. Symptomatic treatment involves the use of mediator antagonists or agents which stabilize the mast cell granules; steroids are effective against late reactions. Courses of antigen injection may desensitize by formation of blocking IgG or IgA antibodies or by turning off IgE production.

Type II—antibody-dependent cytotoxic hypersensitivity

This involves the death of cells bearing antibody attached to a surface antigen. The cells may be taken up by phagocytic cells to which they adhere through their coating of IgG or C3b or lysed by the operation of the full complement system. Cells bearing IgG may also be killed by polymorphs and macrophages or by K-cells through an extracellular mechanism (antibody-dependent cell-mediated cytotoxicity). Examples are: transfusion reactions, haemolytic disease of the newborn through rhesus incompatibility, antibody-mediated graft destruction, auto-immune reactions directed against the formed elements of the blood and kidney glomerular basement membranes, and hypersensitivity resulting from the coating of erythrocytes or platelets by a drug.

Type III—complex-mediated hypersensitivity

This results from the effects of antigen—antibody complexes through (i) activation of complement and attraction of polymorphonuclear leucocytes which release tissue-damaging enzymes on contact with the complex, and (ii) aggregation of platelets to cause microthrombi and vasoactive amine release. Where circulating antibody levels are high, the antigen is precipitated near the site of entry into the body. The reaction in the skin is characterized by polymorph infiltration, oedema and erythema maximal at 3—8 hours (Arthus reaction). Examples are farmer's lung, pigeon fancier's disease and pulmonary aspergillosis where inhaled antigens provoke high antibody levels, reactions to an abrupt increase in antigen caused by microbial cell death during chemotherapy for leprosy or syphilis, and an element of the synovial lesion in rheumatoid arthritis. In relative *antigen excess*, soluble complexes are formed which are removed by binding to the CR1 C3b receptors on red cells. If this system is overloaded or if the classical complement components are deficient, the complexes circulate in the free state and are deposited under circumstances of increased vascular permeability at certain preferred sites, the kidney glomerulus, the joints, the skin and the choroid plexus. Complexes can be detected in tissue biopsies by immunofluorescence and in serum by precipitation with polyethylene glycol, reaction with C1q, changes in C3 and C3c, and binding to the C3 receptor on the Raji cell line. Examples are: serum sickness following injection of large quantities of foreign protein, glomerulonephritis associated with systemic lupus or infections with streptococci, malaria and other parasites, neurological disturbances in systemic lupus and subacute sclerosing panencephalitis, polyarteritis nodosa linked to hepatitis B virus, and haemorrhagic shock in dengue viral infection.

Type IV—cell-mediated or delayed-type hypersensitivity

This is based upon the interaction of antigen with primed T-cells and represents tissue damage resulting from inappropriate cell-mediated immunity reactions. A number of soluble mediators (lymphokines) are released which account for the events which occur in a typical delayed hypersensitivity response such as the Mantoux reaction to tuberculin, namely, the delayed appearance of an indurated and erythematous reaction which reaches a maximum at 24—48 hours and is characterized histologically by infiltration with mononuclear phagocytes and lymphocytes. Another subpopulation of T-cells is activated by class I major histocompatibility antigens to become directly cytotoxic to target cells bearing the appropriate antigen. *In vitro* tests for cell-mediated hypersensitivity include macrophage migration inhibition and assessment of blast cell transformation. Examples are: tissue damage occurring in bacterial (tuberculosis, leprosy), viral (smallpox, measles, herpes), fungal (candidiasis, histoplasmosis) and parasitic (leishmaniasis, schistosomiasis) infections, contact dermatitis from exposure to chromates and poison ivy, and insect bites. Continuing provocation of delayed hypersensitivity by persisting antigen leads to formation of chronic granulomata.

Table 12.2. *Comparison of different types of hypersensitivity.*

		I Anaphylactic	II Cytotoxic	III Complex-mediated	IV Cell-mediated	V Stimulatory
Antibody mediating reaction		Homocytotropic Ab Mast-cell binding	Humoral Ab ± CF*	Humoral Ab ± CF	Receptor on T-lymphocyte	Humoral Ab Non-CF
Antigen		Usually exogenous (e.g. grass pollen)	Cell surface	Extracellular	Associated with MHC antigens on macro- phage or target cell	Cell surface
Response to intra-dermal antigen:	Max. reaction Appearance	30 min (+ late reaction) Wheal and flare	—	3–8 hours Erythema and oedema	24–48 hours Erythema and indura- tion	—
	Histology	Degranulated mast cells; oedema; (late reaction cellular incl. eosinophils)	—	Acute inflammatory reaction; pre- dominant polymorphs	Perivascular inflamma- tion: polymorphs migrate out leaving predominantly mono- nuclear cells	—
Transfer sensitivity to normal subject		◄──────── Serum antibody ────────►			Lymphoid cells Transfer factor	Serum antibody
Examples:		Atopic allergy, e.g. hay fever	Haemolytic disease of newborn (Rh)	Complex glomerulo- nephritis Farmer's lung	Mantoux reaction to TB Granulomatous reaction to schistosome eggs Contact sensitivity	Thyrotoxicosis

* CF = Complement fixation

214

Type V—stimulatory hypersensitivity

This is where the antibody reacts with a key surface component such as a hormone receptor and 'switches on' the cell. An example is the thyroid hyper-reactivity in Graves' disease due to a thyroid-stimulating autoantibody.

Features of the five types of hypersensitivity are compared in table 12.2.

'Innate' hypersensitivity reactions

These reactions involving excessive C3 activation are seen in disseminated intravascular coagulation produced by the Shwartzmann reaction, Gram-negative septicaemia and dengue haemorrhagic shock.

Further reading

Dale M.M. & Foreman J.C. (1984) *Textbook of Immunopharmacology*. Blackwell Scientific Publications, Oxford.

Goetzl E.J. & Kay A.B. (eds) (1982) *Current Perspectives in Allergy*. Churchill Livingstone, UK.

Haeney M. (1985) *Introduction to Clinical Immunology*. Butterworths-Update, London. (In vivid technicolour; suitable for the busy clinician.)

Lachmann P. & Peters D.K. (eds) (1982) *Clinical Aspects of Immunology*, 4th edn. Blackwell Scientific Publications, Oxford.

Lessof M.H. (ed.) (1984) *Allergy: Immunological and Clinical Aspects*. Wiley, Chichester, UK.

Mygind N. (1986) *Essential Allergy*. Blackwell Scientific Publications, Oxford.

Thompson R.A. (ed.) (1985) Laboratory Investigation of Immunological Disorders. *Clinics in Immunology and Allergy*, 5. W.B. Saunders, London.

Thompson R.A. (series ed.) *Recent Advances in Clinical Immunology*. Churchill Livingstone, UK.

Wells J.V. & Nelson D.S. (eds) (1986) *Clinical Immunology Illustrated*. Williams & Wilkins, Sydney.

TRANSPLANTATION

GRAFT REJECTION

The replacement of diseased organs by a transplant of healthy tissue has long been an objective in medicine but has been frustrated to no mean degree by the uncooperative attempts by the body to reject grafts from other individuals. Before discussing the nature and implications of this rejection phenomenon, it would be helpful to define the terms used for transplants between individuals and species:

Autograft—tissue grafted back on to the original donor.

Isograft—graft between syngeneic individuals (i.e. of identical genetic constitution) such as identical twins or mice of the same pure line strain.

Allograft (old term, homograft)—graft between allogeneic individuals (i.e. members of the same species but different genetic constitution), e.g. man to man and one mouse strain to another.

Xenograft (heterograft)—graft between xenogeneic individuals (i.e. of different species), e.g. pig to man.

It is with the allograft reaction that we have been most concerned although it should one day be possible to use grafts from other species. The most common allografting procedure is probably blood transfusion where the unfortunate consequences of mismatching are well known. Considerable attention has been paid to the rejection of solid grafts such as skin and the sequence of events is worth describing. In mice, for example, the skin allograft settles down and becomes vascularized within a few days. Between three and nine days the circulation gradually diminishes and there is increasing infiltration of the graft bed with lymphocytes and monocytes but very few plasma cells. Necrosis begins to be visible macroscopically and within a day or so the graft is sloughed completely (figure 13.1).

Evidence that rejection is immunological

First and second set reactions

It would be expected, if the reaction has an immunological basis, that the second contact with antigen would represent a more explosive event than the first and indeed the rejection of a second graft from the same donor is much accelerated. The initial vascularization is poor and may not occur at all. There is a very rapid invasion by polymorphonuclear leucocytes and lymphoid cells including plasma cells. Thrombosis and acute cell destruction can be seen by three to four days.

Specificity

Second set rejection is not the fate of all subsequent allografts but only of those derived from the original donor or a related strain. Grafts from unrelated donors are rejected as first set reactions.

Role of the lymphocyte

Neonatally thymectomized animals have difficulty in rejecting skin grafts but their capacity is restored by injection of lymphocytes from a syngeneic normal donor, suggesting that T-cells are implicated.

(a)   (b)

Figure 13.1. *Rejection of CBA skin graft by strain A mouse. (a) 10 days after transplantation; discoloured areas caused by destruction of epithelium and drying of the exposed dermis. (b) 13 days after transplantation; the scabby surface indicates total destruction of the graft. (Courtesy Prof. L. Brent.)*

The recipient of T-cells from a donor which has already rejected a graft will give accelerated rejection of a further graft of the same type (figure 13.2) showing that the lymphoid cells are primed and retain memory of the first contact with graft antigens.

Production of antibodies

After rejection, humoral antibodies with specificity for the graft donor may be recognized. In the mouse where the erythrocytes carry transplantation antigens, haemagglutination tests become positive; in the human, lymphocytotoxins are found. A Jerne plaque test using donor strain thymocytes in place of sheep erythrocytes will often demonstrate the presence of antibody-forming cells in the lymphoid tissues of grafted animals.

Genetic control of transplantation antigens

The specificity of the antigens involved in graft rejection is under genetic control. Genetically identical individuals such as mice of a pure strain or uniovular twins have identical transplantation antigens and grafts can be freely exchanged between them. The Mendelian segregation of the genes controlling these antigens has been revealed by interbreeding experiments between mice of different

Figure 13.2. *Graft rejection induces memory which is specific and can be transferred by T-cells. In experiment 1, an A strain recipient of T-cells from another A strain mouse which had rejected a graft from strain B, will give accelerated (i.e. 2nd set) rejection of a B graft. Experiments 2 and 3 show the specificity of the phenomenon with respect to the genetically unrelated third party strain C.*

pure strains. Since these mice breed true within a given strain and always accept grafts from each other, they must be homozygous for the 'transplantation' genes. Consider two such strains A and B with allelic genes differing at one locus. In each case paternal and maternal genes will be identical and they will have a genetic constitution of, say, A/A and B/B respectively (by convention, the genes are expressed in italics and the antigens they encode in normal type). Crossing strains A and B gives a first familial generation (F1) of constitution A/B. Now all F1 mice accept grafts from either parent showing that they are tolerant to both A and B. By intercrossing the F1 generation one would expect an average distribution of genotypes for the F2s as shown in figure 13.3; only 1 in 4 would have no A genes and would therefore reject an A graft because of lack of tolerance, and 1 in 4 would reject B grafts for the same reason. Thus for each locus, 3 out of 4 of the F2 generation will accept parental strain grafts. Extending the analysis, if instead of one locus with a pair of allelic genes there were n loci, the fraction of the F2 generation accepting parental strain grafts would be $(3/4)^n$. In this way an estimate of the number of loci controlling transplantation antigens can be made.

In the mouse around 40 such loci have been established, but as we have seen much earlier, the complex locus termed H-2 predominates in the sense that it controls the 'strong' transplantation antigens which provoke intense allograft reactions and we have looked at the structure (cf. figure 3.16, p. 45) and biology of this *major histocompatibility locus* in some detail in previous chapters. The non-H-2 or 'minor' transplantation antigens such as the male H-Y are recognized in (loose?) association with the MHC molecules on the cell surface by T-cells but not at all readily by B-cells. Presumably, entities like the insulin receptor which seem to have a flirtatious interaction with MHC molecules (p. 48) could function as minor transplantation antigens provided they existed in polymorphic forms. One should not be misled by the term 'minor' into thinking that these antigens do not give rise to serious rejection problems, albeit more slowly than the MHC.

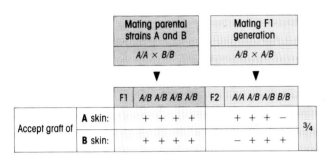

Figure 13.3. *Inheritance of genes controlling transplantation antigens. A represents a gene expressing the A antigen and B the corresponding allelic gene at the same genetic locus. The pure strains are homozygous for A/A and B/B respectively. Since the genes are co-dominant, an animal with A/B genome will express both antigens, become tolerant to them and therefore accept grafts from either A or B donors. The illustration shows that for each gene controlling a transplantation antigen specificity, three-quarters of the F2 generation will accept a graft of parental skin. For n genes the fraction is ($^{3}/_{4}$)^{n}. If F1 A/B animals are back-crossed with an A/A parent, half the progeny will be A/A and half A/B; only the latter will accept B grafts.*

Some other consequences of H-2 incompatibility

Class II MHC differences produce a mixed lymphocyte reaction (MLR)

When lymphocytes from strains of mice of different class II haplotype are cultured together, blast cell transformation and mitosis occurs (MLR), the T-cells of each population of lymphocytes reacting against class II 'Ia' determinants on the surface of the other population. For the 'one-way MLR', the stimulator cells are made unresponsive by treatment with mitomycin C or X-rays and then added to the responder lymphocytes from the other donor. The responding cells belong predominantly to a subpopulation of Ly1 positive T-lymphocytes and are stimulated by the Ia determinants present mostly on B-cells, macrophages and especially dendritic antigen-presenting cells. Thus, the MLR is inhibited by antisera to class II determinants on the stimulator cells.

Cell-mediated lympholysis (CML)

The involvement of class II MHC antigens in the provocation of transplantation rejection has been brought into some focus by the discovery of the phenomenon of CML which was developed as a possible test for histocompatibility. The principle is illustrated in figure 13.4. In short, responder cells activated by the class II-induced MLR help in the generation of cytotoxic T-cells directed to the H-2D/K determinants; in essence, the recognition of class II molecules helps to generate effectors against the class I molecules, in some ways reminiscent of the carrier-hapten system in T−B collaboration with class II equivalent to carrier and class I to hapten.

The graft-vs-host reaction (g.v.h.)

When competent T-cells are transferred from a donor to a recipient which is incapable of rejecting them, the grafted cells survive and have time to recognize the host antigens and react immunologically against

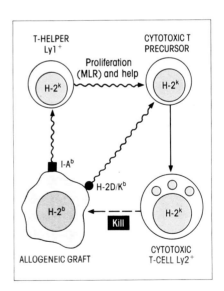

Figure 13.4. *Cell-mediated lympholysis: generation of H-2^{k} T-cells cytotoxic for H-2^{b} grafts. T-helpers respond to I-A^{b} on the graft cells by proliferating (mixed lymphocyte reaction) and are then able to help cytotoxic T-cell precursors specific for the H-2D^{b} or H-2K^{b} antigens of the graft to become cytotoxic effectors.*

217

them. Instead of the normal transplantation reaction of host against graft, we have the reverse, the so-called graft-vs-host (g.v.h.) reaction. In the young rodent there can be inhibition of growth (runting), spleen enlargement and haemolytic anaemia (due to production of red cell antibodies). In the human, fever, anaemia, weight loss, rash, diarrhoea and splenomegaly are observed. The 'stronger' the transplantation antigen difference, the more severe the reaction. Where donor and recipient differ at HLA or H-2 loci, the consequences can be fatal, although it should be noted that reactions to dominant minor transplantation antigens, or combinations of them, may be equally difficult to control.

Two possible situations leading to g.v.h. reactions are illustrated in figure 13.5. In the human this may arise in immunologically anergic subjects receiving bone marrow grafts, e.g. for combined immunodeficiency (p. 228), for red cell aplasia after radiation accidents or as a possible form of cancer therapy. Competent T-cells in blood or present in grafted organs given to immunosuppressed patients may give g.v.h. reactions; so could maternal cells which adventitiously cross the placenta, although in this case there is as yet no evidence of diseases caused by such a mechanism in the human.

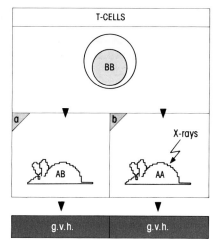

Figure 13.5. *Graft-vs-host reaction. When competent T-cells are inoculated into a host incapable of reacting against them, the grafted cells are free to react against the antigens on the host's cells which they recognize as foreign. The ensuing reaction may be fatal. Two of many possible situations are illustrated: (a) the hybrid AB receives cells from one parent (BB) which are tolerated but react against the A antigen on host cells; (b) an X-irradiated AA recipient restored immunologically with BB cells cannot react against the graft and a g.v.h. reaction will result.*

Mechanisms of graft rejection

Lymphocyte-mediated rejection

A great deal of the work on allograft rejection has involved transplants of skin or solid tumours because their fate is relatively easy to follow. In these cases there is little support for the view that humoral antibodies are instrumental in destruction of the graft although, as we shall see later, this is not necessarily so with transplants of other organs such as the kidney. Whereas passive transfer of *serum* from an animal which has rejected a skin allograft cannot usually accelerate the rejection of a similar graft on the recipient animal, injection of *lymphoid cells* (particularly recirculating small lymphocytes) is effective in shortening graft survival (cf. figure 13.2).

A primary role of lymphoid cells in first set rejection would be consistent with the histology of the early reaction showing infiltration by mononuclear cells with very few polymorphs or plasma cells (figure 13.6). The dramatic effect of neonatal thymectomy in prolonging skin transplants, as mentioned earlier, and the long survival of grafts on children with thymic deficiencies implicate the T-lymphocytes in these reactions. In the chicken, homograft rejection and g.v.h. reactivity are influenced by neonatal thymectomy but not bursectomy. More direct evidence has come from *in vitro* studies showing that T-cells taken from mice rejecting an allograft could kill target cells bearing the graft antigens *in vitro*. Recent work on the importance of murine $Ly1^+2^-$ and human $T4^+$ cells as effectors has cast some doubt, probably wrongly, on the role of cytotoxic cells in graft rejection *in vivo*; although these subsets have sometimes been shown to have cytotoxic potential for class II targets, as a rule they are associated with helper activity, in this case particularly for cytotoxic T-cell precursors, and with the production of lymphokines mediating delayed hypersensitivity reactions. Perhaps they act to encourage access of cytotoxic T-cells to their targets?

The role of humoral antibody

It has long been recognized that isolated allogeneic cells such as lymphocytes can be destroyed by cytotoxic (type II) reactions involving humoral antibody. However, although earlier experience with skin and solid tumour grafts suggested that they were not

Figure 13.6. *Acute early rejection of human renal allograft 10 days after transplantation showing dense cellular infiltration of interstitium by mononuclear cells (pyronin stain). (Courtesy Prof. K. Porter.)*

219

readily susceptible to the action of cytotoxic antibodies, it is now clear that this does not hold for all types of organ transplants. Consideration of the different ways in which kidney allografts can be rejected illustrates the point.

1 *Hyperacute rejection* within minutes of transplantation, characterized by sludging of red cells and microthrombi in the glomeruli, occurs in individuals with pre-existing humoral antibodies—either due to blood group incompatibility or presensitization to class I MHC through blood transfusion.

2 *Acute early rejection* occurring up to 10 days or so after transplantation is characterized by dense cellular infiltration (figure 13.6) and rupture of peritubular capillaries and appears to be a cell-mediated hypersensitivity reaction involving T-lymphocytes.

3 *Acute late rejection*, which occurs from 11 days onwards in patients suppressed with prednisone and azathioprine, is probably caused by the binding of immunoglobulin (presumably antibody) and complement to the arterioles and glomerular capillaries where they can be visualized by immunofluorescent techniques. These immunoglobulin deposits on the vessel walls induce platelet aggregation in the glomerular capillaries leading to acute renal shutdown (figure 13.7). The possibility of damage to antibody-coated cells through antibody-dependent cell-mediated cytotoxicity must also be considered.

4 *Insidious and late rejection* associated with subendothelial deposits of immunoglobulin and C3 on the glomerular basement membranes which may sometimes be an expression of an underlying im-

TRANSPLANTATION

220

Figure 13.7. *Acute late rejection of human renal allograft showing platelet aggregation in a glomerular capillary induced by deposition of antibody on the vessel wall (electron micrograph). (Courtesy Prof. K. Porter.)*

mune complex disorder (originally necessitating the transplant) or possibly of complex formation with soluble antigens derived from the grafted kidney.

The complexity of the action and interaction of cellular and humoral factors in graft rejection is therefore considerable and an attempt to summarize the postulated mechanisms involved is presented in figure 13.8.

There are also circumstances when antibodies may actually *protect* a graft from destruction and this important phenomenon of *enhancement* will be considered further below.

THE PREVENTION OF GRAFT REJECTION

Matching tissue types on graft donor and recipient

Since MHC differences provoke the most vicious rejection of grafts, a prodigious amount of effort has gone into defining these antigen specificities in an attempt to minimize rejection by matching graft and recipient in much the same way that individuals

CHAPTER 13

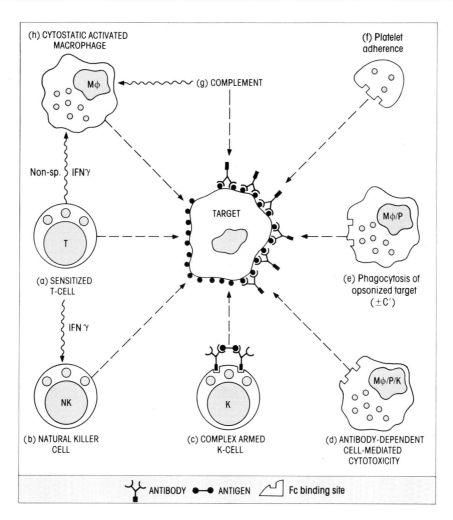

Figure 13.8. *Mechanisms of target cell destruction. Mφ =
macrophage; P = polymorph; K = K cell. (a) Direct killing by
cytotoxic T-cells binding through specific surface receptors.
Indirect tissue damage through release of lymphokines from
delayed-type hypersensitivity T-cells. (b) Killing by NK cells
(p.233) enhanced by interferon. (c) Specific killing by immune-
complex-armed K-cell which recognizes target through free
antibody valencies in the complex. (d) Attack by antibody-
dependent cell-mediated cytotoxicity (in a−d the killing is
extracellular). (e) Phagocytosis of target coated with
antibody (heightened by bound C3). (f) Sticking of platelets to
antibody bound to surface of graft vascular endothelium
leading to formation of microthrombi. (g) Complement-
mediated cytotoxicity. (h) Macrophages activated non-
specifically by agents such as BCG, endotoxin, poly-I: C,
T-cell macrophage activating factor and possibly C3b are
cytostatic and sometimes cytotoxic for dividing tumour cells,
perhaps through extracellular action of peroxide and O₂⁻-
derived radicals generated at the cell surface (p.7). In some
situations in vitro, sensitized B-cells secrete antibody which
coats the target rendering it susceptible to attack by ADCC.*

are cross-matched for blood transfusions (incidentally, the ABO group provides strong transplantation antigens).

Methods for tissue typing

Alleles (tissue types) at the three class I loci, HLA-
A, -B and -C (cf. figure 3.18, p. 46) are identified by
complement-dependent cytotoxic reactions using
operationally monospecific sera which are selected
from patients transfused with whole blood and
multigravidas who often become immunized with
fetal antigens with specificities defined by paternally derived genes absent from the mother's genome.
An individual is typed by setting up his lymphocytes against a panel of such sera in the presence of
complement, cell death normally being judged by
the inability to exclude trypan blue or eosin (figure
13.9a). Different antigens are arbitrarily assigned
numerical specificities (figure 13.10); an individual

heterozygous at each locus must express four *major* class I HLA specificities and two minor ones (HLA-C) derived from both the maternal and paternal chromosomes.

The original class II locus, *HLA-D*, was defined by the mixed lymphocyte reaction (MLR) using homozygous stimulating cells for typing; if an individual failed to respond to a given typing cell then his own lymphocytes must already have borne that specificity (figure 13.9b). As serological reagents were developed it transpired that the *D* locus could be split into *DR* and *DQ* each encoding heterodimer class II molecules with homology for murine *I-E* and *I-A* respectively. Subsequently a new locus, *HLA-DP*, was discovered by the selective action of cytotoxic T-cells (figure 13.9c).

The feasibility of typing by the detection of restriction fragment length polymorphism using DNA probes is under active scrutiny. However, it is vitally important to bear in mind the important distinction between typing based on T-cell discrimination and all other types of analysis because the important initial event for transplantation is the recognition of the graft antigens by *T-cells*, and antibodies do not necessarily define the same epitopes. Thus, individuals bearing the serologically defined DR4 specifi-

cities, can be subdivided by T-lymphocyte typing into five different subgroups.

The polymorphism of the human HLA-system

The latest data on the well-established specificities at the three class I and three class II loci are presented in figure 13.10. Further definition of the DQ and DR specificities with T-cell reagents increases the number even further. With so many alleles at each locus and a total of 12 possible alleles in each individual, it will readily be appreciated that this gives rise to an exceptional degree of polymorphism which is compounded further by the existence of multiple allotypic forms of the class III MHC complement components C2, C4A, C4B and factor B.

This remarkable polymorphism is of great potential value to the species since the need for T-cells to recognize its own individual specificities provides a defence against microbial molecular mimicry in which a whole species might be put at risk by its inability to recognize as foreign an organism which displays determinants similar in structure to these crucial MHC conformations. It is also possible that in some way the existence of a high degree of polymorphism helps to maintain the diversity of

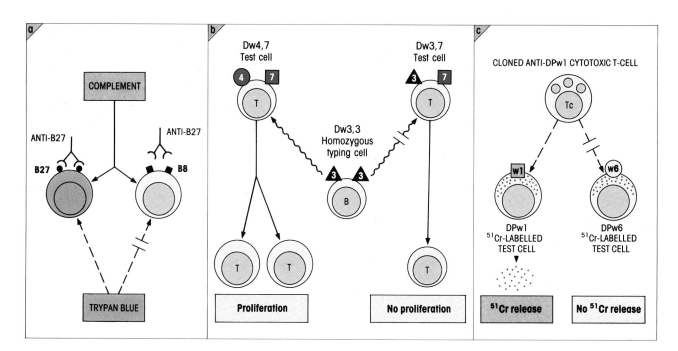

Figure 13.9. *Tissue typing. (a) Serological testing. Complement-mediated killing by mono-specific antibody allows entry of Trypan Blue. (b) Mixed lymphocyte reaction. Cells bearing the HLA-D specificity of the homozygous typing cell are tolerant to that antigen and do not respond. Cells* lacking this specificity give a proliferative response measured by incorporation of [³H]thymidine. (c) Cytotoxic T-cell typing. Cloned reagents are now used. Cytotoxicity is measured by the release of radioactivity from mitogen-stimulated target test cells prelabelled with ⁵¹Cr.

HLA-LOCUS	ALLELES
DP	w1–6
DQ	w1–3
DR	1–5, w6–14
B	5, 7, 8, 12, 13, 14, 15, 17, 18, 27, 35, 37, 38, 39, 40, 49, 51
C	w1–8
A	1, 2, 3, 9, 10, 11, 25, 26, 28, 29, 30, 31, 32

Figure 13.10. *HLA specificities and their inheritance. The complex lies on chromosome 6, the DP locus being closest to the centromere. There are several more specificities at the A and B loci but only the most solidly established are given. The numbers at the A and B loci do not overlap. T-cell reagents subdivide the DQ and DR specificities even further. The small 'w' before a number stands for 'workshop' and indicates that the specificity concerned has not yet been characterized sufficiently for upgrading to full HLA-status. Since there are several possible alleles at each locus, the probability of a random pair of subjects from the general population having identical HLA specificities is low. However, there is a 1:4 chance that two **siblings** will be identical in this respect because each group of specificities on a single chromosome forms a haplotype which will be inherited en bloc giving four possible combinations of paternal and maternal chromosomes. Parent and offspring can only be identical (1:2 chance) if the mother and father have one haplotype in common.*

antigenic recognition within the lymphoid system of a given species and also ensures heterozygosity (hybrid vigour).

The value of matching tissue types

Improvements in operative techniques and the use of drugs such as cyclosporin A have greatly diminished the effects of mismatching HLA specificities on graft survival but, nevertheless, most transplanters favour a reasonable degree of matching especially at the DR locus (see figure 13.10). The concensus is that matching at the DR loci is of greater benefit than the B loci which in turn are of more relevance to graft survival than the A loci.

Because of the many thousands of different HLA phenotypes possible (figure 13.10), it is usual to work with a large pool of potential recipients on a continental basis so that when graft material becomes available the best possible match can be made. The position will be improved when the pool of available organs can be increased through the development of long-term tissue storage banks but techniques are not good enough for this at present except in the case of bone marrow cells which can be kept viable even after freezing and thawing. With a paired organ such as the kidney, living donors may be used; siblings provide the best chance of a good match (cf. figure 13.10). However, the use of living donors poses difficult ethical problems and there has been encouraging progress in the use of cadaver material. Some groups are looking at the possibility of animal organs or mechanical substitutes while some are even trying to prevent the disease in the first place!

Agents producing general immunosuppression

Graft rejection can be held at bay by the use of agents which non-specifically interfere with the induction or expression of the immune response. Because these agents are non-specific, patients on immunosuppressive therapy tend to be susceptible to infections; they are also more prone to develop lymphoreticular cancers.

Lymphoid cell ablation

Thymectomy, splenectomy and lymphadenectomy in adult recipients do not appear to help, although extracorporeal irradiation of blood and thoracic duct cannulation have proved beneficial. More practically, injections of anti-lymphocyte globulin or of monoclonal anti-T3 have successfully reversed acute kidney graft rejection.

Total lymphoid irradiation (TLI)

Fractionated irradiation focused on the lymphoid tissues with shielding of marrow, lungs and other vital non-lymphoid tissue, has been used in humans to treat Hodgkin's disease for over 20 years. When mice given similar treatment are injected with allogeneic bone marrow, they fully accept the graft and show no signs of graft-vs-host disease which would normally occur. Furthermore, the chimaerism (coexistence of both donor and host cells) is permanent and such mice will accept grafts of other tissue from the bone marrow donor strain. The irradiation induces the formation of large granular lymphocytes lacking T, B and macrophage markers which non-specifically suppress the antigen-specific cytolytic arm of allogeneic immune reactions while at the same time facilitating the development of antigen-specific suppressors which maintain tolerance. The successful application to the human is awaited with interest.

Immunosuppressive drugs

The development of an immunological response requires the active proliferation of a relatively small number of antigen-sensitive lymphocytes to give a population of sensitized cells large enough to be effective. Many of the immunosuppressive drugs now employed were first used in cancer chemotherapy because of their toxicity to dividing cells. Aside from the complications of blanket immunosuppression mentioned above, these antimitotic drugs are especially toxic for cells of the bone marrow and small intestine and must therefore be used with great care.

One of the most commonly used drugs in this field is *azathioprine* which has a preferential effect on T-cell mediated reactions. It is broken down in the body first to 6-mercaptopurine and then converted to the active agent, the ribotide. Because of the similarity in shape (figure 13.11), this competes with inosinic acid for enzymes concerned in the synthesis of guanylic and adenylic acids; it also inhibits the synthesis of 5-phosphoribosylamine, a precursor of inosinic acid, by a feedback mechanism. The net result is inhibition of nucleic acid synthesis. Another drug, methotrexate, through its action as a folic acid antagonist also inhibits synthesis of nucleic acid. The N-mustard derivative cyclophosphamide probably attacks DNA by alkylation and cross-linking so preventing correct duplication during cell division. These agents appear to exert their damaging effects on cells during mitosis and for this reason are most powerful when administered after presentation of antigen at a time when the antigen-sensitive cells are dividing.

Cyclosporin A, a neutral hydrophobic cyclical peptide containing 11 amino acids, represents an exciting and entirely new class of compound which is having a dramatic impact on the human transplantation scene. It is a very insoluble fungal metabolite which is of particular interest since it penetrates antigen-sensitive T-cells in the G_0 to G_1 phase and selectively blocks the transcription of lymphokine mRNA, possibly competing for a prolactin receptor. Resting cells which carry the vital memory for immunity to microbial infections are spared and there is little toxicity for dividing cells in gut and bone marrow. Some studies also point to an 'exquisite' sensitivity of the dendritic antigen-presenting cells to the drug. What is really striking is that in some cases it has been possible to show that cyclosporin treatment has led to the development of *specific* T-suppressor cells which could actively maintain tolerance (see figure 13.13 for an experimental example). This clearly warrants further study.

There are, of course, side-effects. It has to be used at doses below those causing nephrotoxicity so that blood levels have to be monitored regularly by radioimmunoassay. There is also some cause for

Figure 13.11. *Metabolic conversion of azathioprine through 6-mercaptopurine to the ribotide: similarity to inosinic acid with which it competes.*

concern that cyclosporin may make patients susceptible to EB virus-induced lymphomas since the drug inhibits T-cells which control EB virus transformation of B-cells *in vitro*; however, the latest results suggest that the incidence of lymphoma is relatively low in comparison with that reported for allografted patients on conventional immunosuppressive therapy. Cyclosporin is proving to be of great clinical value (see figure 13.12 as an example of its use in cardiac transplantation), and furthermore it does offer an intriguing new pathway towards the development of agents with selective action against lymphocytes.

Steroids such as prednisone intervene at many points in the immune response, affecting lymphocyte recirculation and the generation of cytotoxic effector cells, for example; in addition, their outstanding anti-inflammatory potency rests on features such as inhibition of neutrophil adherence to vascular endothelium in an inflammatory area and suppression of monocyte/macrophage functions such as microbicidal activity and response to lymphokines.

Figure 13.12. *Efficacy of initial short-term treatment with cyclosporin for the survival of cardiac allografts. After 3 months on cyclosporin A, the first group were then switched to the conventional therapy of azathioprine and steroids used throughout for the control group; 54 patients on cyclosporin, 60 in the other group. Some transplanters use cyclosporin alone as the only form of immunosuppression. (Reproduced from Morris P.J. (1985)* **Transplantation Proceedings XVII,** *1153, with permission.)*

Strategies for antigen-specific depression of allograft reactivity

If the disadvantages of blanket immunosuppression are to be avoided, we must aim at knocking out only the reactivity of the host to the antigens of the graft, leaving the remainder of the immunological apparatus intact. One approach is through the induction of tolerance which in the adult normally means T-suppression. Total lymph node irradiation plus bone marrow (*vide supra*) is known to induce T-suppression in mice, and grafts of skin and heart from the same donor enjoy prolonged survival. As purified histocompatibility antigens become available, it should ultimately not be beyond the wit of *Homo sapiens* to juggle the relative timing and dosages of antigen and various immunosuppressants to produce a specific hyporesponsive state.

On rather a different tack, it has been reported that tolerance between rodent strains can be established by deliberate autoimmunization with the idiotype of the host receptor for donor transplantation antigens. It now appears that the same effect can be achieved more reliably and somewhat unexpectedly by cyclosporin A treatment of rats receiving kidney allografts. The experiments described in figure 13.13a show that spleen T-cells from cyclosporin A-treated rats bearing a long-standing kid-

ney allograft can suppress graft rejection in a naïve animal. The suppressors proliferate *in vitro* when stimulated by blast cells generated by exposure of host strain T-cells to graft antigens and it is concluded that the suppressors are directed to the idiotype of the cells capable of recognizing the graft (figure 13.13c). Another important feature of these experiments is that suppression is only effective when the grafted kidney is one which has been 'parked' for some time in a cyclosporin-treated recipient; fresh kidneys are rejected normally. A likely interpretation is that passenger B-lymphocytes and dendritic accessory cells rich in class II Ia antigens which are far and away the most immunogenic cells in tissue grafts, are eliminated from the 'parked' kidney graft by the cyclosporin. The argument would be that graft antigens presented on donor dendritic cells provoke powerful rejection by direct stimulation of the appropriate T-helpers, whereas in the absence of dendritic cells, the graft antigens would have to be presented after processing by host cells in association with host class II and under the influence of cyclosporin this allows a build-up of inhibitory anti-idiotype T-suppressors.

Rather comparable mechanisms operate in the survival of kidney grafts produced by the technique of *immunological enhancement*. It has long been

Figure 13.13. *Long-term survival of kidney grafts maintained by T-suppressors induced by enhancement or cyclosporin. Naïve rats were injected with spleen cells from rats treated with cyclosporin (a) or enhancing antibodies (b), carrying long-standing kidney allografts. Unless stated as 'fresh', the grafts had been 'parked' in a cyclosporin or enhanced animal to eliminate immunogenic passenger cells. The mechanism (c) is thought to involve loss of passenger cells and generation of anti-idiotypic T-suppressors. (Data in (a) and (b) reproduced from Batchelor J.R. & Ch. Y.L. (1986) In* Progress in Immunology VI *p.1002, Cinader B. and Miller R.G. (eds), Academic Press, with permission.)*

recognized that deliberate immunization of animals with irradiated tumour cells produces enhancing antibodies which prolong the life of the tumour. Somewhat comparable manipulations can also enhance the survival of kidney grafts and again it transpires that, as with cyclosporin, two major events occur, the elimination of immunogenic passenger cells and the generation of anti-idiotype suppressors (figure 13.13b).

It is relevant that thyroid, parathyroid and islets of Langerhans, after culture for several days in 95% oxygen, are readily accepted as allografts and this has been attributed to loss of Ia-positive dendritic cells; such grafts are rapidly rejected if the recipient is injected with as few as 10^3 peritoneal cells of donor origin which potently present allogeneic class I in the context of allogeneic class II.

CLINICAL EXPERIENCE IN GRAFTING

Privileged sites

Corneal grafts survive without the need for immunosuppression. Because they are avascular they do not sensitize the recipient although they become cloudy if the individual has been pre-sensitized. Grafts of cartilage are successful in the same way but an additional factor is the protection afforded the chondrocytes by the matrix. With bone and artery it doesn't really matter if the grafts die because they can still provide a framework for host cells to colonize.

Kidney grafts

Thousands of kidneys have been transplanted and with improvement in patient management there is a high survival rate (figure 13.14). Matching at the HLA-D locus has a strong effect on graft survival but in the long term (5 years or more) the desirability of reasonable HLA-B, and to a lesser extent HLA-A, matching also becomes apparent. It has now been firmly established that multiple blood transfusions prior to grafting have a significant beneficial effect on survival (figure 13.14) but the explanation is still not forthcoming.

DRw6-positive individuals are rather intriguing. They are relatively poor at accepting DRw6-negative grafts while their kidneys survive relatively well as grafts (table 13.1). The conjecture is that in the recipient, DRw6 is a good immune response (Ir) gene for class II antigens and that when DRw6 is present on a graft it is a good inducer of T-suppression.

Patients are partially immunosuppressed at the time of transplantation because uraemia causes a degree of immunological anergy. The combination of azathioprine and prednisone is commonly employed in the long-term management of kidney grafts but replacement of the azathioprine with cyclosporin A looks very promising. If kidney function is poor during a rejection crisis renal dialysis can be used. When transplantation is performed because of immune complex induced glomerulonephritis, the immunosuppressive treatment used may help to prevent a similar lesion developing in the grafted kidney. Patients with glomerular basement membrane antibodies (e.g. Goodpasture's syndrome) are likely to destroy their renal transplants unless first treated with plasmapheresis and immunosuppressive drugs.

Heart transplants

The 1-year survival figure for heart transplants has moved up to around the 80% mark (figure 13.15), helped considerably by the introduction of cyclosporin A therapy. Its nephrotoxicity is a drawback, however, and some groups switch over to conventional treatment with azathioprine plus steroids (cf. figure 13.12). Full HLA matching is of course not practical but single DR mismatches gave 90% survival at 3 years compared with a figure of 65% for two DR mismatches. Aside from the rejection problem it is likely that the number of patients who would benefit from cardiac replacement is much greater than the number dying with adequately healthy hearts. More attention will have to be given

Table 13.1. *HLA-DRw6 and graft survival two years post-transplant.*

RECIPIENT	DR MISMATCHES	DONOR DRw6 POSITIVE	DONOR DRw6 NEGATIVE
DRw6 POSITIVE (n = 303)	0	80%	—
	1	78%	50%
	2	—	50%
DRw6 NEGATIVE (n = 852)	0	—	71%
	1	75%	63%
	2	81%	62%

Note DRw6+ grafts do better than DRw6−, and DRw6− grafts do worse in DRw6+ than in DRw6− unmatched recipients.

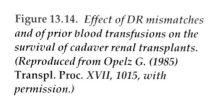

Figure 13.14. *Effect of DR mismatches and of prior blood transfusions on the survival of cadaver renal transplants. (Reproduced from Opelz G. (1985) Transpl. Proc. XVII, 1015, with permission.)*

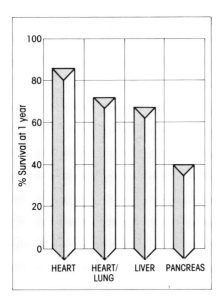

Figure 13.15. *Survival of organ allografts at 1 year. (Data from Batchelor J.R. & Ch. Y.L. (1986) In Progress in Immunology VI, p.1002, Cinader B. and Miller R.G. (eds), Academic Press, with permission.)*

to the possibility of xenogeneic grafts and mechanical substitutes.

Liver transplants

Survival rates for orthotopic liver grafts are broadly in line with those receiving heart transplants (figure 13.15), particularly using combined cyclosporin/steroid therapy. Rejection crises are dealt with by high dose steroids and if this proves ineffective, anti-lymphocyte globulin. Three-quarters of the patients transplanted for hepatic cancer have had recurrence of their tumour within one year.

Experience with liver grafting between pigs revealed an unexpected finding. Many of the animals retained the grafted organs in a healthy state for many months without any form of immunosuppression. The transplanted liver represented a large antigen pool which induced a state of unresponsiveness to grafts of skin or kidney from the same donor. The mechanism is not clear but may involve true tolerance or enhancement. There is as yet no evidence that this highly desirable state can be established by a hepatic transplant in man.

Bone marrow grafting

Patients with certain immunodeficiency disorders and aplastic anaemia are obvious candidates for treatment with bone marrow stem cells as are acute leukaemia patients treated radically with intensive chemotherapy and possibly whole body irradiation in attempts to eradicate the neoplastic cells (table 13.2). Successful results with bone marrow transfers require highly compatible donors if fatal graft-vs-host reactions are to be avoided, and here siblings offer the best chance of finding a matched donor (figure 13.10). Matching for antigens quite distinct from those controlled by the major HLA loci may prove to be essential. The incidence of chronic graft-vs-host disease is reduced if T-cells in the grafted marrow are first removed by a cytotoxic cocktail of anti-T-cell monoclonals and significant improvements have also been reported both for success of primary engraftment and the prevention of g.v.h. disease when patients are treated with cyclosporin A. A curious effect that requires further exploration is the observation that leukaemia patients with g.v.h. disease have a lower incidence of relapse.

DISEASE		PROBABILITY	
TYPE	STAGE	LONG-TERM SURVIVAL	DISEASE RECURRENCE
Acute leukaemia	Relapse	0.1–0.3	0.60
Acute non-lymphocytic leukaemia	1st remission	0.6	0.25
Acute lymphocytic leukaemia	2nd remission	0.3	0.25
Chronic granulocytic leukaemia	Blastic phase	0.2	0.70
Chronic granulocytic leukaemia	Accelerated phase	0.2	0.50
Chronic granulocytic leukaemia	Chronic phase	0.6	0.30
Severe combined immunodeficiency	—	0.5	—
Severe aplastic anaemia	—	0.8	—
Thalassemia major	—	0.7	0.3

Table 13.2. *Bone marrow transplants: summary of survival and relapse data from many centres.*

Other organs

It is to be expected that improvement in techniques of control of the rejection process will encourage transplantation in several other areas—not cases of endocrine disorders where exogenous replacement therapy is convenient, but, for example, in diabetes the number of transplants recorded is rising rapidly and the current success rate is around 40% (figure 13.15). One looks forward in particular to the successful transplantation of skin for lethal burns.

ASSOCIATION OF HLA TYPE WITH DISEASE

An impressive body of data is accumulating which links specific HLA antigens with particular disease states in the human (table 13.3) and even more

Table 13.3. *Association of HLA with disease.*

DISEASE	HLA ALLELE	RELATIVE RISK
a Class II associated		
Hashimoto's disease	DR5	3.2
Rheumatoid arthritis	DR4	5.8
Dermatitis herpetiformis	DR3	56.4
Chronic active hepatitis (autoimmune)	DR3	13.9
Coeliac disease	DR3	10.8
Sjögren's syndrome	DR3	9.7
Addison's disease (adrenal)	DR3	6.3
Insulin-dependent diabetes	DR3	5.0
	DR4	6.8
	DR3/4	14.3
	DR2	0.2
Thyrotoxicosis (Graves')	DR3	3.7
Primary myxoedema	DR3	5.7
Goodpasture's syndrome	DR2	13.1
Tuberculoid leprosy	DR2	8.1
Multiple sclerosis	DR2	4.8
b Class I, HLA-B27 associated		
Ankylosing spondylitis	B27	87.4
Reiter's diesase	B27	37.0
Post-salmonella arthritis	B27	29.7
Post-shigella arthritis	B27	20.7
Post-yersinia arthritis	B27	17.6
Post-gonococcal arthritis	B27	14.0
Uveitis	B27	14.6
Amyloidosis in rheumatoid arthritis	B27	8.2
c Other class I associations		
Subacute thyroiditis	Bw35	13.7
Psoriasis vulgaris	Cw6	13.3
Idiopathic haemochromatosis	A3	8.2
Myasthenia gravis	B8	4.4

(Data mainly from Ryder et al.: see legend to figure 13.16.)

striking relationships may be uncovered as the complexity of the HLA-D region is unravelled. The relationships are influenced by *linkage disequilibrium*, a state where closely linked genes on a chromosome tend to remain associated rather than undergo genetic randomization in a given population, so that the frequency of a pair of alleles occurring together is greater than the product of the individual gene frequencies (figure 13.16a). This could result from natural selection favouring a particular haplotype or from insufficient time elapsing since the first appearance of closely located alleles to allow them to become randomly distributed throughout the population. Be that as it may, a significant association between a disease and a

(a)

HLA GENES	SINGLE GENE	PAIRED GENES	
		EXPECTED	OBSERVED
A1	16	1.6	8.8
B8	10		
A3	13	1.3	2.8
B7	10		

GENE FREQUENCY %

(b)

Figure 13.16. *Linkage disequilibrium and the association between HLA and disease. (a) Two examples of linkage disequilibrium. The expected frequency for a pair of genes is the product of each individual gene frequency. B8 and DR3 are in linkage disequilibrium as are B7 and DR2; thus the haplotypes A1, B8, DR3 and A3, B7, DR2 are* **relatively** *common. (b) Influence of linkage disequilibrium on disease association. *Relative risk: the increased chance of contracting the disease for individuals bearing the antigen relative to those lacking it. (Data from Ryder L.P., Andersen E. & Svejgaard A. (1979) HLA and disease Registry 1979.* **Tissue Antigens,** *Supplement.)*

given HLA specificity does not imply that we have identified the disease susceptibility gene because we might find an even better correlation with another HLA gene in linkage disequilibrium with the first. To take an example: in multiple sclerosis, an association with the B7 allele was first established but when patients were typed for the D locus, a much stronger correlation with DR2 emerged (figure 13.16b). The initial correlation with B7 resulted from linkage disequilibrium between B7 and DR2. We still cannot be sure that DR2 itself is the disease susceptibility gene since, carrying the argument a stage further, one cannot exclude the possibility of finding an even greater association with another closely linked gene.

With the odd exception such as idiopathic haemochromatosis and congenital adrenal hyperplasia resulting from a 21-hydroxylase deficiency, HLA-linked diseases are intimately bound up with immunological processes. By and large, the HLA-D related disorders are autoimmune with a tendency for DR3 to be associated with organ-specific diseases involving cell surface receptors. The question of some link between DR3 and these receptors has been mooted, though not with much confidence. It has also been suggested that HLA antigens might also affect the susceptibility of a cell to viral attachment or infection, thereby influencing the development of autoimmunity to associated surface components.

Inevitably, because class II genes are dominant in these relationships (for the time being), the temptation is to think in terms of immune response genes controlling the nature of the reaction to the relevant autoantigen or to whatever might be a causative agent. On this basis, DR3 and DR4 must influence separate but synergistic immune responses which mediate the onset of insulin-dependent diabetes. In both that disease and in rheumatoid arthritis, the DR2 allele is under-represented and DR2-positive patients have less severe disease, implying that DR2 might be considered a poor-responder gene. In the case of multiple sclerosis where DR2 is a major risk factor, it is conceivable that these individuals are poor T-cell responders to measles since defective cell-mediated immunity to this virus is to date the only major immunological abnormality recognized. However, the B7 allele also correlates positively with an increased incidence of paralytic polio and with relatively poor T-cell activity *in vitro* for heterologous target cells. This raises another interpretation of this phenomenon, which does not necessarily exclude some contribution from immune response genes, in which it is postulated that individual DR alleles control overall cellular interactions and reactivity rather than individual antigenic specificities.

The association with HLA in ankylosing spondylitis is quite extraordinary; up to 95% of patients are of B27 phenotype as compared with around 5% in controls. The incidence of B27 is also markedly raised in other conditions when accompanied by sacro-iliitis, e.g. Reiter's disease, acute anterior uveitis, psoriasis and other forms of infective sacro-iliitis such as yersinia, gonococcal and salmonella arthritis. The very close association with B27 makes it unlikely that as good a correlation with any other gene will be found. The involvement of infective agents may provide a clue: does molecular similarity to B27 imply a tolerance to certain microbial antigens, or is there some more subtle interaction with microbial products? Reports by Ebringer and colleagues of a cross-reaction of B27 with *Klebsiella pneumoniae* and a higher faecal carriage rate for these organisms in patients with active disease are certainly provocative in this respect.

Deficiencies in C4 and C2, which are MHC class III molecules, clearly predispose to the development of immune complex disease (p. 205) and so it would be expected that the inheritance of null genes or alleles coding for the less active complement allotypes would increase the risk of rheumatological disorders and add yet further complexity to the correlations between HLA types and disease.

THE IMMUNOLOGICAL RELATIONSHIP OF MOTHER AND FETUS

A further consequence of polymorphism in an outbred population is that mother and fetus will almost certainly have different MHCs. Some examples of selection for heterozygotes (where maternally and paternally derived haplotypes are different) over homozygotes (both fetal haplotypes identical with the mother's) in viviparous animals suggest that this is beneficial. Likewise, the placentae of F1 offspring are larger than normal when mothers are preimmunized to the paternal H-2 haplotype and smaller when mothers are tolerant to these antigens.

The threat posed to the fetus as a potential graft due to the possession of paternal transplantation antigens so intrigued Lewis Thomas that he was moved to suggest that rejection of the fetus might initiate parturition, although it would be difficult to account for the normal birth of female offspring to pure-strain mating pairs where fetus and mother would have identical histocompatibility antigens without further postulating a placenta-specific surface antigen.

None the less, in the human haemochorial placenta, maternal blood with immunocompetent lymphocytes does circulate in contact with the fetal trophoblast and we have to explain how the fetus avoids allograft rejection, despite the development of an immunological response in a proportion of mothers as evidenced by the appearance of anti-HLA antibodies and cytotoxic lymphocytes. In fact, prior sensitization with a skin graft fails to affect a pregnancy, showing that trophoblast cells are immunologically protected. Some of the many speculations which have been aired on this subject are summarized in figure 13.17.

Undoubtedly, the most important factor is the well-documented lack of both class I and class II MHC antigens on the placental villous trophoblast which protects the fetus from allogeneic attack. It has recently been shown that certain human cytotrophoblast populations in the smooth part of the chorion (chorion laeve), and invasive cytotrophoblast in the placental bed, throughout gestation express class I MHC-related molecules which are products of genes distinct from HLA-A or -B. They could be the human homologue of the Qa-Tla genes in the mouse. They could be involved in suppression of maternal responses. They could be . . . ?

IS THE CANCER CELL LIKE AN ALLOGRAFT?

The ability to reject transplants of tissue may be traced back a long way down the evolutionary tree —back even as far as the annelid worms. Long before the studies on the involvement of self-MHC in immunological responses, Lewis Thomas suggested that the allograft rejection mechanism represented a means by which the body's cells could be kept under *immunological surveillance* so that altered cells with a neoplastic potential could be identified and summarily eliminated. For this to operate, cancer cells must display some new surface structure which can be recognized by the lymphoid cells and examples have been discovered although the phenomenon is not universal.

Changes on the surface of tumour cells (figure 13.18)

(a) Virally controlled antigens

Cells infected with oncogenic viruses usually display two new antigens on their surface, one (V) identical with an antigen on the isolated virion and the other (T), also a product of the viral genome, present only on infected cells; the latter represents a strong transplantation antigen and generates haplotype-restricted cytotoxic T-cells. All syngeneic tumours induced by a given virus carry the same surface antigen, irrespective of their cellular origin, so that immunization with any one of these tumours confers resistance to subsequent challenge with the others.

(b) Expression of embryonic genes

If the uncontrollable cell division of a cancer cell is attributable to the abnormal expression of one of a number of normal differentiation genes (so-called cellular oncogenes), their products or the products encoded by other genes which secondarily might become derepressed could be differentiation antigens normally associated with an earlier fetal stage.

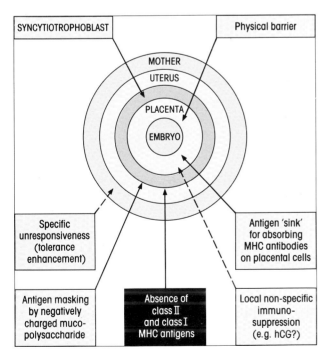

Figure 13.17. *Mechanisms postulated to account for the survival of the fetus as an allograft in the mother. (After L. Brent.)*

Figure 13.18. *Tumour-associated surface changes. Even virally induced tumours may possess idiotypic specificities.*

Thus tumours derived from the same cell type are often found to express such oncofetal antigens which are also present on embryonic cells. Examples would be α-fetoprotein in hepatic carcinoma and carcino-embryonic antigen (CEA) in cancer of the intestine. Certain monoclonal antibodies raised against human melanoma cells also react with tumours of neural crest origin and fetal melanocytes. Another monoclonal antibody defines the SSEA-1 antigen found on a variety of human tumours and early mouse embryos but absent from adult cells with the exception of human granulocytes and monocytes.

Changes have quite frequently been observed in the expression of class I MHC molecules. Diminished or absent expression has been reported, in most cases associated with increased metastatic potential. Sometimes it has proved possible to identify an alien specificity not present on the host class I molecules and attributed by some to gene conversion events with silent class I genes somewhere in the Qa/Tla region in the mouse; there is even evidence that such genes themselves may be transcribed to replace the normal class I expression.

(c) Changes on the surface of cycling cells

The carbohydrate moiety of surface membrane glycoproteins may change during cell division. For example, Thomas found that the density of surface sugar determinants cross-reacting with blood group H fell as murine mastocytoma cells moved into the G_1 phase of the division cycle while, reciprocally, group B determinants increased. We have found that surface components binding the lectin, wheat-germ agglutinin, are abundant on myeloid cells (polys and macrophages) but poorly represented on resting T- and B-cells; however, within 24 hours of stimulation by lymphocyte polyclonal activators and before DNA synthesis begins, high concentrations of lectin binding sites appear on the surface. Transferrin receptors are also abundant on dividing cells which presumably are keen to take more iron on board.

(d) Unique ('idiotypic') determinants

Tumours induced by chemical agents, benzopyrene for example, also possess specific transplantation antigens, but each tumour produced by a given chemical carcinogen has its own individual idiotypic antigen; even when a carcinogen produces two different primary tumours in the same animal, they do not exhibit the same antigenic specificities and do not confer cross-resistance by immunization. In the light of the potentially exciting observation that a retroviral gp 70 molecule on the surface of a methylcholanthrene-induced tumour behaved as a tumour-specific transplantation antigen, it is conceivable that this tumour individuality could be based on diversity in gp 70 produced by some form of random recombination events. Perhaps the nearest one can get to a really tumour-specific antigen is the Ig idiotype on the surface of chronic lymphocytic leukaemic cells.

Immune response to tumours

When present, these antigens can provoke immune responses in experimental animals which lead to resistance against tumour growth but they vary tremendously in their efficiency and in their ability to activate T-suppressors. Powerful antigens associated with tumours induced by oncogenic viruses or ultraviolet light generate strong resistance while chemically induced tumours are weaker and somewhat variable; disappointingly, tumours which arise spontaneously in animals produce little or no response. This would seem to reason against the immune surveillance theory, although it might be argued that most tumours were silenced at their inception by immunological control and that only the very few which lacked a provocative surface component were 'successful'. However, athymic nude mice have a normal incidence of spontaneous tumours and this makes a single, exclusively T-cell surveillance system most unlikely. Furthermore, the only increase in cancer reported in immunosuppressed patients was related to the lymphoreticular system which could have been the direct target for the drugs employed; one exception was the considerable increase in skin cancer in immunosuppressed patients living in high sunshine regions north of Brisbane and we have already noted the 'antigen strength' of such tumours provoked in experimental animals.

Returning to the idea of cancer as a potential allograft, it has been argued that since normal class I MHC molecules would be needed to present neo-antigens on tumours to cytotoxic T-cells, their absence from the cell surface may enable the tumours to escape from surveillance. Accordingly, one group transfected a functional class I gene into highly tumorigenic adenovirus-transformed cells which originally failed to express class I antigens; the treated cells not only expressed the H-2L^d transfected gene but also were no longer oncogenic.

Perhaps in speaking of immunity to tumours, one too readily thinks in terms of acquired responses whereas it is highly possible that innate mechanisms will prove to be of greater significance. Macrophages taken from BCG-infected animals, or activated by a diversity of factors, bacterial lipopolysaccharide, double-stranded RNA, T-cell lymphokine and so forth, destroy tumour cells in tissue culture through the copious production of hydrogen peroxide, a cytolytic protease and tumour necrosis factor (TNF). There is an uncommon flurry of interest in the natural killer (NK) cells which are spontaneously cytolytic for certain, but by no means all, tumour lines in culture. A related cell type lacking the conventional T- and B-cell markers, on activation by IL-2 is capable of killing a variety of fresh tumour cells *in vitro*. The range of specificity for tumours and the ability to kill *fresh* cancer cells distinguish these so-called 'lymphokine-activated killer' (LAK) cells from the NK set. Their use in the therapy of cancer will be discussed below. It is surmised that the target of NK and LAK cells might be altered carbohydrates on the surface membrane glycoproteins, but there is no hard evidence to substantiate this.

Approaches to cancer immunotherapy

On one point all are agreed, if immunotherapy is to succeed, it is essential that the tumour load should first be reduced by surgery, irradiation or chemotherapy, since not only is it unreasonable to expect the immune system to cope with a large tumour mass, but considerable amounts of antigen released by shedding would tend to prevent the generation of any significant response in some cases due to the stimulation of T-suppressors. This leaves the small secondary deposits as the proper target for immunotherapy.

Exploitation of acquired immune responses

For active immunization we need antigen. Based on the not unreasonable belief that certain forms of cancer (e.g. lymphoma) are caused by oncogenic viruses, attempts are being made to isolate the virus and prepare a suitable vaccine from it. In fact, large-scale protection of chickens against the development of Marek's disease lymphoma has been successfully achieved by vaccination with another herpes virus native to turkeys. In the human, patients with Burkitt's lymphoma develop antibodies which react with antigens on cells of their own and other Burkitt tumours which are controlled by a herpes group organism, the Epstein—Barr (EB) virus. The unique idiotype on monoclonal B-cell tumours with surface Ig also offers a potentially feasible target for immunotherapy and successful treatment of one patient has had wide publicity. Immunologists have for long been bemused by the idea of eliminating tumour cells by specific antibody linked to a killer molecule. Not surprisingly, the 'magic bullet' devotees were greatly encouraged by experiments in which guinea-pig B lymphoma cells were killed *in vitro* by anti-idiotype conjugated with ricin, a toxin of such devastating potency that one molecule entering the cell is lethal (those readers who still maintain contact with the outside world will recollect that minute amounts of ricin on the end of a pointed walking stick provide a favourite weapon for the liquidation of unwanted intelligence agents). There is optimism that by using monoclonal antibodies, it may be feasible to apply this approach to the human. It should be mentioned that differentiation antigens present on leukaemic cells but absent from bone-marrow stem cells, even though not tumour-specific, can be used to prepare tumour-free autologous stem cells to restore function in patients treated with chemotherapy or X-irradiation

233

which destroys both their tumour cells and their haematopoietic tissue (figure 13.19).

Despite reports of cytotoxic antibodies in a proportion of patients with malignant melanoma and cytotoxic leucocytes from patients with neuroblastoma or bladder cancer, which indicate that some form of immunological response to tumour antigens is possible, it must be said that attempts to control human cancer by immunization with tumours plus adjuvants have had very mixed and in many ways somewhat disappointing results. Presumably we can only expect results from this approach with those tumours which possess some potential antigen such as the oncofetal proteins. Many attempts are being made to boost the inherently weak autoantigenicity of these cells by infection with viruses, membrane insertion of chemical haptens or fusion with highly immunogenic, allogeneic or xenogeneic normal cells. Another interesting attack is suggested by the finding of two different groups that a proportion of tumour cells after treatment with mutagenic drugs and cloning can be shown to have acquired new antigens which induce an immunological response conferring resistance to the parent tumour.

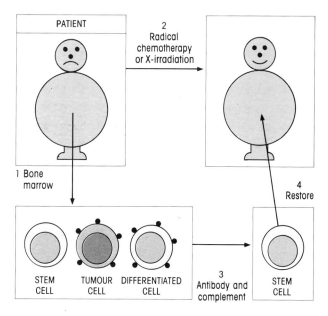

Figure 13.19. *Treatment of leukaemias by autologous bone marrow rescue. By using cytotoxic antibodies to a differentiation antigen (●) present on leukaemic cells and even on other normal differentiated cells, but absent from stem cells, it should be possible to obtain a tumour-free population of the latter which can be used to restore haematopoietic function in patients subsequently treated radically to destroy the leukaemic cells. However, techniques to clean up the marrow effectively are still improving.*

Harnessing innate immunity

With respect to putatively non-antigenic tumours, there have been numerous, not very successful, attempts to boost 'non-specific' effector mechanisms mediated by macrophages and NK cells through the injection of BCG or *C. parvum*. Intimate contact of the adjuvant with the tumour itself can produce dramatic results and one hopeful study records the beneficial effects of intrathoracic BCG in lung cancer. However, significant advances are undoubtedly being made as a result of the availability of recombinant tumour necrosis factor and biological response modifiers such as IL-2, IFNγ and colony stimulating factors.

Immunotherapy based on systemic administration of lymphokine-activated killer (LAK) cells and recombinant interleukin-2

Patients are leucopheresed and the cells cultured for several days with IL-2 to allow LAK cells to develop. Administration of autologous LAK cells together with high doses of IL-2 has led, in one study, to more than 50% reduction in evaluable tumour in 14 out of 41 cancer patients. Renal cancers (figure 13.20), some melanomas and some colorectal cancers are sensitive to this treatment whereas sarcomas appear to be unresponsive (figure 13.21). Although the treatment is cumbersome and there are significant side-effects, there is certainly promise in this approach.

Interferon therapy

At the time of writing, most trials had used IFNα and IFNβ as the γ-form had not been available long enough for evaluation. Overall, a 10–15% objective response rate was seen in patients with renal carcinoma, melanoma and myeloma, an approximate 20% response rate among patients with Kaposi's sarcoma, about 40% positive responders in patients with various lymphomas and a remarkable response rate of 80–90% among patients with hairy cell leukaemia and mycosis fungoides.

With regard to the mechanisms of the antitumour effects, in certain tumours interferons may serve primarily as anti-proliferative agents; in others, activation of NK cells and macrophages may be important, while augmenting the expression of class I MHC molecules may make the tumours more susceptible to control by immune effector mechanisms. In some circumstances the anti-viral effect could be contributory.

CHAPTER 13

Figure 13.20. *Regression of renal-cell cancer metastases in the lung following treatment with autologous LAK cells and rIL-2. X-ray films of multiple pulmonary nodules before (left) and after (right) treatment. All nodules regressed markedly,* *and most resolved completely. The remaining lesions were continuing to regress at 3½ months. (Reproduced from Rosenberg S.A. et al. (1985) N. Eng. J. Med. 313, 1485, with permission from the New England Journal of Medicine.)*

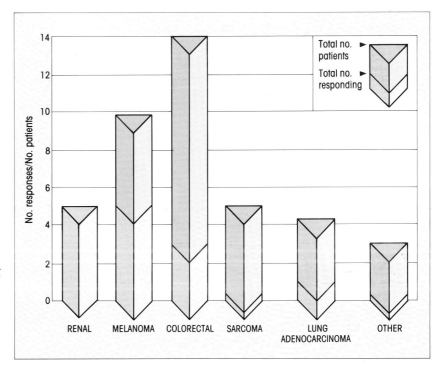

Figure 13.21. *Response of cancer patients to therapy with autologous LAK cells and IL-2. Other cancers included 1 oesophageal adenocarcinoma, 1 lymphoma and 1 gastrinoma. A positive response was reduction of tumour size by ≥ 50%. (Data from Rosenberg S.A. et al. (1986) Surgery 100, 262.)*

TRANSPLANTATION

For diseases like renal cell cancer and hairy cell leukaemia, IFNs have induced responses in a significantly higher proportion of patients than conventional therapies. However, in the wider setting, most investigators consider that their role will be in combination therapy, e.g. with various chemotherapeutic agents where synergistic action has been observed in murine tumour systems. IFNα and β synergize with IFNγ and the latter synergizes with tumour necrosis factor. α-Interferon acts as a radiation sensitizer and its ability to increase the expression of oestrogen receptors on cultured breast cancer cells suggests the possibility of combining IFN with anti-oestrogens in this disease.

Colony stimulating factors

Normal cell development proceeds from an immature stem cell with the capacity for unlimited self renewal, through committed progenitors to the final lineage-specific differentiated cells with little or no potential for self-renewal. Therapy aimed at inducing tumour cell differentiation is founded on the idea that the induction of cell maturation decreases and possibly abrogates the capacity of the malignant clone to divide. Along these lines, the colony stimulating factor which promotes the formation of granulocyte/macrophage colonies in bone marrow cultures (GM-CSF) has been shown to enhance the differentiation, decrease the self-renewal capacity and suppress the leukaemogenicity of murine myeloid leukaemias. Gene cloning of the human analogue and testing the recombinant products in human disease is the obvious pathway forward.

Immunodiagnosis

Analysis of blood for the oncofetal antigens, α-fetoprotein in hepatoma and carcinoembryonic antigen in tumours of the colon has provided valuable diagnostic information, but enthusiasm has been slightly curtailed by the knowledge that there is a high incidence of so-called 'false positives'. Reappearance of these proteins after surgical removal of the primary is strongly indicative of fresh tumour growth. The GM1 monosialoganglioside has been demonstrated in the blood of 96% of patients with pancreatic carcinoma and 64% of colorectal carcinomas as against 2% in normal subjects. Identification of the cell type by surface markers is of increasing value for the diagnosis and treatment of childhood leukaemias such as non-T, non-B-ALL (p. 144).

Preliminary results on the localization of tumours *in vivo* by scanning after injection of radio-labelled monoclonal antibodies to oncofetal antigens holds promise that the technique will one day provide a useful adjunct to existing imaging techniques, particularly if genetically tailor-made novel antibody molecules are created, although it is more likely to challenge the computerized axial tomography (CAT) scans for tumours of the abdomen than the lungs where there is high density contrast.

SUMMARY

Graft rejection is an immunological reaction: it shows specificity, the second set response is brisk, it is mediated by lymphocytes, and antibodies specific for the graft are formed. In each vertebrate species there is a major histocompatibility complex (MHC) which is responsible for provoking the most intense graft reactions.

Class II (Ia) molecules provoke a mixed lymphocyte reaction of proliferation and blast transformation when genetically dissimilar lymphocytes interact; this reaction stimulates the formation of helper T-cells required for the generation of cytotoxic T-cells directed against class I determinants (cf. T−B cooperation with carrier-hapten), the process being termed cell-mediated lympholysis. Ia differences are largely responsible for the reaction of tolerated grafted lymphocytes against host antigen (g.v.h.). The MHC in man (HLA) consists of three loci (HLA-A, B and C) for class I antigens and three (HLA-DP, DQ and DR) for the class II. Individuals are typed by cytotoxic antisera, the mixed lymphocyte reaction and cloned cytotoxic T-cells. The very high degree of polymorphism of the MHC may protect a species from molecular mimicry by parasites, maintain diversity of antigenic recognition and ensure heterozygosity ('hybrid vigour'). Siblings have a 1 : 4 chance of identity with respect to MHC.

Grafts are rejected either by sensitized T-cells or by antibody inducing platelet aggregation or type II hypersensitivity reactions (e.g. antibody-dependent cell-mediated cytotoxicity). Rejection may be prevented by: (i) tissue matching including the DR-locus, (ii) anti-mitotic drugs (e.g. azathioprine), anti-inflammatory steroids and anti-lymphocyte globulin which produce general immunosuppression, and a new drug cyclosporin A which is more selective and can produce (iii) antigen-specific depression through tolerance induction as can enhancement by deliberate immunization.

Cornea and cartilage grafts are avascular and comparatively well tolerated. Kidney grafting gives excellent results and has been the most widespread although immunosuppression must normally be continuous. High success rates are also being achieved with heart and liver transplants particularly helped by the use of cyclosporin. Bone marrow grafts for immunodeficiency and aplastic anaemia are accepted from matched siblings but it is difficult to avoid g.v.h. disease with allogeneic marrow although this can be kept more under control with cyclosporin A.

HLA specificities are often associated with particular diseases, e.g. HLA-B27 with ankylosing spondylitis, B8 with myasthenia gravis, DR3 with autoimmune chronic active hepatitis, DR4 with rheumatoid arthritis and DR2 with multiple sclerosis.

Differences between MHC of mother and fetus may be beneficial to the fetus but as a potential graft it must be protected against transplantation attack by the mother; suggested defence mechanisms are (i) most importantly lack of class I and II MHC antigens on syncytiotrophoblast, (ii) mucopolysaccharide coat around trophoblast, and (iii) local production of immunosuppressant.

The immune surveillance theory of cancer postulates that changes in the surface of the neoplastic cell are recognized by the immune system and eliminated. However, although virally coded, idiotypic and oncofetal antigens may be detected on experimentally induced tumour cells together with components linked to cell division, the incidence of spontaneous cancers in immunosuppressed individuals is not generally higher than normal. Examples of immune responses to tumours in human cancer are known but attempts at control by immunization with tumour plus adjuvant have not been encouraging. Other strategies involving non-specific immune mechanisms are looking more promising. These include treatment with autologous lymphokine activated killer (LAK) cells plus recombinant IL-2, interferons and colony stimulating factors.

Further reading

Hogarth P.J. (1982) *Immunological Aspects of Mammalian Reproduction.* Praeger, New York.

Mason D.W. & Morris P.J. (1986) Effector mechanisms in allograft rejection. *Ann. Rev. Immunol.,* **4**, 119.

Mitchison N.A. (1982) Protective immunity (to tumours) *in vivo.* In *Clinical Aspects of Immunology,* 4th edn. P. Lachmann & D.K. Peters (eds). Blackwell Scientific Publications, Oxford.

Slavin S. (1987) Total lymphoid irradiation. *Immunology Today,* **8**, 88.

237

AUTOIMMUNE DISEASES

I – Scope and Aetiology

238 The monumental repertoire of the adaptive immune system has evolved to allow it to recognize and ensnare virtually any shaped microbial molecules either at present in existence or yet to come, and in so doing, has been unable to avoid the generation of lymphocytes which react with the body's own constituents. We have already discussed the mechanisms which exist to prevent these self-components from provoking an immune response but, as with all machinery, there is always a chance that these systems might break down, and the older the individual, the greater the chance of a breakdown. When this happens *autoantibodies* (i.e. antibodies capable of reacting with 'self' components) are produced. Grabar was of the opinion that autoantibodies have a biological function to act as 'transporting' agents for cellular breakdown products thereby aiding their disposal. While antibodies can act in this way, we are here concerned more with autoimmune phenomena which appear in relation to certain defined human diseases. Ideally we wish to apply the term 'autoimmune disease' to those cases where it can be shown that the autoimmune process contributes to the pathogenesis of the disease rather than situations where apparently harmless autoantibodies are formed following tissue damage, e.g. heart antibodies appearing after a myocardial infarction. Yet the role of autoimmunity in many disorders is still not clearly defined, and it is as a matter of convenience that we will refer to all maladies firmly associated with autoantibody formation as 'autoimmune diseases', except where it

can be shown that the immunological phenomena are purely secondary findings.

The spectrum of autoimmune diseases

These disorders may be looked upon as forming a spectrum. At one end we have *'organ-specific diseases'* with organ-specific autoantibodies. Hashimoto's disease of the thyroid is an example: there is a specific lesion in the thyroid involving infiltration by mononuclear cells (lymphocytes, histiocytes and plasma cells), destruction of follicular cells and germinal centre formation, accompanied, as we showed originally, by the production of circulating antibodies with absolute specificity for certain thyroid constituents (Roitt, Doniach & Campbell).

Moving towards the centre of the spectrum are those disorders where the lesion tends to be localized to a single organ but the antibodies are non-organ specific. A typical example would be primary biliary cirrhosis where the small bile ductule is the main target of inflammatory cell infiltration but the serum antibodies present—mainly mitochondrial—are not liver specific.

At the other end of the spectrum are the *'non-organ-specific diseases'* exemplified by systemic lupus erythematosus (SLE) where both lesions and autoantibodies are not confined to any one organ. Pathological changes are widespread and are primarily lesions of connective tissue with fibrinoid necrosis. They are seen in the skin (the 'lupus' butterfly rash on the face is characteristic), kidney glomeruli, joints, serous membranes and blood vessels. In addition, the formed elements of the blood are often affected. A bizarre collection of autoantibodies are found, some of which react with the DNA and other nuclear constituents of all cells in the body.

An attempt to fit the major diseases considered to be associated with autoimmunity into this spectrum is shown in table 14.1.

Autoantibodies in human disease

At this stage in the discussion it may be of value to have a more precise account of the major autoantibodies detected in the different diseases to provide a framework for reference. Table 14.2 documents a list of these antibodies and the methods employed in their detection. The notes following the table amplify specific points while some of the tests are illustrated in figures 14.1, 14.2, 5.15 and 5.16.

Overlap of autoimmune disorders

There is a tendency for more than one autoimmune disorder to occur in the same individual and when this happens the association is often between diseases within the same region of the autoimmune spectrum (cf. table 14.1). Thus patients with autoimmune thyroiditis (Hashimoto's disease or primary myxoedema) have a much higher incidence of pernicious anaemia than would be expected in a random population matched for age and sex (10% as against 0.2%). Conversely, both thyroiditis and thyrotoxicosis are diagnosed in pernicious anaemia patients with an unexpectedly high frequency. Other associations are seen between Addison's disease and autoimmune thyroid disease and in the rare cases of juveniles with pernicious anaemia and polyendocrinopathy which includes Addison's disease, hypoparathyroidism, diabetes and thyroiditis.

There is an even greater overlap in serological findings. 30% of patients with autoimmune thyroid disease have concomitant parietal cell antibodies in their serum. Conversely, thyroid antibodies have been demonstrated in up to 50% of pernicious anaemia patients. It should be stressed that these are not cross-reacting antibodies. The thyroid-specific antibodies will not react with stomach and vice versa. When a serum reacts with both organs it means that two populations of antibodies are present, one with specificity for thyroid and the other for stomach.

Table 14.1. *Spectrum of autoimmune diseases.*

ORGAN SPECIFIC	
	Hashimoto's thyroiditis
	Primary myxoedema
	Thyrotoxicosis
	Pernicious anaemia
	Autoimmune atrophic gastritis
	Addison's disease
	Premature menopause (few cases)
	Male infertility (few cases)
	Myasthenia gravis
	Juvenile diabetes
	Goodpasture's syndrome
	Pemphigus vulgaris
	Pemphigoid
	Sympathetic ophthalmia
	Phacogenic uveitis
	(?? Multiple sclerosis ??)
	Autoimmune haemolytic anaemia
	Idiopathic thrombocytopenic purpura
	Idiopathic leucopenia
	Primary biliary cirrhosis
	Active chronic hepatitis HB_S-ve
	Cryptogenic cirrhosis (some cases)
	Ulcerative colitis
	Sjögren's syndrome
	Rheumatoid arthritis
	Scleroderma
	Dermatomyositis
	Discoid LE
NON-ORGAN SPECIFIC	Systemic lupus erythematosus (SLE)

239

At the non-organ-specific end of the spectrum, SLE is clinically associated with rheumatoid arthritis and several other diseases which are themselves uncommon: haemolytic anaemia, idiopathic leucopenia and thrombocytopenic purpura, dermatomyositis and Sjögren's syndrome. Antinuclear antibodies, non-organ-specific complement fixation reactions, and anti-globulin (rheumatoid) factors are a general feature of these disorders.

Table 14.2. *Autoantibodies in human disease. (IFT = immunofluorescent test; CFT = complement fixation test.)*

DISEASE	ANTIGEN	DETECTION OF ANTIBODY
Hashimoto's thyroiditis Primary myxoedema	Thyroglobulin	Precipitins; passive haemagglutination
	2nd colloid Ag (CA2)	IFT on fixed thyroid
	Cytoplasmic microsomes	IFT on unfixed thyroid; passive haemagglutination
	Cell surface	IFT on viable thyroid cells; C'-mediated cytotoxicity
Thyrotoxicosis	Cell surface TSH receptors	Bioassay — stimulation of mouse thyroid *in vivo*; blocking combination TSH with receptors; stimulation adenyl cyclase
	'Growth' receptors	Induction of cell division in thyroid fragments
Pernicious anaemia[1]	Intrinsic factor	Neutralization; blocking combination with vit-B_{12}; binding to Int.Fact-B_{12} by coprecipitation
	Parietal cell microsomes	IFT on unfixed gastric mucosa
Addison's disease	Cytoplasm adrenal cells	IFT on unfixed adrenal cortex
Premature onset of menopause[2]	Cytoplasm steroid-producing cells	IFT on adrenal and interstitial cells of ovary and testis
Male infertility (some)[3]	Spermatozoa	Sperm agglutination in ejaculate
Insulin-dependent (juvenile) diabetes[4]	Cytoplasm of islet cells	IFT on unfixed human pancreas
	Cell surface	IFT on isolated cells
Type B insulin resistance c̄ acanthosis nigricans	Insulin receptor	Block hormone binding to receptor Radioimmunoassay with purified receptor
Atopic allergy (some)	β-Adrenergic receptor	Blocking radioassay with hydroxybenzylpindolol
Myasthenia gravis	Skeletal and heart muscle	IFT on skeletal muscle
	Acetyl choline receptor	Blocking or binding radioassay with α-bungarotoxin
(Multiple sclerosis)	Brain	Cytotoxic effects on cerebellar cultures by serum and lymphocytes (? secondary to disease)
Goodpasture's syndrome	Glomerular and lung basement membrane	Linear staining by IFT of kidney biopsy with fluorescent anti-IgG Radioimmunoassay with purified Ag
Pemphigus vulgaris	Desmosomes between prickle cells in epidermis	IFT on skin
Pemphigoid	Basement membrane	IFT on skin
Phacogenic uveitis	Lens	Passive haemagglutination
Sympathetic ophthalmia	Uvea	(Delayed skin reaction to uveal extract)
Autoimmune haemolytic anaemia[5]	Erythrocytes	Coombs' antiglobulin test
Idiopathic thrombocytopenic purpura	Platelets	Shortened platelet survival *in vivo*
Primary biliary cirrhosis	Mitochondria (mainly)	IFT on mitochondria-rich cells (e.g. distal tubules of kidney)
Active chronic hepatitis	Smooth muscle, nuclei	IFT (e.g. on gastric mucosa)
(HB_S−ve)	Cell surface lipoprotein	Leucocyte cytotoxicity
Ulcerative colitis	Colon 'lipopolysaccharide'	IFT; passive haemagglutination (cytotoxic action of lymphocytes on colon cells)
Sjögren's syndrome[6]	Ducts, mitochondria, nuclei, thyroid	IFT
	IgG	Antiglobulin (rheumatoid factor) tests
Rheumatoid arthritis[7]	IgG	Antiglobulin tests: latex agglutination, red sheep cell aggln. test (SCAT; commercial product, RAHA test) and radioassay
	RANA[8]	IFT on EB-transformed cell line
	Collagen	Passive haemagglutination
Discoid lupus erythematosus Dermatomyositis Scleroderma[9]	Nuclear	IFT
	IgG	Antiglobulin tests
Mixed connective tissue disease[10]	Extractable nuclear	IFT; countercurrent electrophoresis
Systemic lupus erythematosus	DNA	Radioassay[11]; pptn
	Nucleoprotein	IFT; latex aggln. L.E. cells[12]
	Cytoplasmic sol.Ag	'Non-organ sp.C'-fixation test
	Array of other Ag incl. formed elements of blood, clotting factors, IgG	
	Cardiolipin	Radioassay

Notes:

1 Two major types of antibody to intrinsic factor are detected, viz. blocking and binding (figure 14.1). Binding antibody combines with preformed Int.Fact.—radioactive B_{12} (*B_{12}) complex which can then be precipitated at 50% ammonium sulphate (cf. figure 5.12) and the radioactivity in the precipitate counted. Blocking antibody prevents binding of *B_{12} to Int. Fact. and the uncombined *B_{12} can then be adsorbed to charcoal and counted.

IF B₁₂	Intrinsic factor — vitamin B_{12} complex
IF Ab	Blocking antibody prevents combination B_{12} with IF
Ab IF B₁₂	Binding antibody links to preformed IF.B_{12} complex

Figure 14.1. *Intrinsic factor autoantibodies: sites of determinants for binding and blocking. (Roitt I.M., Doniach D. & Shapland C. (1964)* **Lancet** *ii, 469.)*

Sjögren's syndrome occupies an interesting position (table 14.3); aside from the clinical and serological features associated with non-organ-specific disease mentioned above, characteristics of an organ-specific disorder are evident. Antibodies reacting with salivary ducts are demonstrable and there is an abnormally high incidence of thyroid autoantibodies; histologically the affected lacrimal and salivary glands reveal changes of a similar nature to those seen in Hashimoto's disease, namely a replacement of the glandular elements by patchy lymphocytic and plasma cell granulomatous tissue. Associations between diseases at the two ends of the spectrum have been reported, but, as might be predicted from the serological data (table 14.3), they are not common.

There is still no entirely satisfactory explanation to account for the rare tendency to develop hypo-gammaglobulinaemia and the increased incidence of certain cancers occurring in autoimmune disease. Patients with organ-specific disorders are slightly more prone to develop cancer in the affected organ whereas generalized lymphoreticular neoplasia shows up with uncommon frequency in non-organ-specific disease.

Genetic factors in autoimmune disease

Autoimmune phenomena tend to aggregate in certain families. For example, the first degree relatives (sibs, parents and children) of patients with Hashimoto's disease show a high incidence of thyroid autoantibodies (figure 14.3) and of overt and subclinical thyroiditis. Interestingly there is also an

241

Table 14.2 continued

2 *Antibodies occur in the minority of patients with associated Addison's disease.*

3 *Only small percentage show agglutinins. Spermatozoa may be agglutinated head to head, tail to tail or joined through their mid-piece. Seen also in small percentage of infertile women.*

4 *Most if not all insulin-dependent diabetics have islet cell antibodies at some stage during the first year of onset. In contrast, islet cell antibodies in diabetic patients with an associated autoimmune polyendocrinopathy persist for many years.*

5 *The Coombs' test involves the demonstration of bound antibody on the washed red cell by agglutination with an antiglobulin (cf. figure 12.13). Erythrocyte autoantibodies, which bind well over the temperature range $0-37°C$ ('warm' Ab), are mostly IgG; approximately 60 per cent of cases are primary, the remainder being associated with other autoimmune disorders, e.g. SLE, ulcerative colitis. 'Cold' Ab, which react best over the range $0-20°C$, are mostly IgM and red cells coated with this Ab can often be agglutinated by anti-complement sera; approximately half are primary, the others being associated with* **Mycoplasma pneumoniae** *infection or generalized neoplastic disease of the lymphoreticular tissues.*

6 *Antibodies specifically reacting with the epithelium of salivary gland excretory ducts are demonstrable by immunofluorescence in up to half the cases.*

7 *The main antiglobulin factors react with the Fc portion of IgG which is usually adsorbed on to latex particles (human IgG) or present in an antigen-antibody complex (sheep red cells coated with sub-agglutinating dose of rabbit antibody). In the radioassay test, rabbit IgG is bound to a plastic tube, patient's serum added and the antiglobulin bound assessed by subsequent binding of labelled anti-human IgG or IgM (cf. p.78). Rheumatoid factors specific for human IgG can be detected by this test using human Fcγ to coat the tubes and labelled anti-human Fdγ or IgM for the final stage.*

8 *The rheumatoid arthritis nuclear antigen (RANA) is revealed as speckled staining by IFT using cells transformed by EB virus; normal cells are negative.*

9 *In scleroderma (progressive systemic sclerosis) antinucleolar antibodies are frequently found.*

10 *This syndrome combines features of scleroderma, rheumatoid arthritis, SLE and dermatomyositis. The antigen is an extractable nuclear antigen which gives speckled fluorescence and RNase-sensitive precipitation by counter-current electrophoresis.*

11 *Antibodies to single or double-stranded DNA are assayed by the salt copptn. test (cf. figure 5.12) using labelled Ag, or by a DNA-coated tube test similar to the radioassay for antiglobulins (note 7 above).*

12 *When blood from an SLE patient is incubated at $37°C$, some white cells are damaged and allow the entry of antibodies. Certain of the antibodies combining with the nuclear surface bind complement and attract polymorphs which strip away the cytoplasm and engulf the nucleus. The polymorph containing the engulfed homogenized nucleus is called an LE-cell.*

(a)

(b)

(c)

(d)

(e)

(f)

(g)　　　　　　　　　　　(h)

(i)　　　　　　　　　　　(j)

243

Figure 14.2 facing page and above. *Fluorescent antibody studies in autoimmune diseases. (a) Thyroid microsomal antibodies staining cytoplasm of acinar cells. (b) Human thyroid sections stained for MHC class II: LHS—normal thyroid with unstained follicular cells and an isolated strongly Ia positive dendritic cell; RHS—thyrotoxic (Graves' disease) thyroid with abundant cytoplasmic MHC class II indicative of active synthesis. (c) Viable suspension of islet cells from the diabetic-prone BB/E/H rat stained for surface MHC class II induced by treatment with recombinant IFNγ, then fixed, cytocentrifuged and stained with fluorescein labelled antibodies to reveal intracytoplasmic insulin. Three cells showing abundant induction of surface class II. (d) That these are insulin-producing cells is shown by simultaneous intracytoplasmic green staining for the hormone. (e) Fluorescence of cells in the pancreatic islets of Langerhans*

stained with serum from insulin-dependent diabetic. (f) The same, showing cells stained simultaneously for somatostatin (the yellow cells are stained with rhodamine anti-somatostatin and fluorescein anti-human IgG which localizes the bound patient's autoantibody). (g) Serum of patient with Addison's disease staining cytoplasm of monkey adrenal granulosa cells. (h) Fluorescence of distal tubular cells of the kidney after reaction with mitochondrial autoantibodies. (i) Diffuse nuclear staining on a thyroid section obtained with nucleoprotein antibodies from an SLE patient. (j) Serum of a scleroderma patient staining the nucleoli of SV-40-transformed human keratinocytes (K14) in monolayer culture. ((a), (e), (f), (g), (h) and (i) kindly provided by Dr F. Bottazzo, (b) by Dr R. Pujol-Borrell, (c) and (d) by Dr A. Cooke and (j) by Dr F.T. Wojnarowska.)

increased frequency of 'non-immunological' thyroid disorders, such as non-toxic nodular goitre. The proportion with autoantibodies is higher in those families where more than one member is clinically affected. Parallel studies have disclosed similar relationships in the families of pernicious anaemia patients in that gastric parietal cell antibodies are prevalent in the relatives who are wont to develop achlorhydria and atrophic gastritis. Familial aggregation of mitochondrial antibodies has been observed, albeit to a lesser extent, in primary biliary cirrhosis. Turning to SLE, disturbances of immunoglobulin synthesis and a susceptibility to develop 'connective tissue diseases' have been reported but

there are some conflicting accounts still not resolved.

These familial relationships could be ascribed to environmental factors such as an infective microorganism, but there is evidence that one or more genetic components must be given serious consideration. In the first place, when thyrotoxicosis occurs in twins there is a greater concordance rate (i.e. both twins affected) in identical than in nonidentical twins. Secondly, thyroid autoantibodies are more prevalent in individuals with ovarian dysgenesis having X-chromosome aberrations such as XO and particularly the iso-chromosome X abnormality. Furthermore, there are strong associations between several autoimmune diseases and particu-

DISEASE	% POSITIVE REACTIONS FOR ANTIBODIES TO:			
	THYROID*	STOMACH*	NUCLEI*	IgG†
Hashimoto's thyroiditis	99.9	32	8	2
Pernicious anaemia	55	89	11	
Sjögren's syndrome	45	14	56	75
Rheumatoid arthritis	11	16	50	75
SLE	2	2	99	35
Controls‡	0–15	0–16	0–19	2–5

Table 14.3. *Organ-specific and non-organ-specific serological interrelationships in human disease.*
* *Immunofluorescence test*
† *Rheumatoid factor classical tests*
‡ *Incidence increases with age and females > males.*

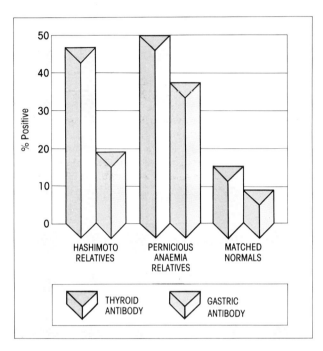

Figure 14.3. *The high incidence of thyroid and gastric autoantibodies in the first degree relatives of patients with Hashimoto's disease or pernicious anaemia. Note the overlap of gastric and thyroid autoimmunity and the higher incidence of gastric autoantibodies in pernicious anaemia relatives. (Data from Doniach D. & Roitt I.M. (1964)* Semin. Haematol. I, *313.)*

chickens with autoimmune thyroiditis and the New Zealand Black (NZB) mouse with autoimmune haemolytic anaemia. The hybrid of NZB with another strain, the New Zealand White (B × W hybrid), actually develops LE-cells, antinuclear antibodies and a fatal immune complex induced glomerulonephritis. Suitable intercross and backcross breeding of these mice has established that a *minimum* of three genes determines the expression of autoimmunity and that the production of both red cell and nuclear antibodies may be under separate genetic control, i.e. there may be different factors predisposing to autoimmunity on the one hand, and to the selection of antigen on the other. This view finds support in the genetic analysis of Obese chickens which has delineated an influence of the MHC, abnormalities in T-cell control and a defect in the thyroid gland.

The facts presented by human autoimmune disease also attest to multifactorial control. The overlaps in autoantibodies and disease discussed above

lar HLA specificities, e.g. DR3 in Addison's disease and DR4 in rheumatoid arthritis (table 13.3, p. 229). Figure 14.4 shows a multiplex family, with insulin-dependent diabetes in which the disease is linked to a particular HLA-haplotype. Since only very restricted determinants on the autoantigenic molecules evoke autoantibodies (e.g. thyroglobulin of molecular weight 650 000, has a valency of only 4), one is tempted to think in terms of Ir genes, it being precisely under such conditions that Ir genes can be recognized.

It is also worthy of note that lines of animals have been bred which spontaneously develop autoimmune disease. In other words, the autoimmunity is genetically programmed. There is an Obese line of

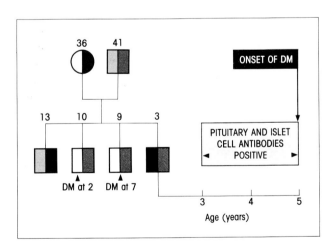

Figure 14.4. *HLA-haplotype linkage and onset of insulin-dependent diabetes (DM). Haplotypes: □ A3, B14, DR6; ■ A3, B7, DR4; ▨ A28, B51, DR4; and ▧ A2, B62, C3, DR4. Disease is linked to possession of the A2, B62, C3, DR4 haplotype. The 3-year-old brother had complement-fixing antibodies to the islet cell surface for 2 years before developing frank diabetes. (From Gorsuch A.N. et al. (1981)* Lancet ii, *1363.)*

point to a general tendency to develop autoimmunity in these individuals and further, the factors which predispose to organ-specific disease must be different from those in non-organ-specific disorders (as judged by the minimal overlap between them). There must be additional factors which are organ related in that relatives of patients with pernicious anaemia are more prone to gastric autoimmunity than members of Hashimoto families (figure 14.3).

Autoantibodies are demonstrable in comparatively low titre in the general population and the incidence of positive results increases steadily with age (figure 14.5) up to around 60–70 years. In the case of the thyroid and stomach at least, biopsy has indicated that the presence of antibody is almost invariably associated with minor thyroiditis or gastritis lesions (as the case may be), and it is of interest that post-mortem examination has identified 10% of middle-aged women with significant degrees of lymphadenoid change in the thyroid similar in essence to that characteristic of Hashimoto's disease.

The point should also be made here that, in general, autoantibodies and autoimmune diseases are found more frequently in women than in men.

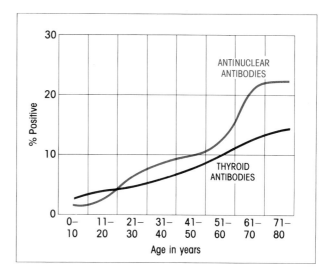

Figure 14.5. *Incidence of autoantibodies in the general population. A serum was considered positive for thyroid antibodies if it reacted at a dilution of 1/10 in the tanned red cell test or neat in the immunofluorescent test and positive for antinuclear antibodies if it reacted at a dilution of 1/4 by immunofluorescence.*

Aetiology of autoimmune responses

How does autoimmunity arise? Our earliest view, with respect to organ-specific antibodies at least, was that the antigens were sequestered within the organ, and through lack of contact with the lymphoreticular system failed to establish immunological tolerance. Any mishap which caused a release of the antigen would then provide an opportunity for autoantibody formation. For a few body constituents this holds true, and in the case of sperm, lens and heart for example, release of certain components directly into the circulation can provoke autoantibodies. But, in general, the experience has been that injection of *unmodified* extracts of those tissues concerned in the organ-specific autoimmune disorders does not readily elicit antibody formation. Indeed detailed investigation of the thyroid autoantigen, thyroglobulin, has disclosed that it is not completely sequestered within the gland but gains access to the extracellular fluid around the follicles and leaves via the thyroid lymphatics (figure 14.6) reaching the serum in normal human subjects at concentrations of approximately 0.01–0.05 μg/ml. In fact, in the majority of cases—e.g. red cells in autoimmune haemolytic anaemia, DNA released from dying cells

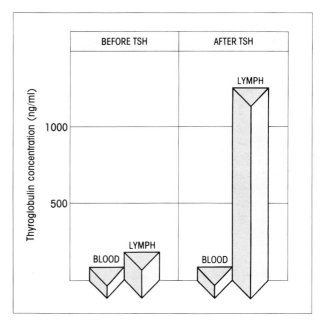

Figure 14.6. *Thyroglobulin in the cervical lymph draining the thyroid in the rat. The concentration of thyroglobulin is increased after injection of pituitary thyroid stimulating hormone (TSH) suggesting that the release from thyroid follicles is linked to the physiological activity of the acinar cells. (From Daniel P.N., Pratt O.E., Roitt I.M. & Torrigiani G. (1967)* Quart. J. Exp. Physiol. *52, 184.)*

in SLE and surface receptors in many cases of organ-specific autoimmunity—the autoantigens are accessible to circulating lymphocytes. None the less, with respect to T-cell recognition, accessibility is not sufficient; there must be an adequate association with class II MHC. Thus, the question must be raised whether these circulating components can achieve a high enough concentration on antigen-presenting cells to be perceived by T-helpers, and indeed whether potential autoantigens on the surface of cells not expressing class II can remain other than silent (cf. p. 131).

There is also mounting evidence that autoreactive B- and T-cells are present normally. A small proportion of the B-cells in normal individuals bind autoantigens such as human thyroglobulin, myelin basic protein and DNA, through their surface receptors. Furthermore, the B-cells in a wide range of vertebrate hosts can be persuaded by various means to synthesize autoantibodies which react with these antigens. Almost certainly the lymphocytes which bind the autoantigens include the population which produces the autoantibodies, a view sustained by 'antigen suicide' experiments in which lymphocytes from thyroglobulin-primed animals fail to make antibodies when challenged in a secondary host if they are allowed to bind thyroglobulin of very high specific radioactivity *in vitro* before transfer; the implication is that cells binding the 'hot' antigen through surface receptors are inactivated by irradiation.

Autoreactive T-cells can also be demonstrated—witness the establishment of T-cell clones and hybridomas, which react specifically with myelin basic protein, thyroglobulin, thyroid surface antigens and other autoantigens such as collagen. The reader may be surprised to learn that in generating T-cell lines it is a not uncommon experience to isolate cells which proliferate and release IL-2 in response to self-class II; even allowing for the fact that the presence of autologous class II positive feeder cells in the cultures will tend to select for these autoreactive cells, it would not have been predicted that cells with such specificity would be permitted to roam around freely in the body. It is also of interest that self-reactive effector T-cells have been generated when lymphocytes have been cultured with a variety of autologous tissues in the presence of an agent such as a mitogenic lectin or fetal calf serum. The message then is that we are all sitting on a minefield of potentially self-reactive cells, with access to their respective autoantigens, but since autoimmune disease is more the exception than the rule, the body must have homeostatic mechanisms to prevent them being triggered under normal circumstances. Accepting its limitations, figure 14.7 provides a framework for us to examine ways in which these mechanisms may be circumvented to allow autoimmunity to develop. It is assumed that the key to the system is control of the autoreactive T-inducer/helper cell. Presumably these cells are unresponsive because of clonal deletion, T-suppression or failure of autoantigen presentation.

T-inducer bypass mechanisms leading to autoimmunity

Provision of new carrier determinant

Allison and Weigle argued independently that if autoreactive T-cells are tolerized and thereby unable to collaborate with B-cells to generate autoantibodies, provision of new carrier determinants to which no self-tolerance had been established would bypass this mechanism and lead to autoantibody production (figure 14.8).

(i) Modification of the autoantigen

A new carrier could arise through some modification to the molecule, for example by defects in

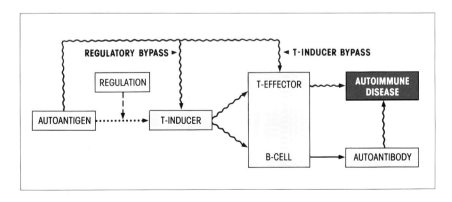

Figure 14.7. *Autoimmunity arises through bypass of the control of autoreactivity. The constraints on the stimulation of self-reactive inducer/helper T-cells by autoantigen can be circumvented either through bypassing the inducer cell or by disturbance of the regulatory mechanisms.*

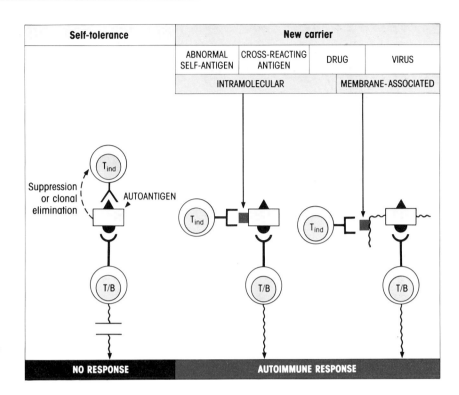

Self-tolerance	New carrier			
	ABNORMAL SELF-ANTIGEN	CROSS-REACTING ANTIGEN	DRUG	VIRUS
	INTRAMOLECULAR		MEMBRANE-ASSOCIATED	

Figure 14.8. *T-inducer bypass through new carrier determinant generates autoimmunity.*

synthesis or by an abnormality in lysosomal break-down yielding a split product exposing some new groupings. Experimentally it has been found that large proteolytic fragments of thyroglobulin are autoantigenic when injected alone but no evidence for such a mechanism has yet been uncovered in man. In fact many studies on spontaneous autoimmune disease have failed to reveal an abnormality in the antigen. Consider the following as an illustration. Neonatal thyroidectomy prevents the spontaneous development of thyroglobulin autoantibodies in Obese strain chickens; however, these animals will now make autoantibodies if injected with thyroglobulin prepared from *normal* chickens suggesting that the immunological response rather than the antigen is abnormal. None the less, there may be defects in the iodine metabolism of the gland itself and recent work has shown that the severity of thyroiditis is ameliorated when the birds are put on a low iodine diet. There might also be more subtle changes in glycosylation patterns which are not picked up by the available serological reagents, the most exciting example being the defect in galactosylation of the Fcγ sugar chains in rheumatoid arthritis, to be discussed later.

Incorporation into Freund's complete adjuvant frequently endows many autologous proteins with the power to induce autoallergic disease in labora-tory animals. It is conceivable that the physical constraints on the proteins at the water–oil interface of the emulsion provide the required alteration in configuration of the 'carrier portions' of the molecules.

Modification can also be achieved through combination with a drug. The autoimmune haemolytic anaemia associated with administration of α-methyl dopa might be attributable to modification of the red-cell surface in such a way as to provide a carrier for stimulating B-cells which recognize the rhesus *e* antigen. This is normally regarded as a 'weak' antigen and would be less likely to induce B-cell tolerance than the 'stronger' antigens present on the erythrocyte. Isoniazid may produce arthritis associated with nuclear antibodies and unlike most other cases of drug-induced autoimmunity, synthesis of these antibodies is said to continue after cessation of drug therapy. A high proportion of patients on continued treatment with procainamide develop nuclear antibodies and 40% present with clinical signs of SLE. Myasthenia gravis and symptoms of pemphigus have been described in some patients on penicillamine. It is not clear in every case whether the drug provides carrier help through direct modification of the autoantigen or of some independent molecule concerned in associative recognition.

(ii) Cross-reactions

Many examples are known in which potential auto-antigenic determinants are present on an exogenous cross-reacting antigen which provides the new carrier that provokes autoantibody formation. Post-rabies vaccine encephalitis is thought to result from an autoimmune reaction to brain initiated by heterologous brain tissue in the vaccine (cf. experimental allergic encephalomyelitis below). Some micro-organisms carry determinants which cross-react with the human and this may prove to be an important way of inducing autoimmunity. In rheumatic fever, antibodies produced to the streptococcus also react with heart, and the sera of 50% of children with the disease who develop Sydenham's chorea give neuronal immunofluorescent staining which can be absorbed out with streptococcal membranes. Colon antibodies present in ulcerative colitis have been found to cross-react with *Escherichia coli* 014. There is also some evidence for the view that antigens common to *Trypanosoma cruzi* and cardiac muscle provoke some of the immunopathological lesions seen in Chagas' disease.

(iii) Associative recognition

I have applied the term in the present context to the phenomenon in which one membrane component may provide help for the immune response to another. In the context of autoimmunity, a new helper determinant may arise through drug modification as mentioned above, or through the insertion of viral antigen into the membrane of an infected cell (figure 14.9d). That this can promote a reaction to a pre-existing cell component is clear from the studies in which infection of a tumour with influenza virus elicited resistance to uninfected tumour cells. The appearance of cold agglutinins often with blood group I specificity after *Mycoplasma pneumonia* infection could have a similar explanation.

Idiotype bypass mechanisms

A substantial body of evidence argues for the view that a regulatable idiotype network appears early in life, possibly related to Ly1$^+$ B-cells and to autoantibody formation (cf. p. 139 and 141). This raises the possibility of involving autoreactive lymphocytes with responses to exogenous agents through idiotype network connections, particularly since most autoimmune diseases are characterized by major cross-reactive idiotypes.

Thus, knowing that T-helpers with specificity for the idiotype on a lymphocyte receptor can be instrumental in the stimulation of that cell, it is conceivable that an environmental agent such as a parasite or virus which triggered antibody carrying a public idiotype (CRI) which happened to be shared with the receptor of an autoreactive T- or B-cell, could provoke an autoimmune response (figure 14.9b). Similarly, if it is correct that the germ-line idiotypes on autoantibodies generate a whole range of anti-idiotypes which mediate the response to exogenous antigens, then by the same token, it is conceivable that antibodies produced in response to an infection may react with the corresponding idiotype on the autoreactive lymphocyte (figure 14.9b). For example, a hybridoma from a myasthenia gravis patient secreted an anti-Id to an acetylcholine receptor autoantibody; this anti-Id was found to react with the bacterial product 1,3-dextran. Similarly, immunization with rheumatoid factor (autoantibody to IgG) gave rise to peptidoglycan antibodies although this could also be explained by an alternative mechanism in which the microbial epitope would be assumed to be similar in shape to the autoantibody Id (figure 14.9a). Finally, it is possible for Id network interactions to allow a viral infection to give rise to auto-antibodies reacting with the viral receptor (figure 14.9c). Since viruses all bind to specific complementary receptors on the cells they infect, this sequence of events may have serious consequences; we note for example that β-adrenergic receptors are the surface targets for certain reoviruses and that rabies virus binds to the acetylcholine receptor.

Polyclonal activation

Microbes often display adjuvant properties through their possession of polyclonal lymphocyte activators such as bacterial endotoxins which act by providing a non-specific inductive signal for B-cell stimulation, so bypassing the need for specific T-cell help (figure 14.10). This can occur by direct interaction with the B-lymphocyte or indirectly through stimulating the secretion of non-specific factors from T-cells or macrophages. A good example is the thymus-dependent production of auto-antibodies by injection of mice with thyroglobulin and endotoxin lipopolysaccharide (LPS). The variety of autoantibodies detected in cases with infectious mononucleosis must surely be attributable to the polyclonal activation of B-cells by EB virus. They are seen also in lepromatous leprosy where the

248

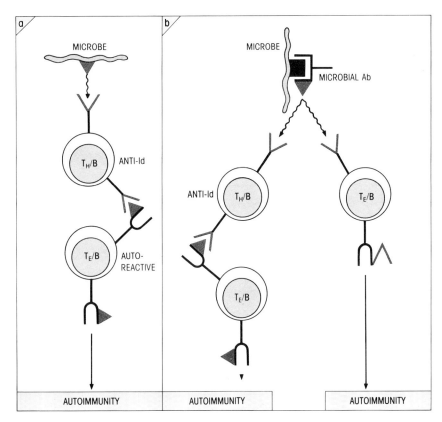

Figure 14.9. *Idiotypic mechanisms leading to autoimmunity.* (a) *Microbial antigen cross-reacts with autoreactive lymphocyte Id.* (b) *Microbial antibodies either share Id's with or are anti-Id to autoreactive lymphocytes.* (c) *Anti-virus generates anti-Id which is autoantibody to viral receptor (Plotz).* (d) *Viral protein provides T-help to activate anti-hormone/anti-receptor network.*

abundance of mycobacteria reproduces some of the features of Freund's adjuvant. However, unlike the usual situation in human autoimmune disease, these autoantibodies tend to be IgM and, in addition, do not persist when the microbial components are cleared from the body. Curiously, lymphocytes from mice with spontaneous autoimmunity (e.g. NZB and BXSB) produce abnormally large amounts of IgM when cultured *in vitro* as if they were under polyclonal activation; so do lymphocytes from many patients with SLE. On the other hand, the failure of

neonatally thyroidectomized Obese strain chickens to make thyroglobulin autoantibodies (p. 246) implies that autoantigen itself is needed for the induction of autoimmunity, in organ-specific disease at least, although the possible requirement for spontaneous production of accessory signals as in the thyroglobulin/LPS experiment just cited, cannot be excluded.

Non-organ-specific autoantibodies directed to autoantigens like DNA and red cells which have repeating antigenic determinants capable of cross-

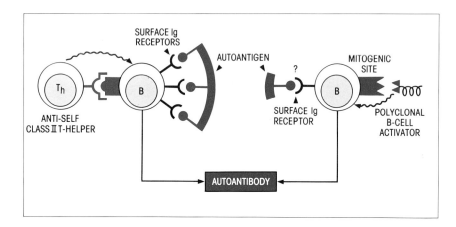

Figure 14.10. *Production of autoantibody by polyclonal activation. Microbial polyclonal activators may not require any signal through the surface Ig receptors. The restriction of autoantibodies generated by graft-vs-host reaction due to allogeneic T-cells, to autoantigens with repeating determinants such as red cells and DNA, make it likely that additional surface Ig signalling in the manner indicated is required for triggering by T-helpers reacting with self-class II.*

linking surface Ig receptors, are produced by a graft-vs-host reaction in which allogeneic T-cells react with host class II molecules on the B-cell. This form of cooperative polyclonal activation could arise if the self-reactive class II specific T-cells mentioned earlier took the place of the allogeneic T-cells (figure 14.10).

Autoimmunity arising through bypass of regulatory mechanisms

Suppressor circuits may not work

It should be emphasized that these T-inducer by-pass mechanisms for the induction of autoimmunity do not by themselves ensure the continuation of the response, since normal animals have been shown to be capable of damping down autoantibody production through T-suppressor interactions as, for example, in the case of red cell autoantibodies induced in mice by injection of rat erythrocytes (figure 14.11). When T-suppressor activity is impaired by low doses of cyclophosphamide or if strains like the SJL which have prematurely ageing suppressors are used, autoimmunity is prolonged and more severe.

In general, manipulations which reduce T-suppressors encourage the development of autoantibodies. Thus, irradiated mice reconstituted with spleen cells deprived of Lyt 2 positive T-cells produce antibodies to thyroglobulin, nuclei and lymphocytes. When rats were thymectomized at a few weeks of age and given divided doses of X-rays, they developed thyroglobulin autoantibodies and thyroiditis. Neonatal thymectomy which greatly depletes the T-suppressor population, induces or

exacerbates spontaneous autoimmune states in susceptible animals—autoimmune haemolytic anaemia in NZB mice and thyroiditis in Obese strain chickens and Buffalo rats. Coombs' positivity (i.e. the state in which circulating red cells are coated with antibody) can be transferred with the spleen cells of a Coombs' positive NZB to a young negative mouse of the same strain, but the continued production of red cell antibodies is short lived unless the recipient's T-cells are first depleted by pretreatment

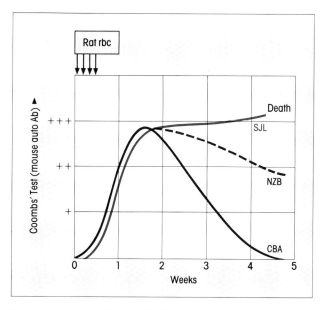

Figure 14.11. *Regulation of self-reactivity. When CBA mice are injected with rat red cells, autoantibodies are produced by this cross-reacting antigen (p.248) which coat the host erythrocytes and are detected by the Coombs' test (p.241). The SJL strain, in which suppressor activity declines rapidly with age, is unable to regulate the autoimmune response and develops particularly severe disease. The response is also prolonged in the autoimmune NZB strain (after A. Cooke & P. Hutchings).*

with anti-lymphocyte serum. Other changes seen with age in the NZB are an increasing resistance to the induction of tolerance to soluble proteins and a sudden fall in the plasma concentration of the thymic peptide thymulin before the onset of disease (note: thymulin is said to inhibit the autoreactive response of spleen cells to syngeneic fibroblasts in culture). Thus, there is a widely held view that one defect in the NZB is a progressive loss of T-suppressors with age and it is relevant that Ly1,2 cells which are needed for the induction of suppressors are low in diseased mice.

Defects are possible at various other control points in the regulatory mechanism: for example, the NOD mouse which spontaneously develops autoimmune diabetes fails to express I-E. Cross-breeding with the C3H strain shows the failure to be recessive and linked to the development of disease. It could be that T-suppressors are generated by a response to I-E in this system (cf. p. 120) and fail to develop if it is not expressed. Another mutant mouse strain with a spontaneous SLE-like syndrome, the MRL/l, has ample numbers of effective Ly1,2 cells but Ly1 helpers are resistant to their suppressor action due, it is said, to excessive *contrasuppressor* activity by a subpopulation of $Ly1^+2^-$ T-cells with binding sites for the lectin *Vicia villosa*. While this area is still relatively unexplored, it requires no gigantic leap of imagination to realize that undue activity by such cells will lower the threshold for autoimmunity (figure 14.12).

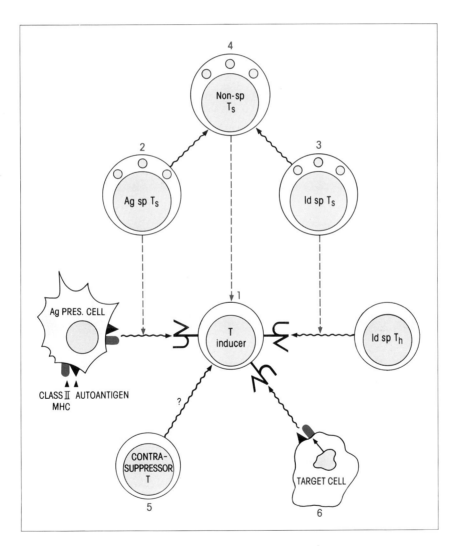

Figure 14.12. *Bypass of regulatory mechanisms leads to triggering of autoreactive T-inducer cells through defects in (1) ability to respond to or induce T-suppressors, or (2) expression of antigen-specific, (3) idiotype-specific or (4) non-specific T-suppressors, or through (5) stimulation of contrasuppressors or (6) derepression of class II genes with inappropriate cellular expression of Ia.*

AUTOIMMUNE DISEASE — SCOPE

We have previously drawn attention to the distinctive properties of the murine Ly1 B population with respect to its propensity to synthesize IgM autoantibodies and its possible intimate relationship to the setting up of the regulatory idiotype network (cf. p. 248) and one must seriously entertain the hypothesis that unregulated activity by these cells could be responsible for certain autoimmune disorders. The pitifully named moth-eaten strain is heavily into autoimmunity, and the mice make masses of anti-DNA and anti-polymorphs and die with intense pneumonitis, often before they have tasted the fruits of life. Their IgM levels rise to a staggering level of 25—50 times normal and—this is quite bizarre—their B-cells are nearly all Ly1 positive. This population is also raised in the NZB and largely accounts for the production of the IgM autoantibodies in this strain. Since pathogenic autoantibodies often tend to be IgG, one is prompted to ask whether these Ly1 B-cells have escaped regulatory control and undergo an unrestrained isotype switch to IgG as a basis for production of disease. Indirect evidence for their participation in the disease process comes from breeding experiments with CBA/N mice with the X-linked immune deficiency (xid) trait which includes an inability to develop Ly1 B-cells. Crossing a female CBA/N with a male NZB gives F1 animals which do express the xid defect and *do not* develop autoimmune haemolytic anaemia, whereas (male CBA/N × female NZB) F1s do not have the xid defect, do make Ly1 B-cells and do develop autoimmune disease.

Less is known of regulatory circuits in man although there is increasing evidence that non-specific T-suppressor function in SLE may be poorly regulated. B-lymphocytes from patients with active disease secrete larger amounts of Ig when cultured *in vitro* than normal B-cells. Concanavalin A-induced non-specific suppressors are reduced or absent and T-cells with Fcγ receptors, which suppress pokeweed mitogen-stimulated lymphocytes (p. 118) are low, the defect being greater the more active the disease. The production of thymulin and of interleukin-2 is also depressed in these patients. A significant proportion of clinically unaffected close relatives also demonstrate abnormally low levels of non-specific suppressors indicating that the deficit in SLE patients is not a consequence of the illness or its treatment and that additional factors must be implicated in the causation of disease.

In any case, it is difficult to account for the antigenic specificity of different autoimmune disorders on the basis of a generalized depression of non-specific suppressors alone, without invoking defects in either antigen- or idiotype-specific suppressor T-cells (p. 120). There is, however, a further possibility which is both novel and exciting.

Inappropriate expression of class II molecules

The majority of organ-specific autoantigens normally appear on the surface of the cells of the target organ in the context of class I but not class II MHC molecules. As such they cannot communicate with T-inducers and are therefore immunologically silent. Pujol-Borrell, Bottazzo and colleagues reasoned that if the class II genes were somehow derepressed and Ia molecules were now synthesized, they would endow the surface molecules with potential autoantigenicity (figure 14.12). Indeed, they have been able to show that human thyroid cells in tissue culture can be persuaded to express HLA-DR (Ia) molecules on their surface after stimulation with γ-interferon, and, further, that the cytoplasm of epithelial cells from the glands of patients with Graves' disease (thyrotoxicosis) stains strongly with anti-HLA-DR reagents, indicating active synthesis of class II polypeptides (figure 14.2b). Inappropriate class II expression has also been reported on the bile ductules in primary biliary cirrhosis and on endothelial cells and some β-cells in the diabetic pancreas both in the human and in the BB rat model (figure 14.2c and d). Whether adventitious expression of class II on these cells by something like virally induced interferon is responsible for *initiating* the autoimmune process by priming autoreactive T-helpers, or whether reaction with *already activated* T-cells induces class II by release of IFNγ and makes the cell a more attractive target for provoking subsequent tissue damage, is still an unresolved issue.

Undoubtedly, the autoimmune diseases have a multifactorial aetiology. Perhaps most, if not all, the defects we have discussed may contribute in different combinations to different disorders. Although these defects individually may be not uncommon, their origin remains obscure. They might be the consequence of some subtle virus infection, perhaps of the target organ in the case of organ-specific disease and of the lymphoid system at the non-organ-specific pole; the shedding of tremendous amounts of a C-type oncornavirus from NZB T-cell lines may be of relevance to this. Or one may be dealing with some ageing process affecting the thymus or the lymphoid stem cells. Sex hormones may also contribute to the increased frequency of auto-

252

immunity in females. Thus, oopherectomy and testosterone treatment alleviate the disease in female (NZB × NZW)F1 hybrids.

SUMMARY

Autoimmunity is associated with certain diseases which form a spectrum. At one pole, exemplified by Hashimoto's thyroiditis, the autoantibodies and the lesions are *organ specific* with the organ acting as the target for autoimmune attack; at the other pole are the *non-organ-specific* diseases such as systemic lupus erythematosus where the autoantibodies have widespread reactivity and the lesions resemble those of serum sickness relating to deposition of circulating immune complexes. There is a tendency for organ-specific disorders such as thyroiditis and pernicious anaemia to overlap in given individuals while overlap of rheumatological disorders is greater than expected by chance. Multifactorial genetic factors increase predisposition to autoimmune disease: these include HLA tissue type and factors affecting the immune system and possibly the potential autoantigens.

Autoantigens are for the most part accessible to circulating lymphocytes which normally include autoreactive T- and B-cells. It is assumed that the key to the system is control of autoreactive T-inducer/helper cells which are normally unresponsive because of clonal deletion, T-suppression or failure of autoantigen presentation. Autoimmunity might arise by several mechanisms involving bypass of these key T-inducer cells. These would include the provision of new carrier determinants on the autoantigen either through abnormal modification through synthesis or breakdown, through cross-reaction with exogenous antigens, or by associative recognition with viral or administered drug determinants. T-inducers could also be bypassed by idiotype network interactions with cross-reactions between public idiotypes on autoantibodies and microbial antibodies or microbes themselves, or by antibodies formed to anti-viral idiotypes which behaved as internal images of the virus and reacted with the cell surface viral receptor. Finally, B-cells can be stimulated directly by polyclonal activators such as EB virus or lipopolysaccharides, or by an expansion of naturally occurring autoreactive anti-self class II T-helpers.

T-inducer bypass alone may be insufficient to *maintain* autoimmunity and it is generally considered that, in addition, a regulatory defect is required. This could occur through an inability of the central T-inducer cell to respond to or induce T-suppressors. It could also arise through defects in the antigen-specific, idiotype-specific and non-specific T-suppressor systems. Other possibilities would be a stimulation of contrasuppressor cells, and an exciting new development, the derepression of class II genes giving rise to inappropriate cellular expression of Ia so breaking the 'silence' between cellular autoantigen and autoreactive T-inducer.

Suggestions for further reading are given at the end of the following chapter.

CHAPTER 15

AUTOIMMUNE DISEASES

II – Pathogenesis, Diagnosis and Treatment

254

PATHOGENIC MECHANISMS IN AUTOIMMUNE DISEASE

We have mentioned that despite certain exceptions as, for instance, myocardial infarction or damage to the testis, traumatic release of organ constituents does not in general elicit antibody formation. Destruction of thyroid tissue by therapeutic doses of radio-iodine does not initiate thyroid autoimmunity, nor does damage to the liver in alcoholic cirrhosis result in the synthesis of mitochondrial antibodies, to give but two examples. We should now look at the evidence which bears directly on the issue of whether autoimmunity, however it arises, plays a *primary* pathogenic role in the production of tissue lesions in the group of diseases labelled as 'autoimmune'.

Effects of humoral antibody

Blood

The erythrocyte antibodies play a role in the destruction of red cells in autoimmune haemolytic anaemia. Normal red cells coated with autoantibody eluted from Coombs' positive erythrocytes have a shortened half-life after reinjection into the normal subject. Platelet antibodies are apparently responsible for idiopathic thrombocytopenic purpura (ITP). IgG from a patient's serum when given

to a normal individual causes a depression of platelet counts and the active principle can be absorbed out with platelets. The transient neonatal thrombocytopenia which may be seen in infants of mothers with ITP is explicable in terms of transplacental passage of IgG antibodies to the child.

Some children with immunodeficiency associated with very low white cell counts have a serum lymphocytotoxic factor which requires complement for its activity. Lymphopenia occurring in patients with SLE and rheumatoid arthritis may also be a direct result of antibody since non-agglutinating antibodies coating the white cells have been reported in such cases.

Thyroid

Cytotoxic antibodies

The serum of patients with Hashimoto's disease is cytotoxic for human thyroid cells growing in monolayer culture after dispersal by trypsin. This is a typical complement-mediated antibody reaction directed against a cell surface antigen which is identical with the microsomal antigen revealed by intracytoplasmic staining of thyroid sections with sera from Hashimoto patients. Curiously, this antigen is expressed only on the apical portion of the follicular cells in contact with the colloid so that it is not normally accessible to circulating antibody. This explains why simple fragments of thyroid which have intact follicles are unaffected by incubation in the presence of medium containing cytotoxic antibody and complement, and also why there is no evidence that infants born to Hashimoto mothers have defective thyroid function despite the presence of the antibody in their serum. None the less, antibody can be detected on the inner surface of thyroid follicles in tissue removed from patients with autoimmune thyroiditis, and it seems necessary to postulate that thyroid damage only occurs when there is collaboration with other factors such as immune complex deposition, sensitized T-cell effectors or mechanisms which bring about a reversal of polarity of the epithelial cells.

Thyroid-stimulating antibodies

Under certain circumstances antibodies to the surface of a cell may stimulate rather than destroy (cf. type V sensitivity; Chapter 12). This would seem to be the case in thyrotoxicosis (Graves' or Basedow's disease). There has long been indirect evidence suggesting a link between autoimmune processes and this disease: thyroid antibodies are detectable in up to 85% of thyrotoxic patients and histologically the majority of the glands removed at operation show varying degrees of thyroiditis and local antibody formation in addition to the characteristic acinar cell hyperplasia; thyrotoxicosis is found with undue frequency in the families of Hashimoto patients; there is an association with gastric autoimmunity in that 30% have gastric antibodies and up to 10% pernicious anaemia. The direct link came with the discovery by Adams and Purves of thyroid stimulating activity in the serum of thyrotoxic patients. Using a new bioassay they found that the serum caused a stimulation of the thyroid gland of the recipient animal which was considerably prolonged relative to the time course of action of the physiological thyroid stimulating hormone (TSH) from the pituitary; it was ultimately shown that this was due

to the presence of thyroid stimulating antibodies (TSAb). These antibodies can block the binding of TSH to thyroid membranes and seem to act in the same manner as TSH, probably by stimulating the identical receptors (cf. figure 12.20). Both operate through the adenyl cyclase system as indicated by the potentiating effect of theophylline, and both produce similar changes in ultrastructural morphology in the thyroid cell, but it is one of Nature's 'passive transfer experiments' which links TSAb most directly with the pathogenesis of Graves' disease. When TSAb from a thyrotoxic mother crosses the placenta it is associated with the production of neonatal hyperthyroidism (figure 15.1), which resolves after a few weeks as the maternal IgG is catabolized.

There is a good correlation between the titre of TSAb and the severity of hyperthyroidism. Because TSAb act independently of the pituitary−thyroid axis, iodine uptake by the gland is unaffected by administration of thyroxine or tri-iodothyronine, whereas normally this would cause feedback inhibition and suppression of uptake; this forms the basis of an important diagnostic test for thyrotoxicosis.

There is reason to believe that enlargement of the thyroid in this disorder is due to the action of antibodies which react with a 'growth' receptor and directly stimulate cell division as distinct from metabolic hyperactivity (figure 15.2a). In contrast, sera from patients with primary myxoedema contain antibodies capable of blocking the mitogenic action of TSH (figure 15.2b) thereby preventing the regeneration of follicles which is a feature of the enlarged Hashimoto goitre. We see now that there is considerable diversity in the autoimmune response to the thyroid leading to tissue destruction, metabolic stimulation, growth promotion or mitotic inhibition which in different combinations account for the variety of forms in which autoimmune thyroid disease presents (figure 15.3).

255

Figure 15.1. *Neonatal thyrotoxicosis. (a) The autoantibodies which stimulate the thyroid through the TSH-receptors are IgG and cross the placenta. (b) The thyrotoxic mother therefore gives birth to a baby with thyroid hyperactivity which spontaneously resolves as the mother's IgG is catabolized. (Photograph courtesy of Dr A. MacGregor.)*

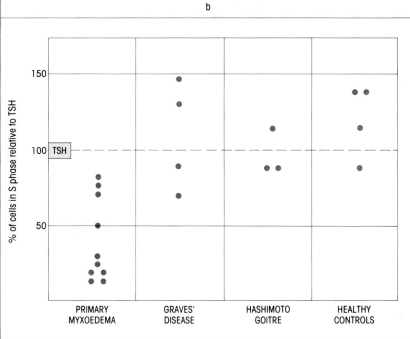

Figure 15.2. *Autoantibodies affecting thyroid growth. (a) Stimulating antibodies in goitrous Graves' disease and autoimmune colloid goitre shown by the increase of cells entering the DNA synthetic (S) phase of the cell cycle in thyroid fragments treated with IgG from the patient's serum. p values relate to differences from results with normal Ig. (b) Blocking antibodies in primary myxoedema revealed by the ability of patient's IgG to inhibit the growth stimulation caused by TSH. Each point represents the value for an individual patient's serum. (Data from Drexhage H.A., Bottazzo G.F., Doniach D., Bitensky L. & Chayen J. (1980)* Lancet ii, *287 and from (1981)* Nature 289, 594.)*

Intrinsic factor

Autoantibodies to this product of gastric mucosal secretion were first demonstrated in pernicious anaemia patients by oral administration of intrinsic factor, vitamin B_{12} and the serum from a patient with this disease. The serum was found to prevent intrinsic factor from mediating the absorption of B_{12} into the body, and further studies showed the active principle to be an antibody. Circulating antibody does not seem to be capable of neutralizing the physiological activity of intrinsic factor; a patient immunized parenterally with hog intrinsic factor in complete Freund's adjuvant had high serum antibody levels and good cell-mediated skin

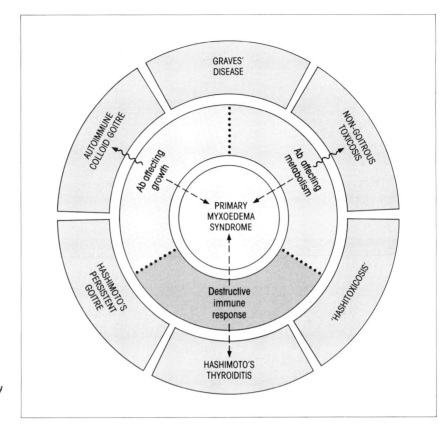

Figure 15.3. *Relationship of different autoallergic responses to the circular spectrum of autoimmune thyroid diseases. Responses involving thyroglobulin and the microsomal/ surface microvillous antigen lead to tissue destruction whereas other autoantibodies can stimulate or block metabolic activity or thyroid cell division. 'Hashitoxicosis' is the down-to-earth term used by our Scots' colleagues to describe a gland showing Hashimoto's thyroiditis and thyrotoxicosis simultaneously (courtesy of Prof. D. Doniach and Dr G.F. Bottazzo).*

257

responses but still absorbed B_{12} well when fed with hog intrinsic factor. These data imply that the antibodies have to be present within the lumen of the gastro-intestinal tract to be biologically effective, and indeed they can be identified in the gastric juice of these patients, synthesized by plasma cells in the gastritic lesion.

Sperm

In some infertile males, agglutinating antibodies cause aggregation of the spermatozoa and interfere with their penetration into the cervical mucus.

Glomerular basement membrane (gbm)

With immunological kidney disease the experimental models preceded the finding of parallel lesions in the human. Injection of cross-reacting heterologous gbm preparations in complete Freund's adjuvant produces glomerulonephritis in sheep and other experimental animals. Antibodies to gbm can be picked up by immunofluorescent staining of biopsies from nephritic animals with anti-IgG. The antibodies are largely, if not completely, absorbed

out by the kidney *in vivo* but they appear in the serum on nephrectomy and can passively transfer the disease to another animal of the same species.

An entirely analogous situation occurs in man in certain cases of glomerulonephritis, particularly those associated with lung haemorrhage (Goodpasture's syndrome). Kidney biopsy from the patient shows *linear* deposition of IgG and C3 along the basement membrane of the glomerular capillaries (figure 12.14a). After nephrectomy, gbm antibodies can be detected in the serum. Dixon and his colleagues eluted the gbm antibody from a diseased kidney and injected it into a squirrel monkey. The antibody rapidly fixed to the gbm of the recipient animal and produced a fatal nephritis (figure 15.4). It is hard to escape the conclusion that the lesion in the human was the direct result of attack on the gbm by these complement-fixing antibodies. The lung changes in Goodpasture's syndrome are attributable to cross-reaction with some of the gbm antibodies.

Muscle

The transient muscle weakness seen in a proportion of babies born to mothers with myasthenia gravis

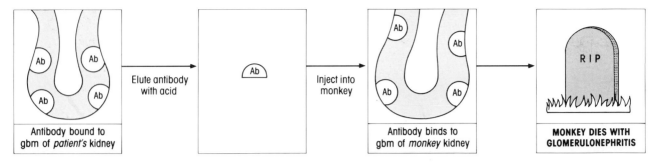

Figure 15.4. *Passive transfer to glomerulonephritis to a squirrel monkey by injection of antiglomerular basement membrane (anti-gbm) antibodies isolated by acid elution* *from the kidney of a patient with Goodpasture's syndrome (after Lerner R.A., Glascock R.J. & Dixon F.J. (1967) J. Exp. Med. 126, 989).*

calls to mind neonatal thrombocytopenia and hyperthyroidism and would certainly be compatible with the transplacental passage of an IgG capable of inhibiting neuromuscular transmission. Strong support for this view is afforded by the consistent finding of antibodies to muscle acetylcholine receptors in myasthenics and the depletion of these receptors within the motor end-plates. In addition, myasthenic symptoms can be induced in animals by injection of monoclonal antibodies to acetylcholine receptors or by active immunization with the purified receptors themselves. None the less, the majority of babies with myasthenic mothers do not display muscle disease and it transpires that they are protecting themselves by producing antibodies directed to idiotypes on the maternal autoantibodies.

Table 15.1 summarizes these direct pathogenic effects of humoral autoantibodies.

Effects of complexes

Systemic lupus erythematosus (SLE)

Where autoantibodies are formed against soluble components to which they have continual access, complexes may be formed which can give rise to lesions similar to those occurring in serum sickness especially when defects in the early classical complement components prevent effective clearance (cf. p. 205). In SLE, complexes of DNA and other nuclear antigens, and possibly C-type viral components, together with immunoglobulin and complement can be detected by immunofluorescent staining of kidney biopsies from patients with evidence of renal dysfunction. The staining pattern with a fluorescent anti-IgG or anti-C3 is punctate or 'lumpy-bumpy' as some would describe it (figure 12.14b) in marked contrast with the linear pattern caused by the gbm antibodies in Goodpasture's syndrome (figure 12.14a; p. 203). The complexes grow in size to become large aggregates visible in the electron microscope as amorphous humps on the epithelial side of the glomerular basement membrane (figure 15.5). During the active phase of the disease, serum complement levels fall as components are affected by immune aggregates in the kidney and circulation. Attempts to detect autoantigens in the circulating complexes have not been conspicuously successful; immunoglobulins and complement components make up the usual tally of constituents which can be identified. Although in a way negative evidence, this is consistent with the possibility that anti-idiotype may perpetuate an autoimmune state once it is initiated (i.e. acts as a surrogate autoantigen) and generate circulating idiotype—anti-idiotype complexes.

Immunofluorescent studies on skin biopsies from patients with the related disease discoid lupus erythematosus also reveal the presence of immune complexes.

Rheumatoid arthritis

Morphological evidence for immunological activity

The joint changes in rheumatoid arthritis are in essence produced by the malign growth of the synovial cells as a pannus overlaying and destroying cartilage and bone (figure 15.6a—f). The synovial membrane which surrounds and maintains the joint space becomes intensely cellular as a result of considerable immunological hyper-reactivity as evidenced by large numbers of T-cells in various stages of activation, usually associated with dendritic cells and macrophages; clumps of plasma

DISEASE	AUTOANTIGEN	LESION
Autoimmune haemolytic anaemia	Red cell	Erythrocyte destruction
Lymphopenia (some cases)	Lymphocyte	Lymphocyte destruction
Idiopathic thrombocytopenic purpura	Platelet	Platelet destruction
Male infertility (some cases)	Sperm	Agglutination of spermatozoa
Pernicious anaemia	Intrinsic factor	Neutralization of ability to mediate B_{12} absorption
Hashimoto's disease	Thyroid surface antigen	Cytotoxic effect on thyroid cells in culture
Goodpasture's syndrome	Glomerular basement membrane	Complement-mediated damage to basement membrane
Myasthenia gravis	Acetylcholine receptor	Blocking and destruction of receptors
Acanthosis nigricans (type B) and ataxia telangiectasia with insulin resistance	Insulin receptor	Blocking of receptors
Atopic allergy (some cases)	β-Adrenergic receptors	Blocking of receptors

Table 15.1. *Direct pathogenic effects of humoral antibodies.*

Figure 15.5. *Renal biopsy of SLE patient with severe immune complex glomerulonephritis and proteinuria. Electron micrograph showing irregular thickening of glomerular capillary walls by subepithelial complexes (a) and subendothelial complexes (b). The mesangial region shows abundant (probably phagocytosed) complexes. (Courtesy of Dr A. Leatham.)*

cells are frequently observed and sometimes even secondary follicles with germinal centres are present as though the synovium had become an active lymph node (figure 15.6g, h and i). Indeed it has been estimated that the synthesis of immunoglobulins by the synovial tissue ranks with that of a stimulated lymph node. There is widespread expression of surface HLA-DR (class II); T- and B-cells, dendritic and synovial lining cells and macrophages are all positive, indicative of some pretty lively action (figure 15.6k). The thesis is that this fiery immunological reactivity provides an intense stimulus to the synovial lining cells which undergo a Dr Jeckyll to Mr Hyde transformation into the invasive pannus which brings about joint erosion through the release of destructive mediators.

AUTOIMMUNE DISEASES – PATHOGENESIS ETC

(a)

(b)

(c)

(d)

(e)

(f)

(g)

(h)

(i)

(j)

(k)

(l)

(m)

(n)

CHAPTER 15

What is provoking this immunological activity?

From the T-cell standpoint, no conventional antigens have yet been identified. There are currently reports of the isolation of T-cell lines from the joint which are driven by EB virus transformed B-cell lines derived from the same lymphocyte populations. This suggests three main possibilities for the T-cell-line specificities: anti-self class II MHC, anti-B-cell idiotype and anti-EBV-determined surface antigens. Although it should not be too difficult to sort out this matter, at the time of writing I do not have the required data. For argument's sake let me plump for the first possibility, namely, that there are large numbers of T-cells which react with autologous class II determinants.

IgG autosensitization

By utilizing the mechanism set out in figure 14.10 (p. 250), these T-cells could stimulate B-lymphocytes which react with autoantigens bearing repeating determinants, in particular, in the context of rheumatoid arthritis, with the multiple Fc regions of IgG within a soluble immune complex. This would lead to the synthesis of autoantibodies to the IgG Fc region, known as antiglobulins or rheumatoid factors, which are the hallmark of the disease being demonstrable in virtually all patients with rheumatoid arthritis. The majority have IgM antiglobulins which react in the classical latex and sheep cell agglutination tests (table 14.2; note 7) and both they and the 'seronegative' patients who fail to react in these tests can be shown to have elevated levels of IgG antiglobulins detectable by solid phase immunoassay (cf. p. 78; figure 15.7).

If, therefore, autosensitization to IgG is an almost universal feature of the disease, most of the plasma cells in the synovium should be synthesizing antiglobulins. But in fact only a relative minority of the plasma cells (say 10–20%) bind fluoresceinated IgG, either in the form of heat-aggregated material (figure 15.6j) or immune complexes (rheumatoid factor is a low affinity antibody and good binding is only seen when multivalent IgG is used as antigen). However, we must take into account a strange and unique feature of IgG antiglobulins; because they are both antigen and antibody at the same time, they are capable of self-association (figure 15.8b) and this hides the majority of free antiglobulin valencies. Cleverly realizing that destruction of the Fc regions by pepsin would liberate these hidden binding sites (figure 15.8c), Munthe & Natvig observed that as many as 40–70% of the plasma cells in the synovium displayed an anti-IgG specificity following treatment with this enzyme.

IgG aggregates, presumably products of these plasma cells, can be regularly detected in the synovial tissues and in the joint fluid where they give rise to typical acute inflammatory reactions with fluid exudates. Analysis shows them to consist almost exclusively of immunoglobulins and complement while a major proportion of the IgG is present as self-associated antiglobulin as shown by binding to an $Fc\gamma$ immunosorbent after treatment with pepsin.

Abnormal glycosylation

One of the most exciting things to hit rheumatoid arthritis in the last few years has been the discovery that the patients' IgG is abnormally glycosylated.

Facing page
Figure 15.6. *Rheumatoid arthritis (RA). (a) Hands of a patient with chronic RA showing classical swan-neck deformities. (b) Diagrammatic representation of a diarthrodial joint showing bone and cartilagenous erosions beneath the synovial membrane derived pannus. (c) Proximal interphalangeal joint depicting marked bony erosion and marginal erosion of the cartilage. (d) Early pannus of granulation tissue growing over the patella. (e) Histology of pannus showing clear erosion of bone and cartilage at the cellular margin. (f) Histology of the pannus stained for macrophage non-specific esterase; note long stained dendritic processes. (g) Chronic inflammatory cells in the deeper layers of the synovium in RA. (h) A hypervillous synovium with well-formed secondary follicles with germinal centres (relatively rare occurrence). (i) A high power view of an area of diseased synovium showing collections of classical plasma cells. (j) Plasma cells isolated from a patient's synovial tissue stained simultaneously for IgM (with fluorescein-labelled*

F(ab')₂ anti-μ) and rheumatoid factor (with rhodamine-labelled aggregated Fcγ). Two of the four IgM-positive plasma cells appear to be synthesizing rheumatoid factors. (k) Rheumatoid synovium showing large numbers of cells stained by anti-HLA-DR (anti-class II). (l) Rheumatoid synovium showing class II positive accessory cells (green) in intimate contact with CD4 positive T-cells (orange). (m) Large rheumatoid nodules on the forearm. (n) Granulomatous appearance of the rheumatoid nodule with central necrotic area surrounded by epithelioid cells, macrophages and scattered lymphocytes. Plasma cells making rheumatoid factor are often demonstrable and the lesion probably represents a response to the formation of insoluble anti-IgG complexes. ((a) kindly given by Dr D. Isenberg, (c), (d), (e), (g), (h) and (i) by Dr L.E. Glynn, (f) by Dr J. Edwards, (j) by Drs P. Youinou and P. Lydyard and (k) and (l) by Prof. G. Janossy.)

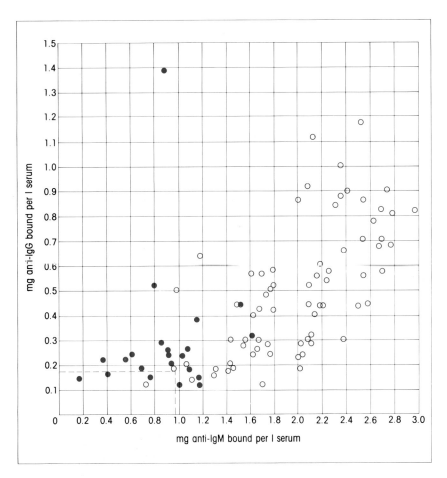

Figure 15.7. *IgM and IgG antiglobulins determined by tube radioassay in patients with seropositive (○) and seronegative (●) rheumatoid arthritis. The dotted lines indicate the 95% confidence limits (mean + 2 S.D.) of the normal group. (From Nineham L., Hay F.C. & Roitt I.M. (1976) J. Clin. Path. 29, 1121.)*

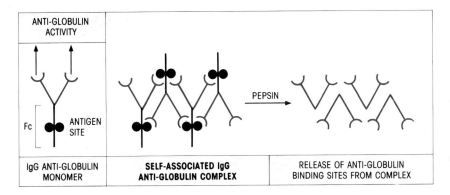

Figure 15.8. *Self-associated complexes of IgG antiglobulins and the exposure of 'hidden' binding sites by pepsin. Although of relatively low affinity, the strength of binding is boosted by the 'bonus effect' of the mutual attachment and, furthermore, such complexes in the joint may be stabilized by IgM antiglobulin and Clq which have polyvalent binding sites for IgG.*

The two C_H2 domains in the Fc region are held apart (cf. p. 39) by two asparagine-linked sugars of the general structure shown in figure 15.9a. The 1,3 arms from each sugar provide a bridge between the domains while the 1,6 sugars are directed towards the protein surface where the terminal sialic acid-galactose lies in a special 'lectin-like' pocket (figure 15.9b and c). Some chains end in N-acetyl-glucosamine and lack the terminal sialic acid-galactose sugars. In normal individuals, some 14% of the IgG Fc sugar groups lack the terminal galactose on *both* chains. What is extraordinary is that the percentage of sugars completely lacking galactose in the IgG of rheumatoid arthritis patients is always higher than in the controls and can go as high as 60% (figure 15.10). This glycosylation defect could lead to conformational change in the Fc structure with two possible consequences:

1   the Fc may have increased autoantigenicity, and
2   self-associated IgG complexes (figure 15.8) would be held together more strongly if the terminal sialic acid-galactose on the Fab sugar of one IgG fits into

Figure 15.9. *The Fc sugars and their role in bridging the two C_H2 domains. (a) Typical structure of each N-linked sugar. Some chains lack terminal galactose-sialic acid. (b) Position of sugar chains in C_H2 domains. (c) Structure of the C_H2 regions and the association between the terminal galactose-sialic acid on the 1,6 arm and the protein surface. The 1,3 arms, one of which must lack galactose, bridge the two domains. (GlcNAc, N-acetylglucosamine; Man, mannose; Gal, galactose; Neu5Ac, sialic acid; Fuc, fucose.)*

the lectin site on C_H2 left vacant by the lack of galactose on the Fc sugar. The glycosylation defect is not seen in SLE but is every bit as abnormal in tuberculosis!

The production of tissue damage

As explained in the legend to figure 15.8, the complexes can be stabilized by the multivalent Fcγ-binding molecules, IgM rheumatoid factor and Clq, and when present in the joint space-they may initiate an Arthus reaction leading to an influx of polymorphs with which they react to release lysosomal enzymes. These include neutral proteinases and collagenase which can damage the articular cartilage by breaking down proteoglycans and collagen fibrils. More damage results if the complexes are adherent to the cartilage since the polymorph

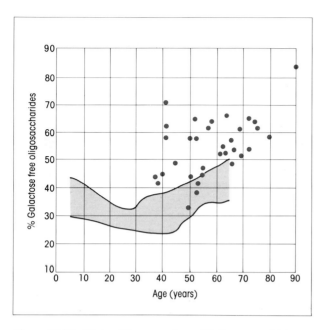

Figure 15.10. *Plots of the percentage of IgG sugars which completely lack terminal galactose showing the abnormal glycosylation of IgG in patients with rheumatoid arthritis. The shaded area indicates the mean ± S.D. of the normal controls. There is preliminary evidence that the defect is less marked when the disease is inactive. (Data from Parekh R.B., Isenberg D.A., Dwek R.A., Roitt I.M., Rook G.A.W. and Rademacher T.W., 1987.)*

can activate osteoclasts to bring about bone resorption which is a further complication of severe disease. Subcutaneous nodules are granulomata (figure 15.6m and n) possibly formed through local production of insolubilized self-associating antiglobulins.

The rheumatological pulse quickened perceptibly a few years ago with the discovery that a high proportion of patients with rheumatoid arthritis have elevated titres of circulating antibodies to a nuclear antigen present in EB virus transformed but absent from normal lymphocytes. This led to the finding that the T-cells in these patients are deficient in the γ-interferon-mediated control of EB virus transformation of B-lymphocytes. Although it is unlikely that this signifies a primary aetiological role for EB virus infection, it could represent a basic regulatory abnormality which results in defective handling of some initiating micro-organism and possibly allows the emergence of anti-self class II T-cells. An overview of the pathogenesis of the disease and speculation on its aetiology are presented in figure 15.11, but it should be emphasized that there are many other conceivable hypotheses, including cross-reactions between microbes and IgG and generation of T-helper anti-Ids, to account for the development of IgG autosensitization.

Cellular hypersensitivity

The inflammatory infiltrate in organ-specific autoimmune disease is usually essentially mononuclear in character and, although not an infallible guide, this has been taken as an expression of cell-mediated hypersensitivity. Direct evidence is still thin. At the time of writing, skin reactions to autoantigens have proved difficult to assess and *in vitro* leucocyte inhibition tests have not been unequivocally accepted, although, for example in autoimmune thyroiditis and thyrotoxicosis, there is a consistent finding of inhibition of leucocyte migration by thyroid microsomes. The killing of colon cells in culture by lymphocytes from patients with ulcerative colitis is encouraging and it has been reported that long-term culture of thyroid target cells with Hashimoto leucocytes leads to significant failure in the metabolic handling of iodine. Firm evidence for a direct participation of T-lymphocytes in any of these reactions has yet to be provided although it must be said that the recent demonstration of the expression of class II molecules on the thyroid cell surface makes it highly likely that T-cell reactions are involved.

binds but is unable to internalize them ('frustrated phagocytosis'); as a result the lysosomal hydrolases are released extracellularly into the space between the cell and the cartilage where they are protected from enzyme inhibitors such as α_2-macroglobulin.

The aggregates may also stimulate the macrophage-like cells of the synovial lining, either directly through their surface receptors or indirectly through phagocytosis and resistance to intracellular digestion. The release of lymphokines from activated T-cells will provide additional macrophage stimulation.

The activated synovial cells grow out as a malign pannus (cover) over the cartilage (figure 15.7d) and at the margin of this advancing granulation tissue, breakdown can be seen (figure 15.7e), almost certainly as a result of the release of enzymes, reactive oxygen intermediates and especially of interleukin-1. Activated macrophages also secrete plasminogen activator and the plasmin formed as a consequence activates a latent collagenase produced by synovial cells. Sensitization to partially degraded collagen may occur and this could lead secondarily to amplification of the lesion. Interleukin-1 and prostaglandin E_2, another product of the stimulated macrophage,

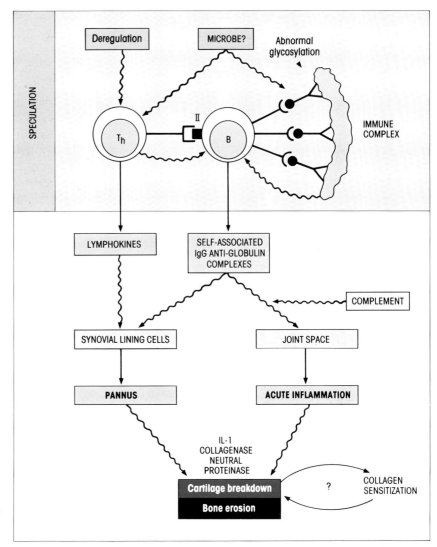

Figure 15.11. *Autoimmune pathogenesis of rheumatoid arthritis and speculation on the induction of autoimmunity.*

One also cannot ignore the possibility of ADCC mechanisms. For example, the destruction of isolated liver cells by leucocytes from patients with HBs-negative active chronic hepatitis can be blocked by antigen (hepatic lipoprotein) or by aggregated normal IgG (which would bind to K-cell Fc receptors), but is not affected by removal of T-cells.

Indirect evidence for a destructive role of the inflammatory cells comes from the observation that high doses of steroids may restore gastric function in certain patients with pernicious anaemia. In one such case studied, biopsy after intensive treatment with prednisone showed a diminution in the cellular infiltrate and new formation of parietal and chief cells in the gastric mucosa; acid and intrinsic factor were now produced after histamine stimulation and the ability to absorb vitamin B_{12} assessed by the Schilling test was restored to near normal values.

The most likely explanation is that attack by the inflammatory cells and attempts to regenerate by mucosal cells were more or less in balance in the atrophic mucosa. Elimination of inflammatory cells by the prednisone allowed the regeneration of gastric mucosal cells to become dominant.

Our views on the pathogenesis of pernicious anaemia may be stated as follows. Autoimmune attack based on the parietal cell antigen gives rise to an atrophic gastritis which in many cases settles down to a dynamic equilibrium where the rate of destruction roughly balances the rate of regeneration; the loss of capacity to make intrinsic factor is evident in tests showing defective B_{12} absorption but sufficient vitamin is absorbed to keep the body in balance. These patients often have parietal cell antibodies and go on for 15 years or so without developing megaloblastic anaemia. However, if they should produce antibodies to intrinsic factor in the lumen of the gastro-intestinal tract, these will neutralize the small amount of intrinsic factor still available and the body will move into negative balance for B_{12}. The symptoms of B_{12} deficiency will then appear some considerable time later as the liver stores become exhausted (figure 15.12). A similar long latent period before the onset of clinical disease is evident in the prospective study of a family with insulin-dependent diabetes documented in figure 14.4 (p. 244) where complement-fixing islet-cell antibodies were detected two years before overt signs of pancreatic deficiency were apparent. Note also that the disease occurs after the auto-immunity pointing yet again to a primary pathogenetic role for the immune process.

The nature of the cellular attack in organ-specific disorders is still not resolved but it is not improbable that cell-mediated hypersensitivity, antibody-mediated cytotoxicity and inflammatory reactions due to immune complexes may operate alone or in concert.

Experimental models of autoimmune disease

If autoimmune processes are pathogenic in human diseases we would expect that the production of autoimmunity should lead to comparable lesions in experimental animals.

Experimental autoallergic disease

When animals are injected with extracts of certain organs emulsified in oil containing killed tubercle bacilli (i.e. in complete Freund's adjuvant), auto-antibodies and destructive inflammatory lesions specific to the organ used for immunization result. Thus, Rose and Witebsky found that rabbits receiving rabbit thyroglobulin in Freund's adjuvant developed antibodies to thyroglobulin and thyroiditis involving invasion of the gland by mononuclear cells of lymphocytic and histiocytic types with destruction of the normal follicular architecture. Histologically there are many points of similarity between this experimental autoallergic lesion and human autoimmune thyroiditis (figure 15.13).

In some of the earliest work in this field it was shown that injection of central nervous tissue produced encephalomyelitis and paralysis in monkeys and guinea-pigs; the parallel with post-rabies vaccine encephalitis is clear since the vaccine contains brain extracts, and optimistic comparisons with multiple sclerosis have been made. Just as with the thyroid, the most convenient model for the production of allergic encephalomyelitis involves immunization with the antigen, in this case myelin basic

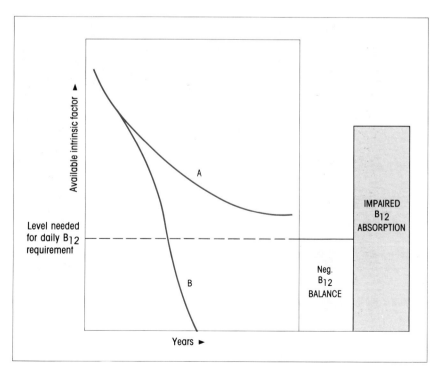

Figure 15.12. *Pathogenesis of pernicious anaemia. Group A: patients with long-standing atrophic gastritis having parietal cell but no intrinsic factor antibodies. Group B: pernicious anaemia patients with intrinsic factor antibodies superimposed upon the atrophic gastritis. (After Doniach D. & Roitt I.M. (1964)* **Semin. Hematol. I, 313.)**

(a) Normal rat thyroid

267

(b) Thyroiditis in the rat

Figure 15.13. *Similarity of lesions in spontaneous human autoimmune thyroiditis and the experimental disease produced by injection of rats with homologous thyroid in complete Freund's adjuvant. Other features of Hashimoto's disease such as the eosinophilic metaplasia of acinar cells (Askenazy cells) and local lymphoid follicles are not seen in this experimental model although the latter occur in the spontaneous thyroiditis of Obese strain chickens.*

(c) Spontaneous human autoimmune thyroiditis

protein, incorporated in complete Freund's adjuvant. Similar lesions can be induced in the adrenal (cf. Addisonian idiopathic adrenal atrophy) and the testis (? model for granulomatous orchitis), while experimental myasthenia gravis can be induced by immunization with acetylcholine receptor. Heterologous glomeruli stimulate the formation of glomerular basement membrane autoantibodies which localize in the kidney of the host to cause severe glomerulonephritis (Steblay model) resembling closely that seen in Goodpasture's syndrome.

The experimental disease can usually be transmitted to syngeneic animals by lymphoid cells from immunized donors and occasionally by serum. In the case of experimental autoallergic orchitis, a synergism between cell-mediated hypersensitivity and antibody was recognized in the transfer studied. Allergic encephalomyelitis can be induced in syngeneic animals by injection of purified T-cells from sensitized donors and in particular by T-cell lines which respond *in vitro* to myelin basic protein. On the other hand, transfer of monoclonal autoantibodies raised to acetylcholine receptors produces the muscle weakness characteristic of myasthenia.

Freund's adjuvant alone without any added antigen produces a migratory polyarthritis in rats, and it has proved possible to transmit the disease to naive animals by injecting a T-cell clone specific for a component of the Freund mycobacterium which cross-reacts with the core protein of cartilage proteoglycan.

The pre-eminent ability of Freund's complete adjuvant to enhance the production of experimental autoallergic disease may depend upon several factors acting concomitantly: modification of antigen, stimulation of T-helpers and (more controversially) disruption of normal T-suppressor feedback perhaps through priming of contrasuppressor cells. Although the precise nature of the events leading to tissue damage has yet to be resolved, it is abundantly clear that the deliberate provocation of an autoallergic state can produce lesions which closely mimic those seen in human organ-specific autoimmune disease and add weight to the notion that the immunological events are directly concerned in the pathogenesis of these disorders.

Spontaneous autoimmune disease

The message from animal models in which autoimmune disease develops spontaneously is the same. Neonatal bursectomy largely prevents the appearance of thyroglobulin antibodies and thyroiditis in Obese strain chickens, so pointing to a primary involvement of thyroid antibodies in the tissue lesions. Immunological control is also implicated by the exacerbation of disease caused by neonatal thymectomy.

The now famous strain of mouse, the New Zealand Black (NZB), consistently develops an autoimmune haemolytic anaemia with positive Coombs' tests (agglutination of antibody-coated erythrocytes by an antiglobulin serum). As discussed earlier, the disease can be provoked in young unaffected NZBs by transfer of spleen cells from a Coombs' positive donor suggesting that it is the production of red cell antibodies which leads to shortened erythrocyte survival and consequent anaemia. A high proportion of these mice, and especially their hybrids with the partially related New Zealand White, (NZB × W)F1, have circulating antinuclear antibodies and an immune complex induced glomerulonephritis. Several other mutant mouse strains which have SLE-like symptoms are also positive for anti-DNA and die with type III hypersensitivity kidney lesions.

DIAGNOSTIC VALUE OF AUTOANTIBODY TESTS

Serum autoantibodies frequently provide valuable diagnostic markers. The most useful routine test is screening of the serum by immunofluorescence on a frozen section prepared from a composite block of unfixed human thyroid and stomach, and rat kidney and liver. This is supplemented by agglutination tests for rheumatoid factors and for thyroglobulin, thyroid microsome and red cell antibodies and by radioassay for antibodies to intrinsic factor, DNA and IgG (see table 14.2). The salient information is summarized in table 15.2.

The tests will also prove of value in screening for people at risk, e.g. relatives of patients with autoimmune disease, thyroiditis patients for gastric autoimmunity and vice versa and ultimately the general population.

TREATMENT OF AUTOIMMUNE DISORDERS

Metabolic control

The majority of approaches to treatment, not unnaturally, involve manipulation of immunological

DISEASE	ANTIBODY	COMMENT
Hashimoto's thyroiditis	Thyroid	Distinction from colloid goitre, thyroid cancer and subacute thyroiditis. Thyroidectomy usually unnecessary in Hashimoto goitre
Primary myxoedema	Thyroid	Tests +ve in 99% of cases. If suspected hypothyroidism assess 'thyroid reserve' by TRH stimulation test
Thyrotoxicosis	Thyroid	High titres of cytoplasmic Ab indicate active thyroiditis and tendency to post-operative myxoedema: anti-thyroid drugs are the treatment of choice although HLA-B8 patients have high chance of relapse
Pernicious anaemia	Stomach	Help in diagnosis of latent PA, in differential diagnosis of non-autoimmune megaloblastic anaemia and in suspected subacute combined degeneration of the cord
Idiopathic adrenal atrophy	Adrenal	Distinction from tuberculous form
Myasthenia gravis	Muscle	When positive suggests associated thymoma (more likely if HLA-B12)
	ACh receptor	Positive in >80%
Pemphigus vulgaris and pemphigoid	Skin	Different fluorescent patterns in the two diseases
Autoimmune haemolytic anaemia	Erythrocyte (Coombs' test)	Distinction from other forms of anaemia
Sjögren's syndrome	Salivary duct cells	
Primary biliary cirrhosis (PBC)	Mitochondrial	Distinction from other forms of obstructive jaundice where test rarely +ve. Recognize subgroup within cryptogenic cirrhosis related to PBC with +ve mitochondrial Ab
Active chronic hepatitis	Smooth muscle anti-nuclear and 20% mitochondrial	Smooth muscle Ab distinguish from SLE
Rheumatoid arthritis	Antiglobulin, e.g. SCAT and latex fixation	High titre indicative of bad prognosis
SLE	High titre antinuclear, DNA; LE-cells	DNA antibodies present in active phase. Ab to double-stranded DNA characteristic
Scleroderma	Nucleolar	
Other 'collagenoses'	Nuclear	

Table 15.2. *Autoantibody tests and diagnosis.*

269

responses (figure 15.14). However, in many organ-specific diseases, metabolic control is usually sufficient, e.g. thyroxine replacement in primary myoedema, insulin in juvenile diabetes, vitamin B_{12} in pernicious anaemia, anti-thyroid drugs for Graves' disease, and so forth. Anticholinesterase drugs are commonly used for long-term therapy in myasthenia gravis; thymectomy is of benefit in most cases and it is conceivable that the gland contains ACh receptors in a particularly antigenic form (? associated with HLA-D expression).

Anti-inflammatory drugs

Patients with severe myasthenic symptoms respond well to high doses of steroids and the same is true for serious cases of other autoimmune disorders such as SLE and immune complex nephritis where the drug helps to suppress the inflammatory lesions.

In rheumatoid arthritis, apart from steroids, anti-inflammatory drugs such as salicylates, indomethacin, phenylbutazone and newer preparations such as fenoprofen and ibuprofen are widely used. Penicillamine, gold salts and antimalarials such as chloroquine all find an important place in therapy but their mode of action is unknown.

Therapeutic blocking of other mediators directly concerned in immunological tissue damage will be feasible if lymphokine and complement antagonists become available.

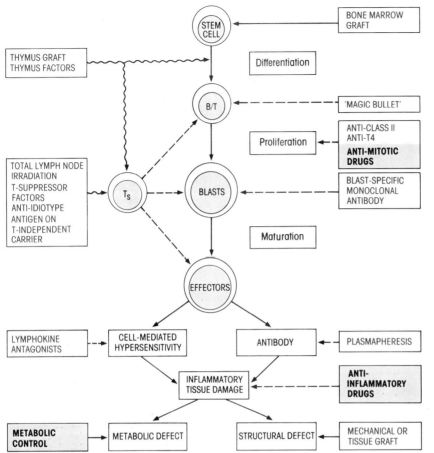

Figure 15.14. *The treatment of autoimmune disease. Current conventional treatments are in bold type; some feasible approaches are given in blue type. (In the case of a live graft, bottom right, the immunosuppressive therapy used may protect the tissue from the autoimmune damage which affected the organ being replaced.)*

Immunosuppressive drugs

In a sense, because it blocks lymphokine secretion by T-cells, cyclosporin A is an anti-inflammatory drug and this seems to be the basis for its control of the uveitis in Behçet's disease; as the drug is withdrawn, the inflammation returns. But since lymphokines like IL-2 are also obligatory for lymphocyte proliferation, cyclosporin is also an anti-mitotic drug and there are preliminary, but not yet proper, trials of its efficacy in insulin-dependent diabetes, SLE and rheumatoid arthritis. There is no evidence yet that administration of the drug during an on-going autoimmune response is likely to establish the type of T-suppression seen in kidney grafting (cf. p. 226).

While awaiting more selective therapy, conventional non-specific anti-mitotic agents such as azathioprine, cyclophosphamide and methotrexate, usually in combination with steroids, have been used effectively in SLE, chronic active hepatitis and autoimmune haemolytic anaemia for example.

Immunological control strategies

Plasma exchange to lower the rate of immune complex deposition in SLE provides only temporary benefit although it may be of value in life-threatening cases of arteritis. Successful results have been obtained in Goodpasture's syndrome when the treatment has been applied in combination with anti-mitotic drugs (figure 15.15), the rationale being an increased tendency for antigen-reactive cells to divide as the negative feedback effect of IgG is lowered following removal of plasma proteins.

It should one day be practical to correct any relevant defects in stem cells or in thymus processing by bone marrow or thymus grafting or perhaps, in the latter case, by thymic hormones.

We have already discussed the possible role of thymic factors in maintaining T-suppressor control of autoimmunity and one anticipates some interesting advances now that purified materials are available. Hybridoma technology or even gene cloning should ultimately provide the clinician with antigen-

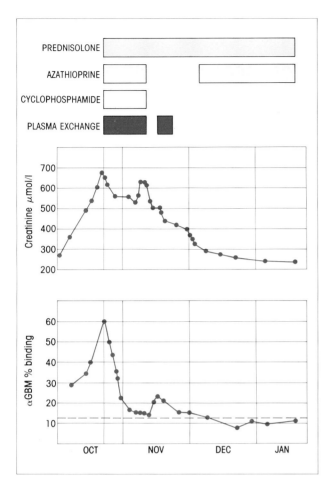

Figure 15.15. *Treatment of a patient with anti-glomerular basement membrane (α-GBM) nephritis with plasma exchange, steroids and immunosuppressive drugs. Kidney function is here monitored by the serum creatinine level. The treatment leads to loss of autoantibody (the dashed line represents the amount of GBM antigen bound in the assay by normal serum) and restoration of kidney function (courtesy of Dr C.M. Lockwood).*

specific suppressor factors. In the meantime, exploration of the therapeutic benefits of total lymph node irradiation (cf. p. 224) is being cautiously undertaken. Another potentially valuable approach for the future involves 'switching off' primed B-cells by presenting hapten linked to a thymus-independent carrier like the copolymer of D-glutamic and D-lysine (D-GL) or isologous IgG particularly when given with high cortisone doses. This has certainly worked well in NZB hybrid mice where anti-DNA levels have been reduced using nucleosides as the haptens: we shall have to see whether man and mouse really are that different.

Injection of monoclonal anti-class II and anti-L3T4 successfully fends off lupus in spontaneous mouse

models and it is relevant to record the preliminary clinical observations that injection of immunoglobulins eluted from placentae, and shown to contain anti-allo-class II, significantly ameliorate the symptoms of rheumatoid arthritis.

The powerful immunosuppressive action of anti-idiotype antibodies has led to much rumination on the feasibility of controlling autoantibody production by provoking appropriate interactions within the immune network. The ability of the newborn children of myasthenic mothers to defend themselves against the pathogenetic effects of maternal acetylcholine receptor antibodies by synthesizing anti-idiotypes, encourages the view that idiotype manipulation might prove to be effective. We have focused previously on the intimate network interactions between hormone receptors, hormones and their respective antibodies (cf. p. 129) and it might be that the autoimmune disorders involving these receptors prove to be especially amenable to idiotype control. There is a growing realization that, in general, more fundamental suppression can be achieved by utilizing the internal elements of the idiotype network rather than anti-idiotype reagents raised in other species. Thus, xenogeneic anti-idiotypes have only achieved transient and partial improvement in the spontaneous thyroiditis of the Buffalo rat and the autoimmune lupus of NZB × W mice presumably due to compensation by idiotype negative clones. On the other hand, much more profound changes have been achieved by treatment with monoclonal autoantibodies (idiotypes) derived from the autoimmune strain in question. Following this line of thought, it has proved possible to protect animals against the induction of experimental allergic encephalomyelitis by immunization with an attenuated T-cell clone specific for myelin basic protein and, even more appealing, to switch off Freund-adjuvant-induced arthritis with an attenuated clone of T-cells generated in response to a mycobacterial constituent of the adjuvant. Although not yet formally proven, the most likely explanation is the induction by the clones of T-suppressors directed to a key idiotype on the pathogenetic T-cells.

Other features of regulatory bypass mechanisms such as excessive contrasuppressor activity or inappropriate HLA-DR expression may also become feasible targets for therapy one day. And last, back to the Holy Grail business, several groups are trying to evolve a strategy based upon the 'magic bullet', the essence of which is to fashion different types of cytotoxic weaponry by coupling bacterial toxins

271

or lots of radioactivity to the antigen which selectively homes on to the lymphocytes bearing specific surface receptors. Something good has got to come out of all this!

SUMMARY

There are many examples which would attribute the pathogenesis of autoimmune disorders to the autoimmune response. Antibodies to erythrocytes and to platelets shorten the half-lives of these cells and transplacental passage of platelet antibodies produces a transient neonatal thrombocytopenia. Different thyroid autoantibodies can cause tissue destruction, stimulation or suppression of thyroid hormone production and stimulation or suppression of thyroid cell division; the various forms in which thyroid autoimmunity presents can be interpreted in terms of different combinations of these antibodies. Antibodies to intrinsic factor and to sperm inhibit their biological actions. Elution of glomerular basement membrane autoantibodies from the kidney of a patient with Goodpasture's syndrome produced a fatal glomerulonephritis when injected into monkeys. Acetylcholine receptor autoantibodies evoke a transient neonatal muscle weakness in a proportion of babies born to myasthenic mothers.

Immune complexes, usually with bound complement, appear in the kidneys, skin and joints of patients with SLE, associated with lesions in the corresponding organs. Most patients with rheumatoid arthritis produce autoantibodies to IgG (rheumatoid factors) as a result of immunological hyper-reactivity in the deeper layers of the synovium. The IgG rheumatoid factors self-associate to form complexes. These give rise to acute inflammation in the joint space and, together with activated (? anti-self class II) T-cells, stimulate the synovial lining cells to grow as a malign pannus which produces erosions in the underlying cartilage and bone through the release of interleukin-1, PGE_2, collagenase, neutral proteinase and reactive oxygen intermediates. The IgG

ORGAN-SPECIFIC (e.g. THYROIDITIS, GASTRITIS, ADRENALITIS)	NON-ORGAN SPECIFIC (e.g. SYSTEMIC LUPUS ERYTHEMATOSUS)
DIFFERENCES	
Antigens only available to lymphoid system in low concentration	Antigens accessible at higher concentrations
Antibodies and lesions organ-specific	Antibodies and lesions non-organ-specific
Clinical and serologic overlap — thyroiditis, gastritis and adrenalitis	Overlap SLE, rheumatoid arthritis, and other connective tissue disorders
Familial tendency to organ-specific autoimmunity	Familial connective tissue disease ? Abnormalities in immunoglobulin synthesis in relatives
Lymphoid invasion, parenchymal destruction by ? ± cell-mediated hypersensitivity ? ± antibodies	Lesions due to deposition of antigen–antibody complexes
Therapy aimed at controlling metabolic deficit	Therapy aimed at inhibiting inflammation and antibody synthesis
Tendency to cancer in organ	Tendency to lymphoreticular neoplasia
Antigens evoke organ-specific antibodies in normal animals with complete Freund's adjuvant	No antibodies produced in animals with comparable stimulation
Experimental lesions produced with antigen in Freund's adjuvant	Diseases and autoantibodies arise spontaneously in certain animals (e.g. NZB mice and hybrids and some dogs) or after injection of parental lymphoid tissue into F_1 hybrids
SIMILARITIES	
Circulating autoantibodies react with normal body constituents	
Patients often have increased immunoglobulins in serum	
Antibodies may appear in each of the main immunoglobulin classes	
Greater incidence in women	
Disease process not always progressive; exacerbations and remissions	
Association with HLA	
Spontaneous diseases in animals genetically programmed	
Autoantibody tests of diagnostic value	

Table 15.3. *Comparison of organ-specific and non-organ-specific diseases.*

in rheumatoid arthritis shows defective galactosylation of the Fc sugars.

Cellular hypersensitivity must play a role in the chronic inflammatory changes of many autoimmune disorders, particularly if one considers the phenomenon of inappropriate class II MHC expression, but it has been difficult to pin-point the exact mechanisms.

Autoallergic disease can be deliberately induced in the thyroid, brain, adrenal, testis and joints of rodents by immunization with the relevant antigen in complete Freund's adjuvant. Spontaneous thyroiditis, diabetes, haemolytic anaemia and lupus have all been observed in certain pure-bred animal strains and the importance of autoimmunity for pathogenesis is shown by the amelioration of symptoms whenever the immune response is suppressed.

A wide range of serum autoantibodies now provide valuable diagnostic markers. Routine immunofluorescent screening is carried out on composite sections of human thyroid and stomach and rat kidney and liver, supplemented by agglutination tests for rheumatoid factors, thyroid and red cell antibodies, and by radioassays for intrinsic factor, DNA and IgG antibodies.

Therapy conventionally involves metabolic control and the use of anti-inflammatory and immunosuppressive drugs. Plasma exchange may be of value especially in combination with anti-mitotic drugs. A whole variety of potential immunological control therapies are under intensive investigation.

The accompanying comparison of organ-specific and non-organ-specific autoimmune disorders (table 15.3) gives an overall view of many of the points raised in these last two chapters.

Further reading

Bottazzo G.F., Pujol-Borrell R., Hanafusa T. & Feldmann M. (1983) Hypothesis: role of aberrant HLA-DR expression and antigen presentation in the induction of endocrine autoimmunity. *Lancet*, **ii**, 1115.

Brochier J., Clot J. & Sany J. (eds) (1986) Anti-Ia antibodies in treatment of autoimmune disease. *Immune Intervention*, **2**. Academic Press, London.

Haeney M. (1985) *Introduction to Clinical Immunology*. Butterworths-Update, London. (In vivid technicolour; suitable for the busy clinician.)

Ivanyi L. (ed.) (1986) *Immunological Aspects of Oral Disease*. MTP Press, Lancaster, UK.

Lachmann P.J. & Peters D.K. (eds) (1982) *Clinical Aspects of Immunology*, 4th edn. Blackwell Scientific Publications, Oxford.

McGregor A.M. (ed.) (1986) *Immunology of Endocrine Diseases*. MTP Press, Lancaster, UK.

Morrow J. & Isenberg D.A. (1987) *Autoimmune Rheumatic Disease*. Blackwell Scientific Publications, Oxford.

Parekh R.B., Dwek R.A., Sutton B.J., Fernandes D.L., Leung A., Stanworth D. & Rademacher T.W. (1985) Association of rheumatoid arthritis and primary osteoarthritis with changes in the glycosylation pattern of total serum IgG. *Nature*, **316**, 452.

Roitt I.M. & Cooke A. (1987) Idiotypes and autoimmunity. In *Progress in Immunology*, **VI**. Cinader B. & Miller R.G. (eds). Academic Press, Orlando, USA.

Schindler R. (ed.) (1985) *Ciclosporin in Autoimmune Diseases*. Springer-Verlag, Berlin.

Thompson R.A. (ed.) (1985) Laboratory Investigation of Immunological Disorders. *Clinics in Immunol. & Allergy*, **5**. W.B. Saunders, London.

Thompson R.A. (series ed.) *Recent Advances in Clinical Immunology*. Churchill Livingstone, UK.

Triger D.R. (ed.) (1986) *Clinical Immunology of Liver and Gastrointestinal Tract*. Wright, Bristol, UK.

Wells J.V. & Nelson D.S. (eds) (1986) *Clinical Immunology Illustrated*. Williams & Wilkins, Sydney.

273

INDEX

Page references in *italics* refer to figures, tables, or
the legends accompanying them.

277

(CEA) 232, 236
Carrier molecules, for haptens *55*
Carrier priming, and secondary
  response to hapten *96*
Cartilage grafts 227, 237
Cartilage proteoglycan 268
Cascade phenomenon 7
Cathepsin G 5
CBA graft 129, *130, 131*
CD3 (T3) 93, 99
  antibodies to 212
CD4 (T4) 93, 111, 118
  and AIDS virus binding 188, 191
  and lymphokine release 111, 114
CD5 (T1), B-cell 139, 151
CD8 (T8) 94
  $CD8^+$ ($T8^+$) cells 119−20
Cell depletion 83
Cell-mediated immunity *see under*
  immunity
Cell-mediated lympholysis (CML) *217*
Cell separation techniques 81−3, 84
'Cell shutdown' 87
Cell sorting
  by panning *83*
  by rosetting *83*
  cytotoxicity techniques *83*
  fluorescence activated cell sorter *81,
    82−3*
Cell wall, bacterial 154, *155*
  lesions 8, *16*
C_λ gene 49
Chagas' disease 248
  and autoimmunity 169
Chediak−Higashi disease 183
Chemiluminescent labels 76
Chemotherapy, and immune-complex
  mediated reactions 207, 213
Chicken bursa 139
Chicken pox 172
Chickens, V genes 149−50
Chloroquine 65
Chlorpromazine 204
Cholera 158
  toxin 177
  vaccine 177
Chondroitin sulphate A *13*
Chorionic gonadotrophin, and
  population control 84
Choroid plexus 208
Chromatography, affinity *76, 77*
Chromosome translocations, in
  lymphoproliferative
  disorders 143
Chronic granuloma 211
Chronic granulomatous disease 183
Chronic inflammation 160, *161*
Chronic lymphocytic leukaemia 143,
  144, 146, 147
Circadian rhythms 128
Circulating complexes 207−9
Classical complement pathway 12
  and viruses 162
  compared to 'alternative
    pathway' 16, *17*
  deficiencies 204
  initiation 15−16
Clonal expansion 21
Clonal selection 21, *23*, 103
Clostridium difficile 2

Clostridium welchii 154
Clotting system 11
c−myc
  deregulation 142, 152
  lymphocyte activation 142
Cobra venom factor 92
Colony stimulating factors 134
  and cancer therapy 236
  GM-CSF 111, 112, 236
Colostral immunoglobulins, maternally
  derived 172
Common acute lymphoblastic
  leukaemia antigen
  (CALLA) 144, *147*
Complement
  alternative pathway *see* alternative
    complement pathway
  and immune-complex
    hypersensitivity 204
  and the acute inflammatory
    reaction 10−11, *12*
  classical pathway *see* classical
    complement pathway
  deficiencies 183−4
  fixation on tissue sections 80
  functions 9−10, 27
  insoluble complex inhibition 204,
    205
  receptors 40
  see also specific factors under C1, etc.
Complete Freund's adjuvant 103,
  181−2, 210, 247, 256, 266, 268
Complexes *see* antigen−antibody
  complexes
Conglutinin 155, 209
Contact hypersensitivity 87, *199*, 209,
  211
Contrasuppressor cells 119, 251
Coombs' test *202, 240*
Coproantibodies 156
Corneal grafts 226−7, 237
Corticosteroids 209
  and immunodeficiency 186
Corynebacterium parvum injections 169
Coulombic attraction *60*
CR1 receptors 155
CR2 receptors 155
CR3 receptors 155
C-reactive protein (CRP) 12
  estimation 69
  increase by IL-1 12
  properties 12
Cross-reactive idiotypes 248
'Cross-tolerance' hypothesis 127
C-type retrovirus 143
Cutaneous basophil
  hypersensitivity 210
Cyclophosphamide 130, 224, 270
  impairs T-suppressors 250
Cyclosporin A 223, 224, *225*
  as an anti-inflammatory drug 270
  as an anti-mitotic drug 270
  bone marrow graft maintenance 228
  heart transplant maintenance 227
  kidney graft maintenance 227
  nephrotoxicity 224−5
Cyclosporin/steroid therapy, in liver
  transplants 228
Cytochrome $b_{−245}$ 183
Cytofluorography, flow *81, 82*

Cytokeratin, in carcinomas 144, *146,
  147*
Cytolysin *13*
Cytolytic (killer) T-cells 111, 113, 115
  T8 113, 115
Cytomegalovirus 148, 163
  in AIDS 188
Cytotoxic drugs, and
  immunodeficiency 186
Cytotoxicity techniques, for cell
  depletion 83
Cytotoxic T-cells *see under* T-cells

Danders, animal 195
Decay accelerating factor (DAF) 183
Delayed-type allergic reactions, to
  smallpox 211
Dendritic cells 92, 119
  follicular *90, 91*, 92
  thymus and 137, 151
Dengue haemorrhagic shock 208, 212,
  213
Dengue virus 163
Dental caries 157
Deoxyguanosine 137, *138*, 151
Determinants
  antigen 56, *57*
  discontinuous 178
Determinant selection 127
Diabetes, insulin-dependent *see*
  insulin-dependent diabetes
Diacylglycerol 97, 194, *195*
  breakdown 94
Diapedesis 11
Dick reaction 157
Differentiation, and surface
  markers 136, *137*
Differentiation factors *see under* B-cells;
  T-cells
DiGeorge syndrome *185*
Dinitrophenyl (DNP) 55
  combined with antibodies *31*, 60
Diphtheria *173*
Diphtheria toxin, 'loop' peptide 178
Discoid lupus erythematosus 208, 258
Disodium cromoglycate 209
Disseminated intravascular coagulation,
  in Gram-negative
  septicaemia 212
Disulphide bonds, immunoglobin
  domain 36, *37*
Diversity
  interchain amplification of 50−1
  intrachain amplification 50
DNA, translocation 49
DNP *see* dinitrophenyl
Domains
  anti-parallel β-pleated 151
  see also under immunoglobulins
Dominant epitope clusters 56, *57*, 68
Donath-Landsteiner antibodies,
  anti-blood group P 203
Double diffusion precipitation 69−70,
  71, 72
DR2
  and multiple sclerosis 230
  poor-responder gene 230
DR3
  and organ-specific diseases 230

INDEX

285